Magnesium Intake and Human Health

Magnesium Intake and Human Health

Special Issue Editors

Federica Wolf
Valentina Trapani

MDPI • Basel • Beijing • Wuhan • Barcelona • Belgrade

MDPI

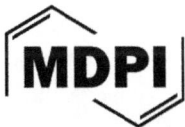

Special Issue Editors
Federica Wolf
Università Cattolica del Sacro Cuore
Italy

Valentina Trapani
Università Cattolica del Sacro Cuore
Italy

Editorial Office
MDPI
St. Alban-Anlage 66
Basel, Switzerland

This is a reprint of articles from the Special Issue published online in the open access journal *Nutrients* (ISSN 2072-6643) from 2017 to 2018 (available at: https://www.mdpi.com/journal/nutrients/special_issues/magnesium_intake1)

For citation purposes, cite each article independently as indicated on the article page online and as indicated below:

LastName, A.A.; LastName, B.B.; LastName, C.C. Article Title. *Journal Name* **Year**, *Article Number, Page Range.*

ISBN 978-3-03897-334-8 (Pbk)
ISBN 978-3-03897-335-5 (PDF)

Contents

About the Special Issue Editors

Federica Wolf, PhD, is Professor of General Pathology at the Catholic University of Sacred Heart of Rome. She has been studying cell magnesium homeostasis throughout her career, focusing on tumor growth, aging, and, more recently, on magnesium channels, including TRPM channels and MagT1. Since 2010, she has been the president of the International Society for the Development of the Research on Magnesium (SDRM, www.sdrmsociety.org). Since 2012, she has been Review Editor for the journal *Magnesium Research* and is currently Co-Editor-in-Chief for the same journal. In 2008, she acted as vice-chairman at the Gordon Research Conference on "Magnesium in Health and Disease" Ventura, California; she has organized several international meetings on Magnesium: 2011, European magnesium Workshop Bologna-Italy; 2016, XIV International Magnesium Symposium, Rome-Italy; and 2018 Workshop Magnesium in Neuroscience, Krakow-Poland. She is organizing the next meeting XV IMS in 2019 at NIH-Bethesda, USA.

Valentina Trapani , PhD, is Assistant Professor of General Pathology at the Catholic University of Sacred Heart of Rome. Moving on from a background in biophysics and cancer biology, she is currently interested in the role of magnesium and magnesium-specific ion channels in diverse pathophysiological processes, in particular inflammation-driven conditions and colon carcinogenesis. Since 2016, she was made a member of the Editorial board of *Magnesium Research*.

Preface to "Magnesium Intake and Human Health"

Magnesium is key for life. In our body, magnesium is an essential and abundant component of all tissues. The biochemistry of magnesium has long been established, and its critical role in human health and disease has become evident, even if incompletely understood at a mechanistic level. Indeed, the complicated homeostatic mechanisms that maintain the concentration of this cation within strict limits testify its importance for normal physiology and metabolism. However, this also explains why its exact role and regulation in specific tissues remain elusive. Only in the last two decades have researchers started to identify the molecular determinants of cell magnesium homeostasis and to study their function. These experimental findings have greatly contributed to our understanding of epidemiological and clinical data, but a lot of work still needs to be done to integrate a body of knowledge that now stretches from nutrition to molecular biology. This book brings together the latest in experimental and clinical magnesium research. We hope that this will foster a deeper understanding of the pathophysiology of diseases in which magnesium homeostasis is deranged and will pave the way for the development of novel, safe, and effective preventive and/or therapeutic strategies, based on supplementation or targeted pharmacological approaches.

Federica Wolf, Valentina Trapani
Special Issue Editors

nutrients

MDPI

Article

Dietary Magnesium and Incident Frailty in Older People at Risk for Knee Osteoarthritis: An Eight-Year Longitudinal Study

Nicola Veronese [1,2,3,*], Brendon Stubbs [4,5,6], Stefania Maggi [3], Maria Notarnicola [1,2], Mario Barbagallo [7], Joseph Firth [8], Ligia J. Dominguez [7] and Maria Gabriella Caruso [1,2]

[1] Ambulatory of Clinical Nutrition, Research Hospital, IRCCS "S. de Bellis", Castellana Grotte, 70013 Bari, Italy; maria.notarnicola@irccsdebellis.it (M.N.); gabriella.caruso@irccsdebellis.it (M.G.C.)

[2] Laboratory of Nutritional Biochemistry, National Institute of Gastroenterology-Research Hospital, IRCCS "S. de Bellis", Castellana Grotte, 70013 Bari, Italy

[3] National Research Council, Neuroscience Institute, Aging Branch, Via Giustiniani, 2, 35128 Padua, Italy; stefania.maggi@in.cnr.it

[4] South London and Maudsley NHS Foundation Trust, Denmark Hill, London SE5 8AZ, UK; brendon.stubbs@kcl.ac.uk

[5] Faculty of Health, Social Care and Education, Anglia Ruskin University, Bishop Hall Lane, Chelmsford CM1 1SQ, UK

[6] Institute of Psychiatry, Psychology and Neuroscience (IoPPN) King's College London, De Crespigny Park, London SE5 8AF, UK

[7] Geriatric Unit, Department of Internal Medicine and Geriatrics, University of Palermo, 90142 Palermo, Italy; mario.barbagallo@unipa.it (M.B.); ligia.dominguez@unipa.it (L.J.D.)

[8] NICM Health Research Institute, University of Western Sydney, Sydney, NSW 2751, Australia; joefirth@gmail.com

* Correspondence: ilmannato@gmail.com; Tel.: +39-049-8218492; Fax: +39-049-8211218

Received: 21 October 2017; Accepted: 12 November 2017; Published: 16 November 2017

Abstract: Inadequate magnesium (Mg) intake is associated with lower physical performance, but the relationship with frailty in older people is unclear. Therefore, we aimed to investigate whether higher dietary Mg intake is associated with a lower risk of frailty in a large cohort of North American individuals. Details regarding Mg intake were recorded through a food-frequency questionnaire (FFQ) and categorized as greater than/equal to Recommended Dietary Allowance (RDA) vs. lower. Frailty was defined using the Study of Osteoporotic Fractures index. Multivariable Cox's regression analyses, calculating hazard ratios (HRs) with 95% confidence intervals (CIs), were undertaken by sex. In total, 4421 individuals with knee osteoarthritis or who were at high risk without frailty at baseline (mean age: 61.3, females = 58.0%) were followed for 8 years. After adjusting for 11 potential baseline confounders, reaching the RDA for Mg lowered risk of frailty among men (total $n = 1857$, HR = 0.51; 95% CI: 0.26–0.93), whilst no significant associations were found in women (total $n = 2564$). Each 100 mg of dietary Mg intake at baseline corresponded to a 22% reduction in men (HR = 0.78; 95% CI: 0.62–0.97; $p = 0.03$), but not in women (HR = 1.05; 95% CI: 0.89–1.23). In conclusion, higher dietary Mg intake appears to reduce the risk of frailty in men, but not in women.

Keywords: frailty; magnesium; older adults; Osteoarthritis Initiative

---

1. Introduction

Frailty is a clinical syndrome that identifies older subjects with increased vulnerability to stress [1]. Frailty is a common condition, with an estimated prevalence of about 10% among community-dwelling older people [2], with even higher numbers reported among older people in long-term care [3].

Frailty has been associated with an increased risk of several deleterious outcomes, including disability, falls, hospitalization, institutionalization, and death [4], but recent literature suggests that frailty might also be associated with a higher risk of metabolic [5], psychiatric [6], and cardiovascular disease [7]. It is widely assumed that early interventions for frailty, particularly in the pre-frailty state, might improve quality of life, reducing adverse outcomes and associated costs of care [8].

The pathophysiology of frailty is complex and multi-factorial. However, nutrition is an important modifiable factor in its onset and therefore a clear target for intervention [9]. It has been reported that frailty is associated with lower levels of several micronutrients, including vitamins and minerals, such as magnesium (Mg) [10]. Mg has a pivotal role in muscle function and it is essential for energy metabolism, transmembrane transport, and muscle relaxation and contraction [11]. In humans, lower Mg levels seem to be associated with a significant lower muscular function [12,13]. This effect could be due to several mechanisms, including higher oxidative stress [14], and inflammatory [15], and insulin-resistance [16] pathways. However, to the best of our knowledge, no longitudinal study has reported a possible association between Mg and the incidence of frailty. Understanding if low Mg is associated with higher risk of frailty is of importance, since the deficiency of Mg is easily reversible with appropriate dietary suggestions or supplementation [17].

Given this background, the aim of the present study was to investigate the association between dietary Mg intake at baseline and the onset of frailty in a large cohort of North American people over a follow-up period of 8 years. Since previous literature has reported that Mg is effective in improving physical function, we hypothesized that subjects with a higher Mg intake would be at lower risk of developing frailty over time.

2. Materials and Methods

2.1. Data Source and Subjects

Data were obtained from the Osteoarthritis Initiative (OAI) database, available for public access at http://www.oai.ucsf.edu/ [18]. The specific datasets utilized were registered during the baseline and screening evaluations (V00) and each database reported data on frailty until 96 months from baseline (V10). Patients at high risk of knee osteoarthritis (OA) were recruited at four clinical centers (Baltimore, MD, USA; Pittsburgh, PA, USA; Pawtucket, RI, USA; and Columbus, OH, USA) between February 2004 and May 2006.

All the participants provided written informed consent. The OAI study protocol was approved by the institutional review board of the OAI Coordinating Center, University of California, San Francisco.

2.2. Baseline Dietary Magnesium Intake (Exposure)

Dietary Mg intake was obtained through a food frequency questionnaire recorded during baseline visit of the OAI [19]. Since this questionnaire included data on Mg supplementation, this intake was also considered. Then, the population was categorized in two main groups (consumption equal to/greater than or less than the corresponding Recommended Dietary Allowance, RDA) using the cut-offs of 420 mg for men and 320 mg for women, as suggested by the Institute of Medicine (IOM) [20].

2.3. Incident Frailty (Outcome)

The study's outcome of interest was incident frailty. Frailty was assessed as outcome at wave 1 (12 months), 3 (24 months), 5 (36 months), 6 (48 months), 8 (72 months) and 10 (96 months). In agreement with the Study of Osteoporotic Fracture (SOF) index and other studies performed through the OAI [21–25], frailty was defined as the presence of at least 2 of the following 3 criteria: (1) weight loss ≥5% between baseline and any follow-up examination (since no information regarding weight changes were available at baseline, we considered those with a body mass index (BMI) of <20 kg/m^2 to fulfill this criteria only for baseline); (2) the inability to rise from a chair five times without arm support (poor chair stand time); and (3) poor physical performance based on Question 10 of the

SF12 questionnaire, i.e., responding to the question "in the past 4 weeks, did you feel full of energy?" with either "A little of the time" or "none of the time".

2.4. Covariates

Other than the number frailty criteria at baseline (categorized as one vs. none), we identified several potential confounders at baseline in the association between Mg supplementation and frailty, including: daily energy intake (in kcal/day); BMI (measured by a trained nurse); physical activity evaluated using the Physical Activity Scale for the Elderly (PASE) [26]; depressive symptoms evaluated through the Center for Epidemiologic Studies Depression Scale [27]; race (whites vs. others); smoking habits (current/previous vs. never smokers); educational level (college degree vs. below) and yearly income (< or ≥US$50,000 or missing data). Validated general health measures of self-reported comorbidities were assessed using the modified Charlson co-morbidity score [28].

2.5. Statistical Analyses

Since the interaction sex by dietary Mg intake at baseline with incident frailty as outcome was significant ($p < 0.0001$), the data are reported by sex.

Normal distributions of continuous variables were tested using the Kolmogorov–Smirnov test. Data are shown as means ± standard deviations (SD) for quantitative measures, and percentages for all discrete variables. The difference in baseline characteristics between those reaching the corresponding RDA or not was tested by the independent *t*-test for continuous variables and the chi-square test for categorical ones.

Cox's regression analysis was used to assess the strength of the association between Mg intake at baseline and the onset of frailty during follow-up. Significantly different factors with respect to those reaching or not reaching the corresponding RDA in at least one sex or factors significantly associated with incident frailty at univariate analysis in at least one sex were included. Multi-collinearity among covariates was assessed using the variance inflation factor (VIF), with a score of 2 leading to the exclusion of a variable, but no parameter was excluded for this reason.

The basic model was adjusted for age. In the fully-adjusted model the variables used were: age (as a continuous variable); race (whites vs. others); BMI (as a continuous variable); education (college degree vs. below); smoking habits (current and previous smokers vs. others); yearly income (categorized as ≥ or <US$50,000 or missing data); Physical Activity Scale for Elderly score (as a continuous variable); Charlson co-morbidity index (as a continuous variable); Center for Epidemiologic Studies Depression Scale (as a continuous variable); number of frailty indexes at baseline (one vs. none); and total energy intake (in kcal/day). The proportional hazard assumption was verified considering Schoenfeld's residuals of the covariates [29]. Cox's regression analysis estimates were reported as hazard ratios (HRs) with 95% confidence intervals (CIs). A similar analysis was run using Mg intake as continuous variable, with increases in 100 mg.

Several sensitivity analyses were conducted evaluating the interaction between dietary Mg at baseline and selected factors (i.e., age below or greater than/equal to 65 years, overweight/obese vs. normal weight, yearly income, sex, race, education, smoking habits, yearly income, and number of frailty indexes at baseline categorized as one vs. none) in the association with frailty, but only sex emerged as moderator of our findings ($p < 0.05$ for the interaction).

All the analyses were performed using SPSS 17.0 for Windows (SPSS Inc., Chicago, IL, USA). All statistical tests were two-tailed and statistical significance was assumed for a *p*-value < 0.05.

3. Results

3.1. Sample Selection

The OAI dataset initially included a total of 4796 American participants. Among them, 22 participants were excluded since they were already frail at baseline and another 353 were excluded since they did not provide data regarding frailty during follow-up, resulting in a final sample of 4421 participants.

3.2. Descriptive Characteristics

Of the 4421 participants included, 1857 were males and 2564 were females, with a mean age of 61.3 years (±9.2 years; range: 45–79). Only 819 (233 men and 586 women; =18.5% of the baseline population; 12.5 vs. 22.9% in men and women, $p < 0.0001$) reached the corresponding RDA, even though 2991 participants (=67.7%) took Mg supplementation.

Table 1 shows the participants' characteristics by their Mg intake at baseline categorized as reaching the corresponding RDA or not, by sexes. In both men and women, people reporting a dietary Mg intake equal to/greater than the corresponding RDA were more physically active ($p = 0.03$ for both comparisons), whilst no significant differences emerged in terms of co-morbidities or depressive symptoms (Table 1). Finally, no significant differences emerged in terms of people reporting poor physical performance, poor chair stand time, or weight loss between people reaching the Mg RDA or not in both sexes (Table 1).

3.3. Dietary Magnesium Intake and Incident Frailty

During the 8-year follow-up, 362 subjects (120 men and 242 women; 8.2% of the baseline population) developed frailty corresponding to a global incidence rate of 12 (95% CI: 10–13)/1000 persons-year. Among the singular criteria, the most frequent criterion during follow-up was poor chair stand time ($n = 780$, 17.6%), followed by poor physical performance ($n = 503$, 11.4%), and weight loss ($n = 19$, 0.4%).

Table 2 shows the association between dietary Mg intake at baseline and incident frailty at follow-up. In men, the incidence of frailty among those reaching the corresponding RDA was significantly lower than for those not reaching this cut-off (6, 95% CI: 3–12 vs. 10, 95% CI: 8–12/1000 persons-year; $p = 0.03$), whilst no significant differences emerged for women (14, 95% CI: 12–16 vs. 16, 95% CI: 12–20/1000 persons-year; $p = 0.36$). After adjusting for 11 potential confounders at baseline, men reaching the RDA had a significant lower risk of frailty of about 49% (HR = 0.51; 95% CI: 0.26–0.93; $p = 0.03$) (Table 2; Figure 1), whilst no significant differences emerged for women (HR = 1.02; 95% CI: 0.71–1.46; $p = 0.92$) or in the sample as whole (HR = 0.88; 95% CI: 0.65–1.20; $p = 0.43$).

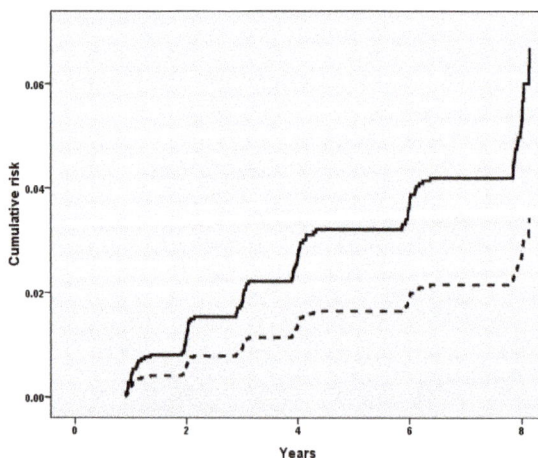

Figure 1. Risk of incident frailty in men by Recommended Dietary Allowance at baseline. Legend: the continuous line represents men not reaching the corresponding RDA at baseline; and the dashed line represents men reaching the RDA.

Table 1. Characteristics of the participants classified according to their baseline dietary magnesium intake.

	Men			Women		
	Greater Than/Equal to RDA (n = 233)	Less than RDA (n = 1624)	p-Value [a]	Greater Than/Equal to RDA (n = 586)	Less than RDA (n = 1978)	p-Value [a]
General characteristics						
Age (years)	61.5 (9.0)	60.9 (9.5)	0.37	62.0 (8.8)	61.4 (9.0)	0.13
Energy intake (kcal/day)	2313 (701)	1488 (523)	<0.0001	1760 (553)	1143 (376)	<0.0001
PASE (points)	187 (96)	174 (86)	0.03	156 (80)	149 (75)	0.03
White race (n, %)	193 (82.8)	1388 (85.6)	0.28	456 (77.9)	1516 (76.6)	0.54
Smoking (previous/current) (n, %)	116 (50.2)	805 (49.8)	0.94	262 (44.9)	894 (45.4)	0.85
Graduate degree (n, %)	87 (37.3)	596 (36.8)	0.89	146 (24.9)	517 (26.2)	0.59
Yearly income (>US$50,000)	79 (33.9)	478 (29.4)	0.17	292 (50.2)	953 (48.2)	0.40
Medical conditions						
BMI (kg/m^2)	28.2 (4.2)	28.9 (4.1)	0.08	28.5 (5.1)	28.6 (5.3)	0.67
CES-D (points)	6.3 (6.7)	5.9 (6.4)	0.35	6.9 (6.9)	7.0 (7.2)	0.61
Charlson co-morbidity index (points)	0.5 (1.1)	0.4 (0.9)	0.22	0.4 (0.8)	0.4 (0.8)	0.94
Frailty items						
Poor physical performance (n, %)	25 (10.8)	146 (9.0)	0.40	68 (11.6)	251 (12.7)	0.52
Poor chair stand time (n, %)	2 (0.9)	10 (0.6)	0.66	7 (1.2)	13 (0.7)	0.19
Weight loss (n, %)	3 (1.3)	11 (0.7)	0.40	23 (3.9)	62 (3.1)	0.36

Notes: The data are presented as means (with standard deviations) for continuous variables and numbers (with percentages) for categorical variables. [a] p values were calculated using the independent t-test for continuous variables and the chi-square test for categorical parameters. Magnesium RDAs were categorized using the cut-offs of 420 mg for men and 320 for women. Abbreviations: CES-D: Center for Epidemiologic Studies Depression Scale; PASE: Physical Activity Scale for the Elderly; BMI: body mass index; RDA: Recommended Dietary Allowance.

Modelling dietary Mg intake as a continuous variable and after adjusting for the potential confounders mentioned before, each increase in 100 mg of dietary Mg intake at baseline corresponded to a significant reduction in frailty incidence of 22% in men (HR = 0.78; 95% CI: 0.62–0.97; p = 0.03), but not in women (HR = 1.05; 95% CI: 0.89–1.23; p = 0.59) or in the population as whole (HR = 0.95; 95% CI: 0.83–1.08; p = 0.40).

Table 2. Association between dietary magnesium intake and incidence of frailty.

	Incidence (95% CI) for 1000 Persons-Year	Basic Adjusted [a] HR (95% CI)	p Value	Fully Adjusted [b] HR (95% CI)	p Value
Men					
Greater than the RDA	10 (8–12)	1 (reference)		1 (reference)	
Greater than/equal to the RDA	6 (3–12)	0.70 (0.38–0.95)	0.03	0.51 (0.26–0.93)	0.03
Women					
Less than the RDA	14 (12–16)	1 (reference)		1 (reference)	
Greater than/equal to the RDA	16 (12–20)	1.13 (0.84–1.51)	0.43	1.02 (0.71–1.46)	0.92

Notes: All the data are presented as hazard ratios (HRs) with their 95% confidence intervals. [a] The basic adjusted model included as a covariate only age. [b] The fully-adjusted model included as covariates: age (as continuous); race (whites vs. others); body mass index (as continuous); education (degree vs. others); smoking habits (current and previous vs. others); yearly income (categorized as ≥ or <US$50,000 and missing data); Physical Activity Scale for Elderly score (as a continuous variable); Charlson co-morbidity index; CES-D: Center for Epidemiologic Studies Depression Scale; number of frailty indexes at baseline (one vs. none); and total energy intake (kcal/day). Abbreviations: CI: confidence interval; HR: hazard ratio; RDA: Recommended Dietary Allowance.

4. Discussion

To the best of our knowledge, the current study is the first to investigate the relationship between dietary and supplementary Mg intake and incident frailty. In summary, the present study involving a large number of persons living in North America found that higher baseline Mg intake is associated with a lower risk of frailty in men, but not in women, after 8 years of follow-up. The risk of frailty in men reaching the RDA was almost halved and each increase in 100 mg of Mg intake decreased the risk of frailty by about 22%.

At baseline, no significant differences emerged between people reaching or not the RDA in both sexes in terms of potential risk factors for frailty, such as age, co-morbidities, or the presence of any frailty item. However, people reporting higher Mg intake were more physically active (as shown by higher PASE scores) and this probably played a role in the lower development of frailty in subjects reaching the corresponding RDA for Mg. However, it should be noted that our analyses were adjusted for this factor, suggesting that appropriate Mg intake can have an additional effect on frailty risk.

Another important consideration is the large number of people not reaching an appropriate intake of Mg. Our data, even if collected in a special population (i.e., people with knee OA or at higher risk of this condition), are similar to those collected in other American surveys. Using data from the NHANES (National Health and Nutrition Examination Survey) study, average intakes of Mg from food alone were higher among users of dietary supplements (350 mg for men and 267 mg for women) than among non-users (268 mg for men and 234 for women), but were still broadly insufficient [30]. Other surveys reported that almost half of the North American population consumed less than the required amount of magnesium from food in 2005–2006, and the figure was down from 56% in 2001–2002 [31]. Collectively, these data suggest that, despite the widespread use of Mg supplements, dietary Mg intake is insufficient in the American population, likely due to low consumption of green leafy vegetables, legumes, nuts, seeds, and whole grains [32], good sources of dietary Mg.

It is widely known that poor nutritional status is associated with the onset of frailty [9,33]. However, the possible association between Mg intake was poorly explored and the data available mainly derived from the literature regarding Mg and physical function [34]. Altogether, the previous findings available showed that higher Mg levels are associated with better physical function [11–13]. However, the design of previous studies (i.e., either cross-sectional or small randomized controlled trials) limits the strength of their findings. Thus, the findings from this longitudinal study involving more than 4000 participants substantially advance our understanding on this topic.

A point of importance is that higher Mg supplementation is associated with lower incidence of frailty in men, but not in women. We can hypothesize that since frailty has different prevalence and incidence between men and women [35,36], the risk factors for frailty (including nutritional factors) are probably different. Unfortunately, there was inadequate data to confirm which specific risk factors may differ between the sexes. However, with regards to Mg, it is known that women have lower Mg intake than men, although it is still debated if a different grade of absorption exists between sexes [37], leading to a different effect on muscle function. Thus, more studies are needed to better identify and understand the different roles of Mg in determining frailty between sexes.

The present findings should be considered within the limitations of the study. First, we had no data about Mg status, except for dietary Mg. Even if the best method for the assessment of Mg status is still equivocal [38,39], it would be interesting to assess if other parameters of Mg status can lead to different results. Second, we used a slightly different definition of frailty at baseline with respect to the one used at the follow-up, particularly with respect to weight loss. Unfortunately, no data regarding weight changes were available in the OAI at baseline and it is possible that some frail individuals at baseline were included in our analysis. Third, the participants of the OAI may not be representative of the general population, due to the inclusion/exclusion criteria of this study. Fourth, the inherent changes of Mg during time were not recorded and, consequently, it is not possible to assess the role of dietary Mg intake over time in the onset of frailty. Finally, the data regarding co-morbidities were self-reported and this can introduce another bias in our results.

5. Conclusions

In conclusions, our data suggests that higher dietary Mg intake is associated with a lower risk of frailty in men, but not in women, suggesting important sex differences in this potential relationship. Since low Mg intake is prevalent in the North American population, other studies are needed to see if Mg supplementation could be associated with lower risk of frailty in older people.

Acknowledgments: The OAI is a public-private partnership comprised of five contracts (N01-AR-2-2258; N01-AR-2-2259; N01-AR-2-2260; N01-AR-2-2261; N01-AR-2-2262) funded by the National Institutes of Health, a branch of the Department of Health and Human Services, and conducted by the OAI Study Investigators. Private funding partners include Merck Research Laboratories; Novartis Pharmaceuticals Corporation, GlaxoSmithKline; and Pfizer, Inc. Private sector funding for the OAI is managed by the Foundation for the National Institutes of Health. This manuscript was prepared using an OAI public use data set and does not necessarily reflect the opinions or views of the OAI investigators, the NIH, or the private funding partners. JF is funded by a Blackmores Institute Fellowship. We did not receive any specific funding for covering the cost for the open access option.

Author Contributions: Study concept and design: N.V., B.S. Data analysis and interpretation: N.V., M.N. Drafting of the manuscript: N.V., B.S., M.B., J.F. Critical revision of the manuscript: S.M., L.J.D., M.G.C. Statistical analysis: N.V.

Conflicts of Interest: The founding sponsors had no role in the design of the study; in the collection, analyses, or interpretation of data; in the writing of the manuscript, and in the decision to publish the results.

References

1. Morley, J.E. Frailty and sarcopenia: The new geriatric giants. *Revista de Investigacion Clinica Organo del Hospital de Enfermedades de la Nutricion* **2016**, *68*, 59–67. [PubMed]
2. Collard, R.M.; Boter, H.; Schoevers, R.A.; Oude Voshaar, R.C. Prevalence of frailty in community-dwelling older persons: A systematic review. *J. Am. Geriatr. Soc.* **2012**, *60*, 1487–1492. [CrossRef] [PubMed]
3. Kojima, G. Prevalence of frailty in nursing homes: A systematic review and meta-analysis. *J. Am. Med. Dir. Assoc.* **2015**, *16*, 940–945. [CrossRef] [PubMed]
4. Clegg, A.; Young, J.; Iliffe, S.; Rikkert, M.O.; Rockwood, K. Frailty in elderly people. *Lancet (Lond. Engl.)* **2013**, *381*, 752–762. [CrossRef]

5. Veronese, N.; Stubbs, B.; Fontana, L.; Trevisan, C.; Bolzetta, F.; De Rui, M.; Sartori, L.; Musacchio, E.; Zambon, S.; Maggi, S.; et al. Frailty is associated with an increased risk of incident type 2 diabetes in the elderly. *J. Am. Med. Dir. Assoc.* **2016**. [CrossRef] [PubMed]

6. Soysal, P.; Veronese, N.; Thompson, T.; Kahl, K.G.; Fernandes, B.S.; Prina, A.M.; Solmi, M.; Schofield, P.; Koyanagi, A.; Tseng, P.T.; et al. Relationship between depression and frailty in older adults: A systematic review and meta-analysis. *Ageing Res. Rev.* **2017**, *36*, 78–87. [CrossRef] [PubMed]

7. Veronese, N.; Cereda, E.; Stubbs, B.; Solmi, M.; Luchini, C.; Manzato, E.; Sergi, G.; Manu, P.; Harris, T.; Fontana, L.; et al. Risk of cardiovascular disease morbidity and mortality in frail and pre-frail older adults: Results from a meta-analysis and exploratory meta-regression analysis. *Ageing Res. Rev.* **2017**. [CrossRef] [PubMed]

8. Morley, J.E.; Vellas, B.; van Kan, G.A.; Anker, S.D.; Bauer, J.M.; Bernabei, R.; Cesari, M.; Chumlea, W.C.; Doehner, W.; Evans, J.; et al. Frailty consensus: A call to action. *J. Am. Med. Dir. Assoc.* **2013**, *14*, 392–397. [CrossRef] [PubMed]

9. Artaza-Artabe, I.; Saez-Lopez, P.; Sanchez-Hernandez, N.; Fernandez-Gutierrez, N.; Malafarina, V. The relationship between nutrition and frailty: Effects of protein intake, nutritional supplementation, vitamin d and exercise on muscle metabolism in the elderly. A systematic review. *Maturitas* **2016**, *93*, 89–99. [CrossRef] [PubMed]

10. Bartali, B.; Frongillo, E.A.; Bandinelli, S.; Lauretani, F.; Semba, R.D.; Fried, L.P.; Ferrucci, L. Low nutrient intake is an essential component of frailty in older persons. *J. Gerontol. Ser. A Biol. Sci. Med. Sci.* **2006**, *61*, 589–593. [CrossRef]

11. Arnaud, M.J. Update on the assessment of magnesium status. *Br. J. Nutr.* **2008**, *99* (Suppl. 3), S24–S36. [CrossRef]

12. Dominguez, L.J.; Barbagallo, M.; Lauretani, F.; Bandinelli, S.; Bos, A.; Corsi, A.M.; Simonsick, E.M.; Ferrucci, L. Magnesium and muscle performance in older persons: The inchianti study. *Am. J. Clin. Nutr.* **2006**, *84*, 419–426. [PubMed]

13. Welch, A.A.; Kelaiditi, E.; Jennings, A.; Steves, C.J.; Spector, T.D.; MacGregor, A. Dietary magnesium is positively associated with skeletal muscle power and indices of muscle mass and may attenuate the association between circulating c-reactive protein and muscle mass in women. *J. Bone Miner. Res.* **2016**, *31*, 317–325. [CrossRef] [PubMed]

14. Hasebe, N. Oxidative stress and magnesium. *Clin. Calcium* **2005**, *15*, 194–202. [PubMed]

15. Barbagallo, M. Role of magnesium in insulin action, diabetes and cardio-metabolic syndrome x. *Mol. Asp. Med.* **2003**, *24*, 39–52. [CrossRef]

16. Veronese, N.; Watutantrige-Fernando, S.; Luchini, C.; Solmi, M.; Sartore, G.; Sergi, G.; Manzato, E.; Barbagallo, M.; Maggi, S.; Stubbs, B. Effect of magnesium supplementation on glucose metabolism in people with or at risk of diabetes: A systematic review and meta-analysis of double-blind randomized controlled trials. *Eur. J. Clin. Nutr.* **2016**, *70*, 1463. [CrossRef] [PubMed]

17. Veronese, N.; Berton, L.; Carraro, S.; Bolzetta, F.; De Rui, M.; Perissinotto, E.; Toffanello, E.D.; Bano, G.; Pizzato, S.; Miotto, F.; et al. Effect of oral magnesium supplementation on physical performance in healthy elderly women involved in a weekly exercise program: A randomized controlled trial. *Am. J. Clin. Nutr.* **2014**, *100*, 974–981. [CrossRef] [PubMed]

18. Peterfy, C.G.; Schneider, E.; Nevitt, M. The osteoarthritis initiative: Report on the design rationale for the magnetic resonance imaging protocol for the knee. *Osteoarthr. Cartil.* **2008**, *16*, 1433–1441. [CrossRef] [PubMed]

19. Veronese, N.; Stubbs, B.; Solmi, M.; Noale, M.; Vaona, A.; Demurtas, J.; Maggi, S. Dietary magnesium intake and fracture risk: Data from a large prospective study. *Br. J. Nutr.* **2017**, *117*, 1570–1576. [CrossRef] [PubMed]

20. Institute of Medicine; Food and Nutrition Board; Standing Committee on the Scientific Evaluation of Dietary Reference Intakes. *Dietary Reference Intakes for Calcium, Phosphorus, Magnesium, Vitamin D, and Fluoride*; The National Academies Press: Washington, DC, USA, 1997; p. 432.

21. Ensrud, K.E.; Ewing, S.K.; Taylor, B.C.; Fink, H.A.; Stone, K.L.; Cauley, J.A.; Tracy, J.K.; Hochberg, M.C.; Rodondi, N.; Cawthon, P.M.; et al. Frailty and risk of falls, fracture, and mortality in older women: The study of osteoporotic fractures. *J. Gerontol. Ser. A Biol. Sci. Med. Sci.* **2007**, *62*, 744–751. [CrossRef]

22. Misra, D.; Felson, D.T.; Silliman, R.A.; Nevitt, M.; Lewis, C.E.; Torner, J.; Neogi, T. Knee osteoarthritis and frailty: Findings from the multicenter osteoarthritis study and osteoarthritis initiative. *J. Gerontol. Ser. A Biol. Sci. Med. Sci.* **2015**, *70*, 339–344. [CrossRef] [PubMed]

23. Veronese, N.; Stubbs, B.; Noale, M.; Solmi, M.; Pilotto, A.; Vaona, A.; Demurtas, J.; Mueller, C.; Huntley, J.; Crepaldi, G.; et al. Polypharmacy is associated with higher frailty risk in older people: An 8-year longitudinal cohort study. *J. Am. Med. Dir. Assoc.* **2017**. [CrossRef] [PubMed]

24. Veronese, N.; Stubbs, B.; Noale, M.; Solmi, M.; Rizzoli, R.; Vaona, A.; Demurtas, J.; Crepaldi, G.; Maggi, S. Adherence to a Mediterranean diet is associated with lower incidence of frailty: A longitudinal cohort study. *Clin. Nutr. (Edinb. Scotl.)* **2017**. [CrossRef] [PubMed]

25. Shivappa, N.; Stubbs, B.; Hebert, J.R.; Cesari, M.; Schofield, P.; Soysal, P.; Maggi, S.; Veronese, N. The relationship between the dietary inflammatory index and incident frailty: A longitudinal cohort study. *J. Am. Med. Dir. Assoc.* **2017**. [CrossRef] [PubMed]

26. Washburn, R.A.; McAuley, E.; Katula, J.; Mihalko, S.L.; Boileau, R.A. The physical activity scale for the elderly (pase): Evidence for validity. *J. Clin. Epidemiol.* **1999**, *52*, 643–651. [CrossRef]

27. Radloff, L.S. The CES-D scale: A self-report depression scale for research in the general population. *Appl. Psychol. Meas.* **1977**, *1*, 385–401. [CrossRef]

28. Katz, J.N.; Chang, L.C.; Sangha, O.; Fossel, A.H.; Bates, D.W. Can comorbidity be measured by questionnaire rather than medical record review? *Med. Care* **1996**, *34*, 73–84. [CrossRef] [PubMed]

29. Grambsch, P.M.; Therneau, T.M. Proportional hazards tests and diagnostics based on weighted residuals. *Biometrika* **1994**, *81*, 515–526. [CrossRef]

30. Bailey, R.L.; Fulgoni, V.L., III; Keast, D.R.; Dwyer, J.T. Dietary supplement use is associated with higher intakes of minerals from food sources. *Am. J. Clin. Nutr.* **2011**, *94*, 1376–1381. [CrossRef] [PubMed]

31. Rosanoff, A.; Weaver, C.M.; Rude, R.K. Suboptimal magnesium status in the united states: Are the health consequences underestimated? *Nutr. Rev.* **2012**, *70*, 153–164. [CrossRef] [PubMed]

32. Veronese, N.; Stubbs, B.; Noale, M.; Solmi, M.; Vaona, A.; Demurtas, J.; Nicetto, D.; Crepaldi, G.; Schofield, P.; Koyanagi, A.; et al. Fried potato consumption is associated with elevated mortality: An 8-year longitudinal cohort study. *Am. J. Clin. Nutr.* **2017**. [CrossRef] [PubMed]

33. Cruz-Jentoft, A.J.; Kiesswetter, E.; Drey, M.; Sieber, C.C. Nutrition, frailty, and sarcopenia. *Aging Clin. Exp. Res.* **2017**, *29*, 43–48. [CrossRef] [PubMed]

34. Bohl, C.H.; Volpe, S.L. Magnesium and exercise. *Crit. Rev. Food Sci. Nutr.* **2002**, *42*, 533–563. [CrossRef] [PubMed]

35. Hubbard, R.E. Sex differences in frailty. In *Frailty in Aging*; Karger Publishers: Basel, Switzerland, 2015; Voloume 41, pp. 41–53.

36. Alexandre, T.D.S.; Corona, L.P.; Brito, T.R.P.; Santos, J.L.F.; Duarte, Y.A.O.; Lebrão, M.L. Gender differences in the incidence and determinants of components of the frailty phenotype among older adults. *J. Aging Health* **2016**. [CrossRef] [PubMed]

37. Walker, A.F.; Marakis, G.; Christie, S.; Byng, M. Mg citrate found more bioavailable than other Mg preparations in a randomised, double-blind study. *Magnes. Res.* **2003**, *16*, 183–191. [PubMed]

38. Veronese, N.; Zanforlini, B.M.; Manzato, E.; Sergi, G. Magnesium and healthy aging. *Magnes. Res.* **2015**, *28*, 112–115. [PubMed]

39. Swaminathan, R. Magnesium metabolism and its disorders. *Clin. Biochem. Rev./Aust. Assoc. Clin. Biochem.* **2003**, *24*, 47–66.

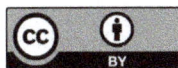

nutrients

Review

Dietary Magnesium and Cardiovascular Disease: A Review with Emphasis in Epidemiological Studies

Nuria Rosique-Esteban [1,2], Marta Guasch-Ferré [1,2,3], Pablo Hernández-Alonso [1,2] and Jordi Salas-Salvadó [1,2,*]

[1] Human Nutrition Unit, Department of Biochemistry and Biotechnology,
    Faculty of Medicine and Health Sciences, University Hospital of Sant Joan de Reus,
    Pere Virgili Institute for Health Research, Rovira i Virgili University, St/Sant Llorenç 21, 43201 Reus, Spain;
    nuria.rosique@urv.cat (N.R.-E.); mguasch@hsph.harvard.edu (M.G.-F.); pablo.hernandez@urv.cat (P.H.-A.)
[2] CIBERobn Physiopathology of Obesity and Nutrition, Institute of Health Carlos III (ISCIII), 28029 Madrid, Spain
[3] Department of Nutrition, Harvard T.H. Chan School of Public Health, Boston, MA 02115, USA
*   Correspondence: jordi.salas@urv.cat; Tel.: +34-977-759-311

Received: 9 January 2018; Accepted: 24 January 2018; Published: 1 February 2018

Abstract: Magnesium (Mg) is an essential dietary element for humans involved in key biological processes. A growing body of evidence from epidemiological studies, randomized controlled trials (RCTs) and meta-analyses have indicated inverse associations between Mg intake and cardiovascular diseases (CVD). The present review aims to summarize recent scientific evidence on the topic, with a focus on data from epidemiological studies assessing the associations between Mg intake and major cardiovascular (CV) risk factors and CVD. We also aimed to review current literature on circulating Mg and CVD, as well as potential biological processes underlying these observations. We concluded that high Mg intake is associated with lower risk of major CV risk factors (mainly metabolic syndrome, diabetes and hypertension), stroke and total CVD. Higher levels of circulating Mg are associated with lower risk of CVD, mainly ischemic heart disease and coronary heart disease. Further, RCTs and prospective studies would help to clarify whether Mg intake and Mg circulating levels may also protect against other CVDs and CVD death.

Keywords: magnesium; cardiovascular; type 2 diabetes; metabolic syndrome; mortality; death; epidemiological studies; inflammation; oxidation

1. Introduction

Magnesium (Mg) is an essential mineral for human health, representing the fourth most abundant mineral in the body. It is involved in important metabolic processes including ATP-dependent biochemical reactions, synthesis of DNA, RNA expression, cell signaling at muscle and nerve levels, and glucose and blood pressure (BP) control, among others (Figure 1) [1]. To guarantee the correct functioning of these processes, humans require a continuous supply of Mg from exogenous sources, i.e., dietary intake. Nuts, seeds, legumes, whole-grain cereals, leafy vegetables or water are well-recognized dietary sources of Mg (Table 1), regular consumption of which enables reaching the recommended dietary allowance currently set in 420 mg/day for adult men and 320 mg/day for adult women [2]. Mg requirements vary across age, sex and physiological situations (Figure 1). Dietary surveys in Europe and United States have shown that daily allowance of Mg are unmet in a large proportion of the population, probably as a result of following Western dietary patterns [2]. Several publications and recent meta-analyses have revealed inverse associations of dietary Mg intake with the risk of cardiovascular disease (CVD); cardiovascular (CV) risk factors including type 2 diabetes (T2D), metabolic syndrome (MetS) or hypertension; and total mortality [3]. Similarly, chronic Mg deficiency (defined as circulating $[Mg^{2+}] < 1.8$ mg/dL) has been associated with increased risk of several cardio-metabolic conditions [4,5]. A low inter-correlation between dietary Mg and circulating $[Mg^{2+}]$ has been described [6], possibly as a result of the tight homeostatic regulation of $[Mg^{2+}]$ through renal reabsorption and excretion, although the determinants of variation within the normal physiologic range are not well understood. For instance, genetic variations in single nucleotide polymorphisms may account for less than 2% of the variance in serum $[Mg^{2+}]$ [7], and the understanding of the influence of endocrine factors on Mg homeostasis need to be clarified [8]. Additionally, serum Mg only represents a minimal proportion of the Mg present in the entire body and thus intracellular $[Mg^{2+}]$ may be a more accurate method reflecting Mg status yet with additional difficulties to be measured [9]. Despite of this, and their low inter-correlation, both Mg intake and circulating $[Mg^{2+}]$ have been repeatedly associated with CV health [3–5], and therefore both are of great research interest.

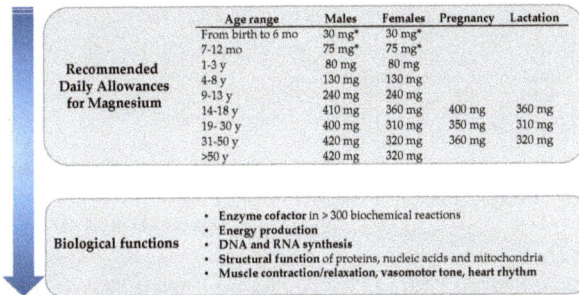

	Age range	Males	Females	Pregnancy	Lactation
	From birth to 6 mo	30 mg*	30 mg*		
	7-12 mo	75 mg*	75 mg*		
Recommended	1-3 y	80 mg	80 mg		
Daily Allowances	4-8 y	130 mg	130 mg		
for Magnesium	9-13 y	240 mg	240 mg		
	14-18 y	410 mg	360 mg	400 mg	360 mg
	19- 30 y	400 mg	310 mg	350 mg	310 mg
	31-50 y	420 mg	320 mg	360 mg	320 mg
	>50 y	420 mg	320 mg		

Biological functions	• Enzyme cofactor in > 300 biochemical reactions • Energy production • DNA and RNA synthesis • Structural function of proteins, nucleic acids and mitochondria • Muscle contraction/relaxation, vasomotor tone, heart rhythm

Figure 1. Summary of current Recommended Daily Allowances (RDAs) for magnesium intake [2] and key biological functions of magnesium. Abbreviations: mo, months; y, years. * indicates Adequate Intake.

Table 1. List of foods and food groups from plant and animal origin with their corresponding magnesium content (mg/100 g edible food).

Food from Plant Origin		Food from Animal Origin	
Nuts and Seeds	Mg mg/100 g	**Dairy and Eggs**	Mg mg/100 g
Pumpkin seeds, dried	592	Parmesan cheese	44
Flaxseed	392	Feta cheese	19
Sesame seeds, roasted	356	Whole-fat milk	13
Almonds, raw	270	Plain whole-fat yogurt	12
Cashew nuts, roasted	260	Whole fresh egg	12
Walnuts	158		
Pistachio nuts, roasted	109		
Legumes		**Fish and seafood**	
Peanuts, roasted	178	Cod, cooked	133
Soybeans, cooked	86	Salmon, cooked	122
Chickpeas, cooked	48	Canned anchovies	69
Kidney beans, cooked	45	Shrimps, cooked	37
Lentils, cooked	36		
Vegetables and fruits		**Meat and meat products**	
Sun-dried tomatoes	194	Chicken breast, cooked	34
Spinach, cooked	87	Turkey, cooked	32
Kale, cooked	57	Veal, cooked	34
Dates	54	Rabbit, cooked	21
Fresh parsley	50		
Baked potatoes with skin	43		
Whole grains			
Buckwheat flour	251		
Amaranth grain	248		
Quinoa grain	197		
Oats	177		
Spelt	136		
Barley	133		

Data obtained from the US Department of Agriculture (USDA), Nutrient Database for Standard Reference, Release 28 [10].

The present review aims to summarize the most up-to-date scientific evidence on dietary Mg intake and circulating Mg, in relation to CVD. To this end, efforts have been made to describe most recent meta-analyses of prospective studies and RCTs on the topic, as well as current literature on Mg intake and CV risk factors. Recent investigations relating circulating Mg and CVD and plausible biological mechanisms underlying the potential beneficial role of dietary Mg intake on CV health have been reviewed. Because the present review is not based on a systematic search, some articles may not have been identified and publication bias should be acknowledged. However, all the authors independently conducted the literature search.

2. Dietary Magnesium and Cardiovascular Disease Risk Factors

Experimental and observational studies have shown that higher Mg intake can exert beneficial effects on CV risk factors by improving glucose and insulin metabolism, enhancing endothelium-dependent vasodilation, ameliorating lipid profile and by its actions as an antihypertensive and anti-inflammatory agent [11].

2.1. Type 2 Diabetes and Metabolic Syndrome

Mg plays an important role in glucose and insulin metabolism, likely via insulin resistance (IR) pathways and directly affecting glucose transporter protein activity 4 (GLUT 4) [12]. A large body of observational literature has suggested that higher Mg intake is associated with a lower risk of T2D and MetS. Indeed, several meta-analyses on this topic have already been conducted. The most recent one included 637,922 individuals with 26,828 T2D cases from twenty-five cohort studies. Results of this meta-analysis indicated that compared with those participants in the lowest Mg consumption category, the risk of T2D was reduced by 17% across all the studies; 19% in women and 16% in men. In addition, a linear dose–response relationship was observed between Mg intake and T2D, such that risk was 8%–13% lower per 100 mg/day increment in intake [13]. Previous meta-analyses evaluating Mg intake and T2D have also found consistent inverse associations [14,15]. More recently, a large prospective cohort study including more than 200,000 participants followed for over 28 years from the Nurses' Health Study (NHS) I, NHS II and Health Professionals' Follow-up study (HPFS) showed that, in pooled analysis across the three cohorts, those with the highest Mg intake (intake ranging from 350 to 500 mg/day) had 15% lower risk of T2D compared to those in the lowest Mg intake group (Hazard Ratio (HR) in the highest vs. the lowest quintile: 0.85 (95% CI 0.80–0.91)) [16]. This evidence has been further confirmed by clinical trials on Mg supplementation indicating beneficial effects of Mg on markers of glucose and insulin metabolism in individuals with and without T2D [17–19]. Findings from a recent meta-analysis of RCTs on the effects of supplemental Mg have demonstrated a significant effect of Mg on the Homeostatic model assessment of insulin resistance (HOMA-IR) index (weighted mean difference (WMD): −0.67, 95% CI: −1.20, −0.14); however, reductions in IR and fasting glucose were only observed when trials had a follow-up larger than four months [17].

IR is indeed one of the underlying causes of a cluster of risk factors for CVD, namely MetS. Evidence exists suggesting that there are potential benefits of dietary Mg in preventing MetS and its components [20,21]. A recent meta-analysis on this topic has summarized the evidence of nine observational studies including 31,876 participants [22]. Results indicated that higher consumption of Mg was associated with a lower risk of MetS (Odds Ratio (OR): 0.73, 95% CI, (0.62–0.86)) compared to participants in the lowest categories of Mg consumption. However, this meta-analysis combined the estimates from cross-sectional and prospective cohort studies altogether, and the association between components of the MetS and Mg intake was not assessed because it was not reported in the majority of the included studies [22]. However, for example, in a study conducted in a sample of 535 participants, Mg intake was inversely associated not only with the MetS but significant inverse relationships were observed between Mg intake, and body mass index (BMI) (OR: 0.47, 95% CI: 0.22–1.00, *p* for trend = 0.03), and fasting glucose (OR: 0.41, 95% CI 0.22–0.77, *p* for trend = 0.005) [23]. Two other review articles published in 2014 also summarized the associations between Mg intake and MetS in several studies [24,25]. Ju et al. [24] found an inverse dose–response association when pooling the data of nine observational studies, and Dibaba et al. [25] also observed consistent inverse associations between Mg intake and MetS when combining the data of six cross-sectional studies.

Overall, data from observational studies suggest a beneficial role of Mg intake in T2D prevention, whereas results from intervention studies have shown beneficial effects on HOMA-IR and fasting glucose. Given that these are surrogate biomarkers, further RCTs of Mg intake should focus on evaluating major endpoints, such as T2D incidence. Findings from studies on dietary Mg and MetS point to an inverse association with the prevalence of MetS, but further larger and long-term prospective studies and RCTs are needed to elucidate the role of Mg intake on MetS and its components.

2.2. Hypertension and Endothelial Function

High blood pressure or hypertension has been established as a strong risk factor for CVD. Among others, a diet rich in Na^+ and an inadequate dietary intake of other minerals including K^+, Ca^+ and Mg has been linked to hypertension [26]. Previous evidence has indicated that Mg deficiency might affect BP, thus leading to hypertension, and oral Mg supplementation may act as a mild antihypertensive agent [27]. In a recent meta-analysis on this topic, the authors have pooled the estimates on dietary Mg and hypertension of six prospective cohort studies including 20,119 cases and 180,566 participants [13]. The summary estimate indicated a statistically significant inverse association between dietary Mg and hypertension risk (pooled RR comparing extreme categories = 0.92; 95% CI: 0.86, 0.98) without apparent evidence of heterogeneity between studies. The range of dietary Mg intake among the included studies was 96–425 mg/day, and the follow-up ranged from 4 to 15 years. In addition, a 100 mg/day increment in Mg intake was associated with a 5% reduction in the risk of hypertension (RR = 0.95; 95% CI: 0.90, 1.00) [13]. These findings were consistent with those from RCTs examining the effect of Mg supplementation on BP. The most recent meta-analysis has identified eleven RCTs including 543 participants with preclinical or non-communicable diseases who were followed for a range of 1–6 months [28]. The weighted overall effects indicated that the group who was supplemented with oral Mg had a significantly greater reduction in both systolic BP (Standardized Mean Difference (SMD): −0.20; 95% CI: −0.37, −0.03) and diastolic BP (SMD: −0.27; 95% CI: −0.52, −0.03) than did the control group. Mg supplementation resulted in a mean reduction of 4.18 mmHg in systolic BP and 2.27 mmHg in diastolic BP [28]. Previous meta-analysis and systematic reviews on dietary Mg, BP and hypertension have also suggested potential benefits of dietary Mg [29,30], yet showing a more moderate effect, possibly as a result of combining individuals with and without chronic diseases in the pooled analysis.

Hypertension is indeed an important risk factor for endothelial dysfunction, and an essential step in the pathogenesis of atherosclerosis that ultimately may lead to coronary artery disease (CHD). Mg is involved in several essential physiological biochemical and cellular processes regulating CV function; in addition, it plays a crucial role in modulating vascular smooth muscle tone and endothelial function [31]. Several observational studies and clinical trials have evaluated the relationship between dietary Mg and biomarkers of endothelial function. As an illustration, in a cross-sectional study of 657 women of the NHS, in the age-adjusted linear regression analyses, Mg intake was inversely associated with plasma concentrations of E-selectin ($p = 0.001$), and soluble intercellular adhesion molecule 1 (sICAM-1) ($p = 0.03$). After further adjustment for physical activity, smoking status, alcohol use, postmenopausal hormone use, and BMI, dietary Mg intake remained inversely associated with E-selectin [32]. In another report of the Women's Health Initiative Observational Study including 3713 postmenopausal women, dietary Mg intake was inversely associated with plasma concentrations of soluble vascular cell adhesion molecule 1 (sVCAM-1) and E-selectin, independent of known risk factors for metabolic outcomes. Specifically, an increase of 100 mg/day Mg was inversely associated with sVCAM-1 (-0.04 ± 0.02 ng/mL; $p = 0.07$) [33]. Finally, a randomized, double-blind, placebo-controlled trial has indicated that oral Mg supplementation (30 mmol Mg/day) for six months resulted in a significant improvement in endothelium-dependent brachial artery flow-mediated vasodilation in 50 patients with coronary artery disease, indicating a beneficial effect of Mg on endothelial function [34].

In summary, several lines of evidence have suggested a potential beneficial link between high dietary Mg and low blood pressure, particularly among those individuals with either preclinical or non-communicable diseases. Furthermore, Mg intake seems to improve endothelial function but more studies are needed to confirm these associations in the long-term.

2.3. Lipid Profile

Dyslipidemia, one of the components of MetS, is a modifiable risk factor for the development of atherosclerosis and CVD [35]. Besides the potential benefits of dietary and supplemental Mg on IR, BP and endothelial function, several studies have also indicated that dietary Mg may be linked to an improvement in lipid profile including a decrease in low-density lipoprotein (LDL) cholesterol and triglycerides levels and an increase in high-density lipoprotein (HDL) cholesterol [36,37]. In a cross-sectional study, Guerrero-Romero et al. compared 192 individuals with MetS with 384 healthy age- and sex-matched controls. Of all of the MetS components, hypomagnesemia was most closely related with dyslipidemia (OR: 2.8; 95% CI: 1.3, 2.9) and hypertension (OR: 1.9; 95% CI: 1.4, 2.8) [38]. Similarly, in a cross-sectional analysis of the Tehran Lipid and Glucose Study including 2504 participants which evaluated the associations between dietary Mg and MetS and its components, Mg intake (mean intake of 349 mg/day) was inversely associated with triglycerides ($\beta = -0.058$, $P = 0.009$) [39]. In another recent cross-sectional study including 4443 individuals from the European Prospective Investigation into Cancer (EPIC)-Norfolk cohort, higher Mg intake was inversely associated with total cholesterol (p for trend = 0.02 men and 0.04 women) [40]. However, the evidence from longitudinal observational studies on dietary Mg and lipid profile biomarkers is limited. Most of the evidence regarding Mg and blood lipids comes from RCTs on oral Mg supplementation. A recent meta-analysis of RCTs did not show significant effects of Mg on plasma concentrations of total cholesterol, LDL-cholesterol, HDL-cholesterol and triglycerides [41]. The authors suggested that this may be explained by the inter-study heterogeneity due to the different formulations and salts of Mg used across the studies and the heterogeneity of the studied populations [41]. Nonetheless, the authors reported a significant reduction on LDL-cholesterol and triglyceride concentrations after Mg supplementation in a subgroup of studies in participants with hypercholesterolemia and hypertriglyceridemia, respectively. Thus, results suggested that according to the metabolic status, Mg may affect the lipid profile [41]. Moreover, in a randomized trial were 214 participants were administered a Mg-rich diet (1142 ± 225 mg/day) and 216 participants followed their usual diet (438 ± 118 mg/day) for 12 weeks, there was a significant decrease in total serum cholesterol (10.7%), LDL-cholesterol (10.5%) and triglycerides (10.1%) in participants following a Mg-rich diet compared to the baseline concentrations; no such changes were evident in participants following a usual diet. HDL-cholesterol showed a marginal mean decrease of 0.8 mg/dL in the control group and 2.0 mg/dL increase in the intervention group [36].

In conclusion, evidence from RCTs have suggested plausible beneficial effects of oral Mg supplementation for improving some lipid parameters, but improvements were only evident in individuals with dyslipidemia. Therefore, longer and larger trials and prospective cohort studies on this topic are still required.

3. Dietary Magnesium and Cardiovascular Disease

Most of the scientific literature on dietary Mg intake and CVD derive from prospective studies. Recently, an increasing number of meta-analyses have summarized previous literature on this topic, thus providing a more concise and public health-directed overview. The present section focuses on the evidence from epidemiological studies in relation with dietary Mg intake and major CVD events, as well as with CV death.

3.1. Stroke

Current scientific evidence on dietary Mg and the risk of stroke is mostly available from prospective cohort studies in North American, European and, to a lesser degree, from Asian populations. Previous and more recent meta-analyses have exemplified the available data [3,42–44], reporting similar results on the dose-dependent protective effect of Mg intake on stroke risk. While previous meta-analyses have reported between 2% and 13% protection against total stroke for an increment of 100 mg/day intake of dietary Mg [42–44], Fang et al. have confirmed this protective effect in the most updated analysis conducted in 2016, including fourteen prospective cohort studies [3]. In this updated meta-analysis, the authors have also reported 22% lower risk of stroke (RR: 0.88; 95% CI, 0.82, 0.95) in those individuals in the highest vs. the lowest categories of dietary Mg intake, which is in agreement with findings reported in previous studies [43]. It is important to highlight that these meta-analyses have shown null to low heterogeneity between studies, they have found no evidence of publication bias and they included studies adjusting for several potential confounders. Taken together, current evidence from prospective studies in large populations across the world indicated a dose-dependent inverse association between dietary Mg and stroke incidence.

3.2. Coronary Heart Disease

Coronary Heart Disease (CHD) in relation with dietary Mg intake has been extensively investigated in large population cohorts in America and Asia, including the NHS, the HPFS and the Shanghai Women's and Men's Healthy study, among other cohorts [6,45–49]. However, most of these studies did not show a significant association when comparing the highest vs. the lowest category of Mg intake in relation to the risk of CHD in either men or women. For instance, in an analysis of more than 86,000 healthy American nurses, no significant associations were found comparing the highest vs. the lowest quintile of Mg intake on total and non-fatal CHD over a median of 28 years of follow-up [6]. In this study, and similar to other analysis in the same cohort [47], Mg intake included those from food sources and supplements, whereas the rest of the investigations only included Mg intake from foods [45,46,48]. A pooled analysis by Fang and collaborators [3] including nine different prospective cohorts have revealed inverse borderline associations with the highest category of Mg intake on CHD risk (RR: 0.90; 95% CI, 0.80, 0.99), with low heterogeneity across studies. In an additional dose–response analysis, the authors reported non-significant associations for higher Mg intake on CHD, with low to medium heterogeneity among studies. On the contrary, a recently published prospective study conducted in a large cohort of community-based Japanese adults [49] with a total of 1283 cases of CHD has revealed a protection against CHD in men in the fourth (HR: 0.70 95% CI, 0.50, 0.99) and fifth quintile (HR: 0.66 95% CI, 0.44, 0.97) of Mg intake compared to the lowest quintile (*P* for linear trend = 0.036). Overall, current evidence on Mg intake and CHD suggests a non-significant inverse association in most of the populations studied. Nevertheless, additional prospective studies and clinical trials on this topic should focus on addressing plausible age, sex and country differences.

3.3. Heart Failure

Epidemiological evidence on the associations between dietary Mg and heart failure (HF) are currently limited to two independent American and Japanese cohort studies [50,51]. Although large risk reductions in HF incidence have been reported in the highest vs. lowest Mg intake among black American individuals and Japanese women, the associations were non-significant for Japanese men [51]. These differences may be due to the lower Mg intake in Japanese men compared to their American counterparts (294 and 474 mg/day, respectively), or due to biological differences between the study populations. Nevertheless, a recently published meta-analysis [3] including these two independent cohorts has shown a strong inverse association with HF for the highest vs. the lowest categories (RR: 0.69; 95% CI, 0.52, 0.91) and also per an increment of 100 mg/day of Mg intake (RR: 0.78, 95% CI, 0.69, 0.89), both with no apparent heterogeneity. Further data from prospective studies and clinical trials in other countries and ethnicity-specific populations is required to have an extensive insight on the possible role of Mg in preventing HF.

3.4. Atrial Fibrillation

The associations between dietary Mg intake and atrial fibrillation, a common cardiac arrhythmia, have barely been explored in epidemiological and experimental settings. To the best of our knowledge, only one prospective cohort study has, so far, addressed this topic [52]. The authors followed more than 14,000 middle-aged American whites and African American participants from the ARIC study for 20.6 years, reporting 1755 incident cases of atrial fibrillation. Compared to the middle quintile (median dietary Mg: 223.2–264.8 mg/day), those individuals in the highest (median dietary Mg: ≥320.1 mg/day) or the lowest quintile of Mg intake (median dietary Mg < 180.9 mg/day)—exclusively from dietary sources, as assessed by food frequency questionnaire—did not show significantly higher or lower incidence of atrial fibrillation. These results were found regardless of sex or ethnicity, as the authors reported no significant interactions with dietary Mg. Despite these results, previous experimental studies under controlled conditions in individuals with similar characteristics have demonstrated that dietary-induced Mg depletion can induce heart rhythm changes with few participants showing atrial flutter and fibrillation [53], and that subsequent Mg repletion with supplements reverse these heart rhythm changes. These limited and mixed results illustrate the need of more epidemiological and experimental evidences to elucidate the link between dietary Mg intake and atrial fibrillation across different populations.

3.5. Cardiovascular Death

Several epidemiological studies across North American [6,47,54–56], Asian [48,51], and, to a lesser degree, European populations [57] of middle-aged men and women have prospectively evaluated the associations between dietary Mg intake and risk of CV death yielding inconclusive results. With the purpose of summarizing the existing evidence on the topic, two meta-analyses have been published to date [58,59]. In a first meta-analysis, Xu et al. [58] included a total of six prospective studies comprising more than 200,000 men and women with a follow-up ranging between 10 and 26 years. In the pooled analysis, those participants in highest category of Mg intake comparted to those in the lowest category, showed no significant differences regarding total CV death risk, yet high heterogeneity across studies was detected. However, further inspection of subgroup analyses revealed a 29% protection only in women (RR: 0.71; 95% CI, 0.60, 0.84).

In a more recent updated meta-analysis [59] including more than 400,000 adults from different cohorts who were followed for 5 to 28 years, the summary estimate comparing individuals at the higher vs. the lowest categories of dietary Mg intake showed a protection of 14% (HR: 0.86; 95% CI, 0.81, 0.91) against the risk of CV death, with high heterogeneity among studies and no evidence of publication bias. Subgroup analyses revealed that this protection corresponded to 16% in women and 8% in men. Further inspection of the subtypes of CVD death showed that dietary Mg intake was inversely and significantly associated with lower risk for CHD, heart failure and sudden cardiac death. Additional dose–response analysis showed a protection of 25% (HR: 0.75; 95% CI, 0.58, 0.99) in women for the increment of 100 mg/day of Mg intake.

Overall, current evidence in relation to dietary Mg intake and death for total CVD and CV subtypes shows a protective role, particularly in women. Nevertheless, the results derived from meta-analyses should be interpreted with caution given the high heterogeneity found across the studies. Further RCTs on dietary Mg intake should focus on assessing CV hard endpoints to clarify current available evidence aroused from prospective studies.

4. Circulating Magnesium and Cardiovascular Disease

Several prospective studies have analyzed the associations between peripheral levels of Mg or urine Mg excretion (Mg status) and the risk of several CVD including cardiac arrhythmias, congestive HF, CHD, stroke, sudden death and death from all these causes.

Although a poor correlation between dietary Mg and plasma levels of this mineral has been reported in several prospective studies [6,45], evidence exists demonstrating that very low Mg diets may lead to low serum Mg levels, and a recent meta-analysis of RCTs demonstrated significant dose and time responses of circulating $[Mg^{2+}]$ and 24 h urine Mg excretion to oral Mg supplementation [60].

Therefore, in this section, we summarize the epidemiological evidence in the literature analyzing the association between low circulating (serum/plasma) $[Mg^{2+}]$ or urinary Mg excretion and CVDs.

4.1. Cardiovascular Disease, Coronary Disease and Stroke

The most recent systematic review and meta-analysis analyzing the associations between peripheral $[Mg^{2+}]$ and CVD identified significant associations of circulating Mg and risk of CVD events [4]. Circulating $[Mg^{2+}]$ (per 0.2 mmol/L increment) was associated with a 30% lower risk of CVD, with trends towards a lower risk of ischemic heart disease (IHD) and fatal IHD. This meta-analysis, including a total of 313,041 individuals and documenting 4106 CVD, 3215 IHD, and 1528 fatal IHD events, provides the most robust evidence to date of the associations between circulating $[Mg^{2+}]$ across their usual physiologic ranges with CVD risk. However, a moderate heterogeneity between the studies analyzed was reported.

Since then, two additional large prospective studies examining this relation have been conducted. Chiuve et al. [6] conducted a nested case–control analysis in the context of the NHS with 458 cases of incident CHD matched to controls. Higher plasma $[Mg^{2+}]$ was associated in an L-shaped fashion with lower risk of CHD, although this association was not independent of CVD biomarkers. In contrast, in the Prevention of Renal and Vascular End-Stage Disease (PREVEND) study—a prospective population-based cohort study—low urinary Mg excretion was independently associated with a higher risk of IHD incidence. Nevertheless, no significant associations were observed between plasma levels of this mineral and IHD incidence or death [61].

In relation to stroke, several cross-sectional and retrospective case–control studies have reported lower serum $[Mg^{2+}]$ in those individuals with acute stroke compared with healthy controls. However, in these studies Mg was not measured before stroke diagnosis and thus hypomagnesemia may have been a consequence rather than a cause of stroke in these patients. No prospective association between serum $[Mg^{2+}]$ and risk of stroke was reported in the ARIC Study cohort after adjusting by several confounders (based on 577 ischemic stroke cases in men and women with 16 years of follow-up) [62]. In the NHS, plasma Mg levels were not associated with the risk of ischemic stroke in women [63]. However, women with $[Mg^{2+}]$ levels < 0.82 mmol/L had a 57% higher risk of ischemic stroke, and this association remained unchanged after controlling for other factors associated with Mg levels and stroke risk.

4.2. Atrial Fibrillation and Sudden Death

Low serum $[Mg^{2+}]$ has been linked to an increased risk of atrial fibrillation (AF) after cardiac surgery. However, it is unknown whether hypomagnesemia predisposes to AF in the general population. Two prospective studies have analyzed the association between serum $[Mg^{2+}]$ and AF risk in healthy populations and in individuals at risk of CVD. In the context of the Framingham Health Study, low serum $[Mg^{2+}]$ was moderately associated with the development of AF in individuals without previous history of CVD [64]. In the ARIC cohort, an L-shaped association between serum $[Mg^{2+}]$ and incident AF was also identified, with the highest risk of AF in those individuals with low serum $[Mg^{2+}]$, and a lower risk at more normal and elevated $[Mg^{2+}]$ levels [52]. This association, not different among white and African populations, was evident even after adjustment for the most important recognized risk factors of AF.

4.3. Left Ventricular Hypertrophy and Heart Failure

A few lines of evidence suggest that low circulating $[Mg^{2+}]$ may predict left ventricular hypertrophy or HF among population-based individuals. For example, low serum $[Mg^{2+}]$ has been demonstrated to predict higher increase in left ventricular mass over five years of follow-up in the population-based longitudinal Study of Health in Pomerania including 1348 individuals with echocardiographic data [65]. This prognostic impact was regardless of sex, age and traditional CV risk factors including prevalent hypertension. In relation to cardiac insufficiency, in the ARIC Study, a North American population-based cohort, low serum $[Mg^{2+}]$ and high serum phosphorus and calcium concentrations were independently associated with greater risk of incident HF after controlling for several potential confounders, with the association remaining consistent across sex and ethnicity [66]. In a population-based prospective study of middle-aged Finnish men without HF at baseline, the Kuopio Ischemic Heart Disease Study, a decreased risk for incident HF with increasing serum $[Mg^{2+}]$ was also reported [67]. This association persisted after controlling for baseline characteristics, predictors of incident HF, metabolic and renal biomarkers, and other related micronutrients.

4.4. Atherosclerosis and Coronary Artery Calcification

In few epidemiological studies, low circulating $[Mg^{2+}]$ was inversely associated with atherosclerosis and coronary artery calcification. For example, in the ARIC study, decreased serum $[Mg^{2+}]$ were associated with increased mean carotid wall thickness in women [68]. Hashimoto et al. [69] analyzed 728 subjects from the general Japanese population and also found that serum $[Mg^{2+}]$ to be inversely associated with intima-media thickness of the common carotid artery, and with the presence of atherosclerotic plaque. In two recent cross-sectional studies conducted in Korean and Mexican populations free from CVD, low serum $[Mg^{2+}]$ were also associated with coronary artery calcification [70,71].

4.5. Cardiovascular Death

In a systematic review and meta-analysis, using the results of four studies including 27,293 individuals and 1528 cases the association between circulating $[Mg^{2+}]$ and fatal IHD risk has been evaluated [4], showing a trend towards a lower risk in those individuals with lower $[Mg^{2+}]$, with substantial between-study heterogeneity. In secondary analyses using fixed effects, circulating $[Mg^{2+}]$ were associated with a significantly lower risk of fatal IHD. Nevertheless, meta-regression analysis did not show statistically significant sources of heterogeneity, although statistical power to identify heterogeneity was limited because only four studies were included in the analysis.

Peripheral $[Mg^{2+}]$ were also inversely associated with fatal CHD in the NHS [6], and with fatal stroke in the NHANES I Epidemiologic Follow-up Study [72]. Low serum $[Mg^{2+}]$ were also associated with an increased risk of CHD death and sudden cardiac death in a recent European prospective population-based cohort study [73].

Finally, in a recent systematic review and meta-analysis of studies conducted in HF patients, hypermagnesemia with serum $[Mg^{2+}] \geq 1.05$ mmol/L was associated with an increased risk of CVD death and all-cause death, but this was not observed for hypomagnesemia [74]. However, these findings were limited to elderly patients with chronic HF who had reduced left ventricular systolic function.

5. Plausible Mechanisms Connecting Magnesium and Cardiovascular Disease

The inverse association between Mg intake and IR, hyperglycemia, dyslipidemia, hypertension, and markers of inflammation may justify the protective effect of dietary Mg on CVD. As reviewed in previous sections, several RCTs and epidemiological studies have widely indicated that higher dietary Mg intake and/or circulating [Mg^{2+}] are associated with lower risk of CVD, such as IHD and sudden cardiac death. Given the participation of Mg^{2+} in a wide range of biological pathways and outcomes, it is not surprising that alterations in Mg homeostasis may influence different disease status, such as T2D and hypertension, together with CV events (Figure 2). Numerous studies have reported an increased oxidative stress during Mg-deficiency (Mg-D), including enhanced erythrocyte, tissue, and lipoprotein peroxidation, implicated in the early stages and progression of CVDs [75–79].

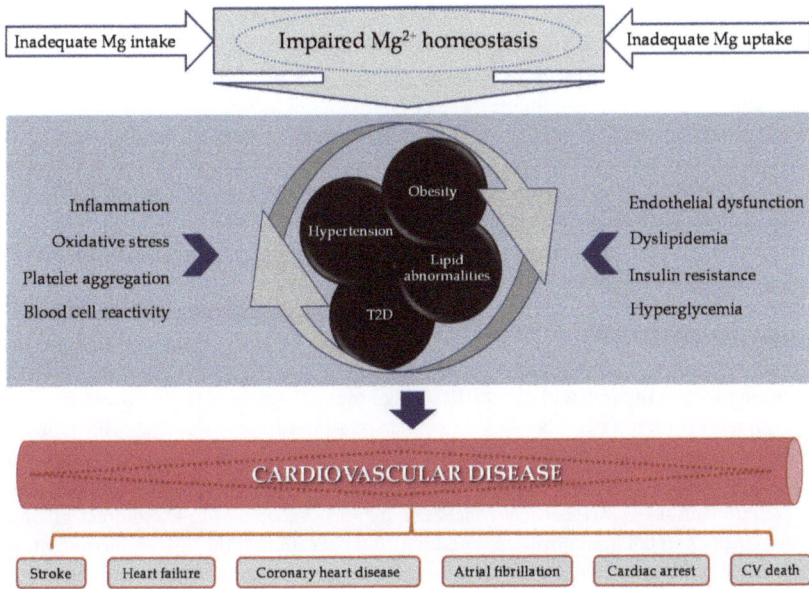

Figure 2. Mechanisms linking magnesium abnormalities (intake or circulating levels) with molecular outcomes leading to CV risk factors that may induce CV disease. Abbreviations: CV, cardiovascular; Mg, magnesium; T2D, type 2 diabetes.

In this paper, we have mainly focused in outcomes related to CVD and/or their risk factors. Studies investigating these mechanisms have mostly focused on the effects of Mg supplementation or circulating [Mg^{2+}] levels on inflammation and/or oxidative processes. However, specific in vitro and/or in vivo research has also been conducted to explore the overall processes affecting CV outcomes or CV risk factors (Figure 2).

5.1. Oxidative and Inflammatory Stress

Already at the beginning of the 20th century, after the discovery of Mg as an essential nutrient, Mg-D was linked to inflammation [80]. It is well-characterized that a previous phase of Mg depletion renders cells—particularly myocardial tissue—more sensitive to oxidative stress [75–77]. However, supplementation with Mg led to an increase in antioxidant blood concentrations [75,81,82]. It has been hypothesized either that Mg-D induces oxidative stress due to its pro-inflammatory effect, or that Mg itself possess antioxidant properties, scavenging oxygen radicals [75,76]. Mg-D may also induce a pro-inflammatory response by modulation of the intracellular Ca^{2+} concentration, release of neurotransmitters, or the activation of nuclear factor-kB implicated in the regulation of immune and inflammatory responses [76].

Freedman and collaborators demonstrated during the nineties the participation of free radicals in Mg-D cardiomyopathy and the incapacity of Mg-deficient animals to withstand an in vivo oxidative stress [78,79]. They evaluated the effect on Syrian hamsters being fed for 14 days with a Mg-deficient diet or a Mg-supplemented control diet, showing that Mg-D increases the susceptibility of the CV system to oxidative stress [79]. However, researchers also found that the concentration of nitric oxide (NO) is markedly increased in plasma of Mg-deficient rats, thus providing an additional cause of oxidative lesions through formation of peroxynitrite [83].

In vitro studies were also performed and the effect of Mg-deficient culture on endothelial cell susceptibility to oxidative stress was examined. Bovine endothelial cells were cultured in either control sufficient (0.8 mM) or deficient (0.4 mM) levels of $MgCl_2$. Results derived from this investigation suggest that in vitro Mg-D enhances free radical-induced intracellular oxidation and cytotoxicity in endothelial cells [84]. To further explore these effects, Wiles et al. examined the exposure of acute Mg-D to this cell type. Decreasing $[Mg^{2+}]$ ($\leq$0.25 mM) significantly increased endothelial cell oxidant production relative to control $[Mg^{2+}]$ (1 mM). This suggested that acute Mg-D is sufficient for the induction of endothelial cells oxidant production, the extent of which may determine, at least in part, the extent of endothelial cells dysfunction/injury associated with chronic Mg-D [85].

Severe dietary Mg restriction (9% of the recommended dietary allowance (RDA) is sufficient to induce a pro-inflammatory neurogenic response in rats [86]. Thus, Kramer and collaborators evaluated in 2003 whether less severe dietary Mg restriction modulates the extent of both the neurogenic/oxidative responses in vivo and ischemia/reperfusion injury in vitro. Male Sprague-Dawley rats maintained on Mg (40% RDA) or Mg (100% RDA) diets during the first three weeks were compared with the 9% RDA Mg group. They found that erythrocyte glutathione and plasma malondialdehyde levels revealed a direct relationship between the severity of oxidative stress and hypomagnesemia. Thus, suggesting that varying dietary Mg intake directly influences the magnitude of the neurogenic/oxidative responses in vivo and the resultant myocardial tolerance to ischemia/reperfusion stress [87]. Because it has been demonstrated that Mg-D promotes inflammation in vivo, Bernardini and collaborators evaluated the effect of different $[Mg^{2+}]$ on microvascular 1G11 cells [88]. They reported that low $[Mg^{2+}]$ inhibits endothelial growth and migration, while it increases some inflammatory- and endothelial-related markers (IL-1a, IL-6, NO and VCAM), whereas high $[Mg^{2+}]$ stimulates cell proliferation and migration. This result demonstrated a direct role of Mg in the modulation of microvascular functions and provided a molecular explanation to the link among Mg, angiogenesis and inflammation observed in in vivo CV models [88].

5.2. Lipid Profile and Peroxidation

Rayssiguier and collaborators demonstrated for the first time in 1993, using Wistar rats, that dietary Mg-D affects susceptibility of lipoproteins and tissues to peroxidation [89]. The destruction of membrane lipids and the end-products of such lipid peroxidation reactions are especially dangerous for the viability of cells and tissues, hence comprising a crucial step in the pathogenesis of several CVD [90]. Several years later, Morrill et al. monitored changes in rat lipid extracts of aortic and cerebrovascular smooth muscle as extracellular $[Mg^{2+}]$ was being reduced. They found, within the pathophysiological range of Mg^{2+}, a progressive reduction in fatty acid chain length and double bond content—which results in fatty acid truncation—as $[Mg^{2+}]$ is lowered. A decrease in lipid oxidation in the presence of elevated $[Mg^{2+}]$ could contribute to the apparent protective role of increased Mg intake on vascular function in humans [91].

Postprandial accumulation of triglyceride-rich lipoproteins (TGRLP) is an important characteristic of hyperlipidemia associated with Mg-D in animal models. Control and Mg-deficient rats were fed for eight days on adequate or Mg-D diets. Researchers tested the susceptibility of TGRLP isolated from control and treated rats to cell-dependent peroxidation and the effect of these lipoproteins on in vitro cultured vascular smooth muscle cells (VSMC). Results showed a higher oxidation in the case of Mg-deficient rats. This outcome warrants the atherogenic properties of Mg-D, which is accompanied by hyperlipidemia and which affects two important linked pathways: lipoprotein peroxidation and VSMC proliferation [92]. Moreover, additional results proved that TGRLP-oxidative damage is not the result of a decrease in vitamin E antioxidant status [93].

Altura and collaborators investigated in vivo the etiology of cardiac diseases. They examined the effects of Mg depletion on myocardial bioenergetic, carbohydrate, lipid and phospholipid metabolism. Rat myocardial biopsies were studied after being fed for 3 months with a dietary Mg restriction (20% normal dietary intake). Dietary Mg-D resulted in a drop in myocardial glycogen, glucose 6-phosphate, glycerol phosphate, as well as the contents of different phospholipids, illustrating impaired phospholipid metabolism and mitochondrial oxidation of long-chain fatty acids. These observations are consistent with the principle that prolonged low [Mg^{2+}] can result in marked reduction in O_2 and substrate delivery to the cardiac myocytes, with concomitant changes in membrane phospholipids (potentially resulting in a pro-oxidant state) probably as a result of coronary vasoconstriction [94].

5.3. Glucose Homeostasis/Type 2 Diabetes

The means whereby hypomagnesemia may promote or worsen existing T2D have not been fully unraveled. It has been suggested that Mg^{2+} regulates cellular glucose metabolism directly as it serves as an important cofactor for various enzymes and acts as a second messenger for insulin [95]. Importantly, it was also observed that insulin enhances intracellular Mg^{2+} uptake and this in turn mediates diverse effects ascribed to insulin [95]. Furthermore, low [Mg^{2+}] may induce altered cellular glucose transport, reduced pancreatic insulin secretion, defective post-receptor insulin signaling and/or altered insulin–insulin receptor interactions [96] and thus aggravate the processes related to IR, important risk factor for CVD [95].

5.4. Endothelial Function, Blood Pressure and Hypertension

In spite of considerable research, the exact underlying causes for altered Mg metabolism in hypertensive individuals remain unclear [97]. It is assumed that inadequate dietary Mg intake or a malfunction on its metabolism can lead to vasospasm and endothelial damage [98]. Therefore, as it has already introduced before, Mg-D might affect BP and/or endothelial function, which may promote hypertension.

In an in vitro study, Maier et al. cultured human umbilical vein endothelial cells for various times in media containing different [Mg^{2+}] (2–10 mM) and compared them to the corresponding controls (1 mM). High [Mg^{2+}] stimulated endothelial proliferation and enhanced the mitogenic response to angiogenic factors. In addition, high [Mg^{2+}] did not modulate the levels of plasminogen activator inhibitor-1, but enhanced the synthesis of NO, in part through the up-regulation of endothelial nitric oxide synthase. Thus, as it induces the synthesis of NO, Mg supplementation could be a helpful management approach in hypertension as well as in preventing thrombosis [99].

The effect of dietary Mg supplementation on BP and CV function has also been evaluated in vivo. Normotensive rats and mineralocorticoid-salt (DOCA-salt) hypertensive rats were fed for 5 weeks with a purified diet containing either a normal or Mg-supplemented diet (1.5 or 10 g/kg diet). Mg supplementation significantly lowered BP levels in hypertensive rats, but not in normotensive rats, and heart rate was not affected in either group. These findings suggested that the lowering effect of Mg supplementation on BP in hypertensive rats may be related to a vascular effect of Mg that reduces vascular tone [100]. To further test the effect of its supplementation on the development of hypertension in spontaneously hypertensive rats (SHR), Touyz et al. designed an in vivo study. Ten-week-old SHR and control Wistar-Kyoto rats (WKY) were divided into four groups which were fed for 17 weeks: WKY, WKY with Mg supplementation (650 mg/L), SHR, and SHR with Mg supplementation (650 mg/L). From 13 weeks of age, BP was significantly elevated in SHR compared with age-matched WKY. BP was significantly reduced in SHR after 10 weeks of Mg supplementation. From 18 weeks of age, serum and intracellular [Mg^{2+}] levels were significantly lower in SHR than in WKY. Mg supplementation was able to normalize intracellular $[Mg^{2+}]$ and $[Ca^{2+}]$ in SHR. Overall, these results showed that mid-term Mg supplementation significantly attenuates, but does not prevent, the development of hypertension in SHR [101]. Importantly, Blache et al. tested the long-term effect of Mg-D. Rats were fed for 22 months with moderately deficient (150 mg/kg), standard (800 mg/kg), or supplemented (3200 mg/kg) Mg diets. Compared to the standard and supplemented diets, Mg-D enriched diet significantly increased BP, plasma IL-6, fibrinogen, and erythrocyte lysophosphatidylcholine. Thus, Mg-D induced a chronic impairment of redox status associated with inflammation, which could significantly contribute to increased oxidized lipids and promote hypertension and vascular disorders with aging. Extrapolating these results to the human situation and considering that Mg-D has been reported to be remarkably common—particularly among elderly individuals—Mg supplementation may be useful as an adjuvant therapy in preventing CVD [77].

5.5. Cardiovascular Disease Events: Arrhythmia and Acute Myocardial Infarction

Probably the most widely accepted and practiced use of Mg in CV medicine is for the prevention and/or treatment of cardiac arrhythmias [31]. Anti-arrhythmogenic properties of Mg may involve changes in the activity of some ionic channels, such as Ca^{2+} and K^+ [102]. Both extracellular and cytosolic Mg^{2+} has significant effects on cardiac ion channels, which in turn may have important consequences on the duration of action potential, cell excitability and contractility [102]. Mg^{2+} exerts its antiarrhythmic effect via modulation of myocardial excitability. However, very few studies have evaluated the effect of Mg^{2+} on cardiac voltage-dependent Na^+ channels. Using inside-out patches from guinea pig ventricular myocytes to measure currents through single cardiac Na^+ channels, Mubagwa et al. [103] showed that $[Mg^{2+}]$ had no effect on inward currents but decreased the outward current amplitude in a concentration and voltage-dependent manner. This suggested that Mg^{2+} primarily exerts only an open channel blocking effect, with little or no direct allosteric modulatory action on the voltage-dependent Na^+ channels.

Data coming from autopsies indicated that patients who had died from IHD had reduced Mg^{2+} levels in myocardium and muscle compared with those who had died from non-cardiac causes. It was observed that during myocardial ischemia, total intracellular Mg^{2+} decreases while free intracellular Mg^{2+} increases [104]. In addition, ischemia per se leads to intracellular Ca^{2+} overload, which compromises myocardial function. It was speculated that Mg^{2+} administration reduces Ca^{2+} overload as a result of the competence between these two elements for the same binding sites. In addition, the effects of Mg^{2+} on vascular tone, its ability to improve endothelial dependent vasodilation, its anticoagulant properties, possibly through improvement of NO release [105], may all exert a beneficial effect in acute myocardial infarction. In accordance with these findings, investigators started to study Mg^{2+} replacement as an adjunctive pharmacotherapy in the context of acute myocardial infarction.

5.6. A Focus on Magnesium Receptors

Research in the mechanisms of control of vascular Mg^{2+} homeostasis revealed two cation channels of the transient receptor potential melastatin (TRPM), TRPM6 and TRPM7, as important Mg^{2+} transporters [105]. They are differentially expressed, with TRPM6 being primarily found in epithelial cells and TRPM7 occurring ubiquitously. Vascular TRPM7 is modulated by vasoactive agents, pressure, stretch, and osmotic changes and may be a novel mechanotransducer. In addition to its Mg^{2+} transporter function, TRPM7 has been implicated as a signaling kinase involved in VSMC growth, apoptosis, adhesion, contraction, important processes involved in vascular remodeling associated with hypertension and other vascular diseases [105]. Overall, TRPM7 has been shown to play an essential role in maintaining cellular Mg^{2+} homeostasis. However, more research is needed to clarify the exact mechanisms of Mg^{2+} regulation in the CV system and the implications of abnormal transmembrane Mg^{2+} transport in the pathogenesis of vascular diseases [106]. In fact, a recent randomized, double-blind clinical trial conducted in pre-hypertensive subjects compared the effect of oral Mg supplementation versus placebo treatment for four month in the expression of different Mg^{2+} transporters in leukocytes. Rodríguez-Ramírez and collaborators reported a significant increase in the TRPM6 mRNA relative expression in leukocytes from pre-hypertensive individuals following the oral Mg supplementation compared to placebo group. Conversely, non-significant differences were reported regarding TRPM7 and solute carrier family 41 member 1 (SLC41A1) mRNA relative expression [107].

Overall, Mg is an essential microelement critical in several biological processes. Its specific role on the CV system has been widely investigated. However, further in vitro and in vivo studies are needed to explore other potential molecular targets and pathways putatively modulated and influenced by dietary and circulating Mg^{2+} levels.

6. Final Conclusions

Taken together, current evidence from epidemiological studies shows that higher Mg intake, either dietary or via supplementation, is associated with a protection against major CV risk factors, including MetS, T2D and hypertension/BP, as well as against stroke and total CVDs. Nevertheless, further prospective studies and RCTs are warranted to elucidate the relation between Mg intake and MetS individual components, endothelial dysfunction, lipid profile and obesity—of which current scientific knowledge remains very scarce—and HF, CHD and CVD death in different populations. Available evidence on circulating Mg and CVDs shows that greater circulating $[Mg^{2+}]$ is also associated with lower risk of CVDs, mainly IHD and CHD, yet further insights are needed to clarify the less consistent results with other CVDs and CV death. Because Mg plays a crucial role in a wide range of biological pathways and outcomes, it is not surprising that alterations in Mg homeostasis may influence different disease status.

Importantly, the fact that Mg intake is determined using indirect methods in epidemiological studies, such as food frequency questionnaires, makes it difficult to separate the observed associations from those of other microelements that may also positively contribute to cardiometabolic health. Thus, a residual effect from the intake of other dietary microelements cannot be discarded despite the efforts for controlling this in multivariate models.

Traditionally, supplement formulations from organic Mg (aspartate, citrate, lactate and chloride) have been considered to be more bioavailable than those with inorganic Mg (oxide and sulfate), as reported by a number of studies [108]. However, this topic is currently under debate given that other studies have found no differences between these formulations, and several factors have been shown to play a role in the complex process of Mg absorption and utilization [109].

The inverse association between Mg intake and IR, hyperglycemia, dyslipidemia, hypertension, and markers of inflammation may justify the protective effect of dietary Mg on CVD. Overall, the current evidence supports the importance of adequate dietary magnesium for lowering CVD risk. In addition, these findings support the importance to increase the consumption of magnesium-rich foods, including fruits, vegetables, legumes, nuts and whole grains for the prevention of chronic diseases.

Acknowledgments: This work was supported in part by the Spanish Ministry of Health (Carlos III Health Institute) through the Fondo de Investigacion para la Salud (FIS), which is co-funded by the European Regional Development Fund. NR.-E is beneficiary of a predoctoral FI-AGAUR fellowship from the Secretaria d'Universitats i Recerca del Departament d'Economia i Coneixement de la Generalitat de Catalunya. Marta Guasch-Ferré was supported by a postdoctoral fellowship granted by the Lilly Foundation European Association of Diabetes (EASD) through the Institut d'Investigacions Sanitàries Pere i Virgili (IISPV), Tarragona, Spain.

Author Contributions: N.R.-E., M.G.-F., P.H.-A. and J.S.S. designed the review; N.R.-E., M.G.-F., P.H.-A. and J.S.S. performed the literature research; N.R.-E., M.G.-F., P.H.-A. and J.S.S. wrote the first draft of the manuscript; and all authors contributed to the editing of the manuscript. All authors approved the final version of the manuscript.

Conflicts of Interest: The authors declare no conflict of interest.

Nutrients **2018**, *10*, 168

Abbreviations

ARIC	Atherosclerosis Risk in Communities
ATP	adenosine triphosphate
BMI	body mass index
BP	blood pressure
Ca^{2+}	calcium
CHD	coronary heart disease
CV	cardiovascular
CVD	cardiovascular disease
DNA	deoxyribonucleic acid
GLUT 4	glucose transporter protein activity 4
HDL	high-density lipoprotein
HF	heart failure
HR	hazard ratio
HOMA-IR	homeostatic model assessment of insulin resistance
IHD	ischemic heart disease
IL	interleukin
IR	insulin resistance
K+	potassium
LDL	low-density lipoprotein
MetS	metabolic syndrome
Mg	magnesium
Mg-D	Mg-deficiency
$[Mg^{2+}]$	magnesium concentrations
Mg^{2+}	intracellular magnesium
Na+	sodium
NO	nitric oxide
O2	oxygen
T2D	type 2 diabetes
TGRLP	triglyceride-rich lipoproteins
TRPM	transient receptor potential melastatin
RCT	randomized control trial
RDA	recommended dietary allowance
RR	Relative Risk
sICAM-1	soluble intercellular adhesion molecule 1
SLC41A1	solute carrier family 41 member 1
SHR	spontaneously hypertensive rats
UVEC	umbilical vein endothelial cells
VCAM	vascular cell adhesion protein 1
VSMC	vascular smooth muscle cells
WKY	Wistar-Kyoto rats

References

1. Gröber, U.; Schmidt, J.; Kisters, K. Magnesium in Prevention and Therapy. *Nutrients* **2015**, 8199–8226. [CrossRef] [PubMed]
2. Standing Committee on the Scientific Evaluation of Dietary Reference Intakes; Food and Nutrition Board; Institute of Medicine (IOM). *Dietary Reference Intakes for Calcium, Phosphorus, Magnesium, Vitamin D, and Fluoride*; National Academies Press: Washington, DC, USA, 1997.
3. Fang, X.; Wang, K.; Han, D.; He, X.; Wei, J.; Zhao, L.; Imam, M.U.; Ping, Z.; Li, Y.; Xu, Y.; et al. Dietary magnesium intake and the risk of cardiovascular disease, type 2 diabetes, and all-cause mortality: A dose—Response meta- analysis of prospective cohort studies. *BMC Med.* **2016**. [CrossRef] [PubMed]

4. Del Gobbo, L.C.; Imamura, F.; Wu, J.H.Y.; Otto, M.C.D.O.; Chiuve, S.E. Circulating and dietary magnesium and risk of cardiovascular disease: A systematic review and meta-analysis of prospective studies. *Am. J. Clin. Nutr.* **2013**, 160–173. [CrossRef] [PubMed]

5. Qu, X.; Jin, F.; Hao, Y.; Li, H.; Tang, T.; Wang, H.; Yan, W.; Dai, K. Magnesium and the Risk of Cardiovascular Events: A Meta-Analysis of Prospective Cohort Studies. *PLoS ONE* **2013**, *8*. [CrossRef] [PubMed]

6. Chiuve, S.E.; Sun, Q.; Curhan, G.C.; Taylor, E.N.; Spiegelman, D.; Willett, W.C.; Manson, J.E.; Rexrode, K.M.; Albert, C.M. Dietary and plasma magnesium and risk of coronary heart disease among women. *J. Am. Heart Assoc.* **2013**, 1–10. [CrossRef] [PubMed]

7. Meyer, T.E.; Verwoert, G.C.; Hwang, S.J.; Glazer, N.L.; Smith, A.V.; van Rooij, F.J.A.; Ehret, G.B.; Boerwinkle, E.; Felix, J.F.; Leak, T.S.; et al. Genome-wide association studies of serum magnesium, potassium, and sodium concentrations identify six loci influencing serum magnesium levels. *PLoS Genet.* **2010**, *6*. [CrossRef] [PubMed]

8. Saris, N.-E.L.E.A. Magnesium An update on phsyiological, clinical and analytical aspects. *Clin. Chim. Acta* **2000**, *294*, 1–26. [CrossRef]

9. Jahnen-Dechent, W.; Ketteler, M. Magnesium basics. *CKJ Clin. Kidney J.* **2012**, *5*. [CrossRef] [PubMed]

10. US Department of Agriculture, Agricultural Research Service, Nutrient Data Laboratory. USDA National Nutrient Database for Standard Reference, Release 28 (Revised). Available online: www.ars.usda.gov/ba/bhnrc/ndl (accessed on 24 January 2018).

11. Shechter, M. Magnesium and cardiovascular system. *Magnes. Res.* **2010**, *23*, 60–72. [CrossRef] [PubMed]

12. Gommers, L.M.M.; Hoenderop, J.G.J.; Bindels, R.J.M.; de Baaij, J.H.F. Hypomagnesemia in Type 2 Diabetes: A Vicious Circle? *Diabetes* **2016**, *65*, 3–13. [CrossRef] [PubMed]

13. Fang, X.; Han, H.; Li, M.; Liang, C.; Fan, Z.; Aaseth, J.; He, J.; Montgomery, S.; Cao, Y. Dose-Response Relationship between Dietary Magnesium Intake and Risk of Type 2 Diabetes Mellitus: A Systematic Review and Meta-Regression Analysis of Prospective Cohort Studies. *Nutrients* **2016**, *8*, 739. [CrossRef] [PubMed]

14. Dong, J.-Y.; Xun, P.; He, K.; Qin, L.-Q. Magnesium Intake and Risk of Type 2 Diabetes: Meta-analysis of prospective cohort studies. *Diabetes Care* **2011**, *34*, 2116–2122. [CrossRef] [PubMed]

15. Schulze, M.B.; Schulz, M.; Heidemann, C.; Schienkiewitz, A.; Hoffmann, K.; Boeing, H. Fiber and magnesium intake and incidence of type 2 diabetes: A prospective study and meta-analysis. *Arch. Intern. Med.* **2007**, *167*, 956–965. [CrossRef] [PubMed]

16. Hruby, A.; Guasch-Ferré, M.; Bhupathiraju, S.N.; Manson, J.E.; Willett, W.C.; McKeown, N.M.; Hu, F.B. Magnesium Intake, Quality of Carbohydrates, and Risk of Type 2 Diabetes: Results from Three U.S. Cohorts. *Diabetes Care* **2017**, *40*, 1695–1702. [CrossRef] [PubMed]

17. Simental-Mendía, L.E.; Sahebkar, A.; Rodríguez-Morán, M.; Guerrero-Romero, F. A systematic review and meta-analysis of randomized controlled trials on the effects of magnesium supplementation on insulin sensitivity and glucose control. *Pharmacol. Res.* **2016**, *111*, 272–282. [CrossRef] [PubMed]

18. Guerrero-Romero, F.; Rodríguez-Morán, M. Magnesium improves the beta-cell function to compensate variation of insulin sensitivity: Double-blind, randomized clinical trial. *Eur. J. Clin. Investig.* **2011**, *41*, 405–410. [CrossRef] [PubMed]

19. Song, Y.; He, K.; Levitan, E.B.; Manson, J.E.; Liu, S. Effects of oral magnesium supplementation on glycaemic control in Type 2 diabetes: A meta-analysis of randomized double-blind controlled trials. *Diabetes Med.* **2006**, *23*, 1050–1056. [CrossRef] [PubMed]

20. Guerrero-Romero, F.; Tamez-Perez, H.E.; González-González, G.; Salinas-Martínez, A.M.; Montes-Villarreal, J.; Treviño-Ortiz, J.H.; Rodríguez-Morán, M. Oral magnesium supplementation improves insulin sensitivity in non-diabetic subjects with insulin resistance. A double-blind placebo-controlled randomized trial. *Diabetes Metab.* **2004**, *30*, 253–258. [CrossRef]

21. He, K.; Liu, K.; Daviglus, M.L.; Morris, S.J.; Loria, C.M.; Van Horn, L.; Jacobs, D.R.; Savage, P.J. Magnesium intake and incidence of metabolic syndrome among young adults. *Circulation* **2006**, *113*, 1675–1682. [CrossRef] [PubMed]

22. Sarrafzadegan, N.; Khosravi-Boroujeni, H.; Lotfizadeh, M.; Pourmogaddas, A.; Salehi-Abargouei, A. Magnesium status and the metabolic syndrome: A systematic review and meta-analysis. *Nutrition* **2016**, *32*, 409–417. [CrossRef] [PubMed]

23. McKeown, N.M.; Jacques, P.F.; Zhang, X.L.; Juan, W.; Sahyoun, N.R. Dietary magnesium intake is related to metabolic syndrome in older Americans. *Eur. J. Nutr.* **2008**, *47*, 210–216. [CrossRef] [PubMed]

24. Ju, S.-Y.; Choi, W.-S.; Ock, S.-M.; Kim, C.-M.; Kim, D.-H. Dietary magnesium intake and metabolic syndrome in the adult population: Dose-response meta-analysis and meta-regression. *Nutrients* **2014**, *6*, 6005–6019. [CrossRef] [PubMed]

25. Dibaba, D.T.; Xun, P.; Fly, A.D.; Yokota, K.; He, K. Dietary magnesium intake and risk of metabolic syndrome: A meta-analysis. *Diabet. Med.* **2014**, *31*, 1301–1309. [CrossRef] [PubMed]

26. Nguyen, H.; Odelola, O.A.; Rangaswami, J.; Amanullah, A. A Review of Nutritional Factors in Hypertension Management. *Int. J. Hypertens.* **2013**, *2013*, 1–12. [CrossRef] [PubMed]

27. Touyz, R.M.; Milne, F.J.; Reinach, S.G. Intracellular Mg^{2+}, Ca^{2+}, Na^{2+} and K^{+} in platelets and erythrocytes of essential hypertension patients: Relation to blood pressure. *Clin. Exp. Hypertens. A* **1992**, *14*, 1189–1209. [CrossRef] [PubMed]

28. Dibaba, D.T.; Xun, P.; Song, Y.; Rosanoff, A.; Shechter, M.; He, K. The effect of magnesium supplementation on blood pressure in individuals with insulin resistance, prediabetes, or noncommunicable chronic diseases: A meta-analysis of randomized controlled trials. *Am. J. Clin. Nutr.* **2017**, *106*, 921–929. [CrossRef] [PubMed]

29. Jee, S.H.; Miller, E.R.; Guallar, E.; Singh, V.K.; Appel, L.J.; Klag, M.J. The effect of magnesium supplementation on blood pressure: A meta-analysis of randomized clinical trials. *Am. J. Hypertens.* **2002**, *15*, 691–696. [CrossRef]

30. Kass, L.; Weekes, J.; Carpenter, L. Effect of magnesium supplementation on blood pressure: A meta-analysis. *Eur. J. Clin. Nutr.* **2012**, *66*, 411–418. [CrossRef] [PubMed]

31. Kolte, D.; Vijayaraghavan, K.; Khera, S.; Sica, D.A.; Frishman, W.H. Role of magnesium in cardiovascular diseases. *Cardiol. Rev.* **2014**, *22*, 182–192. [CrossRef] [PubMed]

32. Song, Y.; Li, T.Y.; van Dam, R.M.; Manson, J.E.; Hu, F.B. Magnesium intake and plasma concentrations of markers of systemic inflammation and endothelial dysfunction in women. *Am. J. Clin. Nutr.* **2007**, *85*, 1068–1074. [PubMed]

33. Chacko, S.A.; Song, Y.; Nathan, L.; Tinker, L.; de Boer, I.H.; Tylavsky, F.; Wallace, R.; Liu, S. Relations of dietary magnesium intake to biomarkers of inflammation and endothelial dysfunction in an ethnically diverse cohort of postmenopausal women. *Diabetes Care* **2010**, *33*, 304–310. [CrossRef] [PubMed]

34. Shechter, M.; Sharir, M.; Labrador, M.J.; Forrester, J.; Silver, B.; Bairey Merz, C.N. Oral magnesium therapy improves endothelial function in patients with coronary artery disease. *Circulation* **2000**, *102*, 2353–2358. [CrossRef] [PubMed]

35. Carr, M.C.; Brunzell, J.D. Abdominal obesity and dyslipidemia in the metabolic syndrome: Importance of type 2 diabetes and familial combined hyperlipidemia in coronary artery disease risk. *J. Clin. Endocrinol. Metab.* **2004**, *89*, 2601–2607. [CrossRef] [PubMed]

36. Singh, R.B.; Rastogi, S.S.; Sharma, V.K.; Saharia, R.B.; Kulshretha, S.K. Can dietary magnesium modulate lipoprotein metabolism? *Magnes. Trace Elem.* **1990**, *9*, 255–264. [PubMed]

37. Geiger, H.; Wanner, C. Magnesium in disease. *Clin. Kidney J.* **2012**, *5*, i25–i38. [CrossRef] [PubMed]

38. Guerrero-Romero, F.; Rodríguez-Morán, M. Low serum magnesium levels and metabolic syndrome. *Acta Diabetol.* **2002**, *39*, 209–213. [CrossRef] [PubMed]

39. Mirmiran, P.; Shab-Bidar, S.; Hosseini-Esfahani, F.; Asghari, G.; Hosseinpour-Niazi, S.; Azizi, F. Magnesium intake and prevalence of metabolic syndrome in adults: Tehran Lipid and Glucose Study. *Public Health Nutr.* **2012**, *15*, 693–701. [CrossRef] [PubMed]

40. Bain, L.K.M.; Myint, P.K.; Jennings, A.; Lentjes, M.A.H.; Luben, R.N.; Khaw, K.-T.; Wareham, N.J.; Welch, A.A. The relationship between dietary magnesium intake, stroke and its major risk factors, blood pressure and cholesterol, in the EPIC-Norfolk cohort. *Int. J. Cardiol.* **2015**, *196*, 108–114. [CrossRef] [PubMed]

41. Simental-Mendía, L.E.; Simental-Mendía, M.; Sahebkar, A.; Rodríguez-Morán, M.; Guerrero-Romero, F. Effect of magnesium supplementation on lipid profile: A systematic review and meta-analysis of randomized controlled trials. *Eur. J. Clin. Pharmacol.* **2017**, *73*, 525–536. [CrossRef] [PubMed]

42. Larsson, S.C.; Orsini, N.; Wolk, A. Dietary magnesium intake and risk of stroke: A meta-analysis of prospective studies. *Am. J. Clin. Nutr.* **2012**, *95*, 362–366. [CrossRef] [PubMed]

43. Nie, Z.-L.; Wang, Z.-M.; Zhou, B.; Tang, Z.-P.; Wang, S.-K. Magnesium intake and incidence of stroke: Meta-analysis of cohort studies. *Nutr. Metab. Cardiovasc. Dis.* **2013**, *23*, 169–176. [CrossRef] [PubMed]

44. Adebamowo, S.N.; Spiegelman, D.; Willett, W.C.; Rexrode, K.M. Association between intakes of magnesium, potassium, and calcium and risk of stroke: 2 Cohorts of US women and updated meta-analyses. *Am. J. Clin. Nutr.* **2015**, *101*, 1269–1277. [CrossRef] [PubMed]

45. Liao, F.; Folsom, A.R.; Brancati, F.L. Is low magnesium concentration a risk factor for coronary heart disease? The Atherosclerosis Risk in Communities (ARIC) Study. *Am. Heart J.* **1998**, *136*, 480–490. [CrossRef]

46. Abbott, R.D.; Ando, F.; Masaki, K.H.; Tung, K.H.; Rodriguez, B.L.; Petrovitch, H.; Yano, K.; Curb, J.D. Dietary magnesium intake and the future risk of coronary heart disease (The Honolulu heart program). *Am. J. Cardiol.* **2003**, *92*, 665–669. [CrossRef]

47. Song, Y.; Manson, J.E.; Cook, N.R.; Albert, C.M.; Buring, J.E.; Liu, S. Dietary magnesium intake and risk of cardiovascular disease among women. *Am. J. Cardiol.* **2005**, *96*, 1135–1141. [CrossRef] [PubMed]

48. Dai, Q.; Shu, X.-O.; Deng, X.; Xiang, Y.-B.; Li, H.; Yang, G.; Shrubsole, M.J.; Ji, B.; Cai, H.; Chow, W.-H.; et al. Modifying effect of calcium/magnesium intake ratio and mortality: A population-based cohort study. *Br. Med. J.* **2013**, *3*, e002111. [CrossRef] [PubMed]

49. Kokubo, Y.; Saito, I.; Iso, H.; Yamagishi, K.; Yatsuya, H.; Ishihara, J.; Maruyama, K.; Inoue, M.; Sawada, N.; Tsugane, S. Dietary magnesium intake and risk of incident coronary heart disease in men: A prospective cohort study. *Clin. Nutr.* **2017**, 1–7. [CrossRef] [PubMed]

50. Taveira, T.H.; Ouellette, D.; Gulum, A.; Choudhary, G.; Eaton, C.B.; Liu, S.; Wu, W.C. Relation of magnesium intake with cardiac function and heart failure hospitalizations in black adults. *Circ. Heart Fail.* **2016**, *9*. [CrossRef]

51. Zhang, W.; Iso, H.; Ohira, T.; Date, C.; Tamakoshi, A. Associations of dietary magnesium intake with mortality from cardiovascular disease: The JACC study. *Atherosclerosis* **2012**, *221*, 587–595. [CrossRef] [PubMed]

52. Misialek, J.R.; Lopez, F.L.; Lutsey, P.L.; Huxley, R.R.; Peacock, J.M.; Chen, L.Y.; Soliman, E.Z.; Agarwal, S.K.; Alonso, A. Serum and Dietary Magnesium and Incidence of Atrial Fibrillation in Whites and in African Americans—Atherosclerosis Risk in Communities (ARIC) Study. *Circ. J.* **2013**, *77*, 323–329. [CrossRef] [PubMed]

53. Nielsen, F.H.; Milne, D.B.; Klevay, L.M.; Gallagher, S.; Johnson, L.A. Dietary magnesium deficiency induces heart rhythm changes, impairs glucose tolerance, and decreases serum cholesterol in post menopausal women. *J. Am. Coll. Nutr.* **2007**, *26*, 121–132. [CrossRef] [PubMed]

54. Deng, X.; Song, Y.; Manson, J.E.; Signorello, L.B.; Zhang, S.M.; Shrubsole, M.J.; Ness, R.M.; Seidner, D.L.; Dai, Q. Magnesium, vitamin D status and mortality: Results from US National Health and Nutrition Examination Survey (NHANES) 2001 to 2006 and NHANES III. *BMC Med.* **2013**, *11*, 187. [CrossRef] [PubMed]

55. Levitan, E.B.; Shikany, J.M.; Ahmed, A.; Snetselaar, L.G.; Martin, L.W.; Curb, J.D.; Lewis, C.E. Calcium, magnesium and potassium intake and mortality in women with heart failure: The Women's Health Initiative. *Br. J. Nutr.* **2013**, *110*, 179–185. [CrossRef] [PubMed]

56. Chiuve, S.E.; Korngold, E.C.; Januzzi, J.L., Jr.; Gantzer, M.L.; Albert, C.M. Plasma and dietary magnesium and risk of sudden cardiac death. *Am. J. Clin. Nutr.* **2011**, 253–260. [CrossRef] [PubMed]

57. Guasch-Ferré, M.; Bulló, M.; Estruch, R.; Corella, D.; Martínez-González, M.A.; Ros, E.; Covas, M.; Arós, F.; Gómez-Gracia, E.; Fiol, M.; et al. Dietary magnesium intake is inversely associated with mortality in adults at high cardiovascular disease risk. *J. Nutr.* **2014**, *144*, 55–60. [CrossRef] [PubMed]

58. Xu, T.; Sun, Y.; Xu, T.; Zhang, Y. Magnesium intake and cardiovascular disease mortality: A meta-analysis of prospective cohort studies. *Int. J. Cardiol.* **2013**, *167*, 3044–3047. [CrossRef] [PubMed]

59. Fang, X.; Liang, C.; Li, M.; Montgomery, S.; Fall, K.; Aaseth, J.; Cao, Y. Dose-response relationship between dietary magnesium intake and cardiovascular mortality: A systematic review and dose-based meta-regression analysis of prospective studies. *J. Trace Elem. Med. Biol.* **2016**, *38*, 64–73. [CrossRef] [PubMed]

60. Zhang, X.; Del Gobbo, L.C.; Hruby, A.; Rosanoff, A.; He, K.; Dai, Q.; Costello, R.B.; Zhang, W.; Song, Y. The Circulating Concentration and 24-h Urine Excretion of Magnesium Dose- and Time-Dependently Respond to Oral Magnesium Supplementation in a Meta-Analysis of Randomized Controlled Trials. *J. Nutr.* **2016**, *146*, 595–602. [CrossRef] [PubMed]

61. Joosten, M.M.; Gansevoort, R.T.; Mukamal, K.J.; Van Der Harst, P.; Geleijnse, J.M.; Feskens, E.J.M. Urinary and plasma magnesium and risk of ischemic heart disease. *Am. J. Clin. Nutr.* **2013**, *97*, 1299–1306. [CrossRef] [PubMed]

62. Ohira, T.; Peacock, J.M.; Iso, H.; Chambless, L.E.; Rosamond, W.D.; Folsom, A.R. Serum and dietary magnesium and risk of ischemic stroke. *Am. J. Epidemiol.* **2009**, *169*, 1437–1444. [CrossRef] [PubMed]

63. Akarolo-Anthony, S.N.; Jiménez, M.C.; Chiuve, S.E.; Spiegelman, D.; Willett, W.C.; Rexrode, K.M. Plasma magnesium and risk of ischemic stroke among women. *Stroke* **2014**, *45*, 2881–2886. [CrossRef]

64. Khan, A.M.; Lubitz, S.A.; Sullivan, L.M.; Sun, J.X.; Levy, D.; Vasan, R.S.; Magnani, J.W.; Ellinor, P.T.; Benjamin, E.J.; Wang, T.J. Low serum magnesium and the development of atrial fibrillation in the community: The framingham heart study. *Circulation* **2013**, *127*, 33–38. [CrossRef] [PubMed]

65. Reffelmann, T.; Dörr, M.; Ittermann, T.; Schwahn, C.; Völzke, H.; Ruppert, J.; Robinson, D.; Felix, S.B. Low serum magnesium concentrations predict increase in left ventricular mass over 5 years independently of common cardiovascular risk factors. *Atherosclerosis* **2010**, *213*, 563–569. [CrossRef] [PubMed]

66. Lutsey, P.L.; Alonso, A.; Michos, E.D.; Loehr, L.R.; Astor, B.C.; Coresh, J.; Folsom, A.R. Serum magnesium, phosphorus, and calcium are associated with risk of incident heart failure: The Atherosclerosis Risk in Communities (ARIC). *Am. J. Clin. Nutr.* **2014**, 756–764. [CrossRef] [PubMed]

67. Kunutsor, S.K.; Khan, H.; Laukkanen, J.A. Serum magnesium and risk of new onset heart failure in men: The Kuopio Ischemic Heart Disease Study. *Eur. J. Epidemiol.* **2016**, *31*, 1035–1043. [CrossRef] [PubMed]

68. Ma, J.; Folsom, A.R.; Melnick, S.L.; Eckfeldt, J.H.; Sharrett, A.R.; Nabulsi, A.A.; Hutchinson, R.G.; Metcalf, P.A. Associations of serum and dietary magnesium with cardiovascular disease, hypertension, diabetes, insulin, and carotid arterial wall thickness: The aric study. *J. Clin. Epidemiol.* **1995**, *48*. [CrossRef]

69. Hashimoto, T.; Hara, A.; Ohkubo, T.; Kikuya, M.; Shintani, Y.; Metoki, H.; Inoue, R.; Asayama, K.; Kanno, A.; Nakashita, M.; et al. Serum magnesium, ambulatory blood pressure, and carotid artery alteration: The ohasama study. *Am. J. Hypertens.* **2010**, *23*, 1292–1298. [CrossRef] [PubMed]

70. Lee, S.Y.; Hyun, Y.Y.; Lee, K.B.; Kim, H. Low serum magnesium is associated with coronary artery calcification in a Korean population at low risk for cardiovascular disease. *Nutr. Metab. Cardiovasc. Dis.* **2015**, *25*, 1056–1061. [CrossRef] [PubMed]

71. Posadas-Sánchez, R.; Posadas-Romero, C.; Cardoso-Saldaña, G.; Vargas-Alarcón, G.; Villarreal-Molina, M.T.; Pérez-Hernández, N.; Rodríguez-Pérez, J.M.; Medina-Urrutia, A.; Jorge-Galarza, E.; Juárez-Rojas, J.G.; et al. Serum magnesium is inversely associated with coronary artery calcification in the Genetics of Atherosclerotic Disease (GEA) study. *Nutr. J.* **2015**, *15*, 22. [CrossRef] [PubMed]

72. Zhang, X.; Xia, J.; Del Gobbo, L.C.; Hruby, A.; Dai, Q.; Song, Y. Serum magnesium concentrations and all-cause, cardiovascular, and cancer mortality among U.S. adults: Results from the NHANES I Epidemiologic Follow-up Study. *Clin. Nutr.* **2017**. [CrossRef] [PubMed]

73. Kieboom, B.C.T.; Niemeijer, M.N.; Leening, M.J.G.; van den Berg, M.E.; Franco, O.H.; Deckers, J.W.; Hofman, A.; Zietse, R.; Stricker, B.H.; Hoorn, E.J. Serum Magnesium and the Risk of Death From Coronary Heart Disease and Sudden Cardiac Death. *J. Am. Heart Assoc.* **2016**, *5*, e002707. [CrossRef] [PubMed]

74. Angkananard, T.; Anothaisintawee, T.; Eursiriwan, S.; Gorelik, O.; McEvoy, M.; Attia, J.; Thakkinstian, A. The association of serum magnesium and mortality outcomes in heart failure patients. *Medicine (Baltimore)* **2016**, *95*, e5406. [CrossRef] [PubMed]

75. Barbagallo, M.; Dominguez, L.J.; Galioto, A.; Ferlisi, A.; Cani, C.; Malfa, L.; Pineo, A.; Busardo', A.; Paolisso, G. Role of magnesium in insulin action, diabetes and cardio-metabolic syndrome X. *Mol. Asp. Med.* **2003**, *24*, 39–52. [CrossRef]

76. Mazur, A.; Maier, J.A.M.; Rock, E.; Gueux, E.; Nowacki, W.; Rayssiguier, Y. Magnesium and the inflammatory response: Potential physiopathological implications. *Arch. Biochem. Biophys.* **2007**, *458*, 48–56. [CrossRef] [PubMed]

77. Blache, D.; Devaux, S.; Joubert, O.; Loreau, N.; Schneider, M.; Durand, P.; Prost, M.; Gaume, V.; Adrian, M.; Laurant, P.; et al. Long-term moderate magnesium-deficient diet shows relationships between blood pressure, inflammation and oxidant stress defense in aging rats. *Free Radic. Biol. Med.* **2006**, *41*, 277–284. [CrossRef] [PubMed]

78. Freedman, A.M.; Atrakchi, A.H.; Cassidy, M.M.; Weglicki, W.B. Magnesium deficiency-induced cardiomyopathy: Protection by vitamin E. *Biochem. Biophys. Res. Commun.* **1990**, *170*, 1102–1106. [CrossRef]

79. Freedman, A.M.; Cassidy, M.M.; Weglicki, W.B. Magnesium-deficient myocardium demonstrates an increased susceptibility to an in vivo oxidative stress. *Magnes. Res.* **1991**, *4*, 185–189. [PubMed]

80. King, D.E. Inflammation and elevation of C-reactive protein: Does magnesium play a key role? *Magnes. Res.* **2009**, *22*, 57–59. [PubMed]

81. Olatunji, L.A.; Soladoye, A.O. Increased magnesium intake prevents hyperlipidemia and insulin resistance and reduces lipid peroxidation in fructose-fed rats. *Pathophysiology* **2007**, *14*, 11–15. [CrossRef] [PubMed]

82. Garcia, L.A.; Dejong, S.C.; Martin, S.M.; Smith, R.S.; Buettner, G.R.; Kerber, R.E. Magnesium reduces free radicals in an in vivo coronary occlusion- reperfusion model. *J. Am. Coll. Cardiol.* **1998**, *32*, 536–539. [CrossRef]

83. Rock, E.; Astier, C.; Lab, C.; Malpuech, C.; Nowacki, W.; Gueux, E.; Mazur, A.; Rayssiguier, Y. Magnesium deficiency in rats induces a rise in plasma nitric oxide. *Magnes. Res.* **1995**, *8*, 237–242. [PubMed]

84. Dickens, B.F.; Weglicki, W.B.; Li, Y.S.; Mak, I.T. Magnesium deficiency in vitro enhances free radical-induced intracellular oxidation and cytotoxicity in endothelial cells. *FEBS Lett.* **1992**, *311*, 187–191. [CrossRef]

85. Wiles, M.E.; Wagner, T.L.; Weglicki, W.B. Effect of acute magnesium deficiency (MgD) on aortic endothelial cell (EC) oxidant production. *Life Sci.* **1997**, *60*, 221–236. [CrossRef]

86. Kramer, J.H.; Mišík, V.; Weglicki, W.B. Magnesium-deficiency potentiates free radical production associated with postischemic injury to rat hearts: Vitamin E affords protection. *Free Radic. Biol. Med.* **1994**, *16*, 713–723. [CrossRef]

87. Kramer, J.H.; Mak, I.T.; Phillips, T.M.; Weglicki, W.B. Dietary magnesium intake influences circulating pro-inflammatory neuropeptide levels and loss of myocardial tolerance to postischemic stress. *Exp. Biol. Med. (Maywood)* **2003**, *228*, 665–673. [CrossRef] [PubMed]

88. Bernardini, D.; Nasulewic, A.; Mazur, A.; Maier, J.A.M. Magnesium and microvascular endothelial cells: A role in inflammation and angiogenesis. *Front. Biosci.* **2005**, *10*, 1177–1182. [CrossRef] [PubMed]

89. Rayssiguier, Y.; Gueux, E.; Bussière, L.; Durlach, J.; Mazur, A. Dietary magnesium affects susceptibility of lipoproteins and tissues to peroxidation in rats. *J. Am. Coll. Nutr.* **1993**, *12*, 133–137. [CrossRef] [PubMed]

90. Mylonas, C.; Kouretas, D. Lipid peroxidation and tissue damage. *In Vivo* **1999**, *13*, 295–309. [PubMed]

91. Morrill, G.A.; Gupta, R.K.; Kostellow, A.B.; Ma, G.Y.; Zhang, A.; Altura, B.T.; Altura, B.M. Mg^{2+} modulates membrane lipids in vascular smooth muscle: A link to atherogenesis. *FEBS Lett.* **1997**, *408*, 191–194. [CrossRef]

92. Bussière, L.; Mazur, A.; Gueux, E.; Nowacki, W.; Rayssiguier, Y. Triglyceride-rich lipoproteins from magnesium-deficient rats are more susceptible to oxidation by cells and promote proliferation of cultured vascular smooth muscle cells. *Magnes. Res.* **1995**, *8*, 151–157. [PubMed]

93. Gueux, E.; Azais-Braesco, V.; Bussière, L.; Grolier, P.; Mazur, A.; Rayssiguier, Y. Effect of magnesium deficiency on triacylglycerol-rich lipoprotein and tissue susceptibility to peroxidation in relation to vitamin E content. *Br. J. Nutr.* **1995**, *74*, 849–856. [PubMed]

94. Altura, B.M.; Gebrewold, A.; Altura, B.T.; Brautbar, N. Magnesium depletion impairs myocardial carbohydrate and lipid metabolism and cardiac bioenergetics and raises myocardial calcium content in-vivo: Relationship to etiology of cardiac diseases. *Biochem. Mol. Biol. Int.* **1996**, *40*, 1183–1190. [CrossRef] [PubMed]

95. Takaya, J.; Higashino, H.; Kobayashi, Y. Intracellular magnesium and insulin resistance. *Magnes. Res.* **2004**, *17*, 126–136. [PubMed]

96. Pham, P.-C.T.; Pham, P.-M.T.; Pham, S.V.; Miller, J.M.; Pham, P.-T.T. Hypomagnesemia in Patients with Type 2 Diabetes. *Clin. J. Am. Soc. Nephrol.* **2007**, *2*, 366–373. [CrossRef] [PubMed]

97. Sontia, B.; Touyz, R.M. Magnesium transport in hypertension. *Pathophysiol. Off. J. Int. Soc. Pathophysiol.* **2007**, *14*, 205–211. [CrossRef] [PubMed]

98. Barbagallo, M.; Dominguez, L.J.; Resnick, L.M. Magnesium metabolism in hypertension and type 2 diabetes mellitus. *Am. J. Ther.* **2007**, *14*, 375–385. [CrossRef] [PubMed]

99. Maier, J.A.M.; Bernardini, D.; Rayssiguier, Y.; Mazur, A. High concentrations of magnesium modulate vascular endothelial cell behaviour in vitro. *Biochim. Biophys. Acta Mol. Basis Dis.* **2004**, *1689*, 6–12. [CrossRef] [PubMed]

100. Laurant, P.; Kantelip, J.P.; Berthelot, A. Dietary magnesium supplementation modifies blood pressure and cardiovascular function in mineralocorticoid-salt hypertensive rats but not in normotensive rats. *J. Nutr.* **1995**, *125*, 830–841. [PubMed]

101. Touyz, R.M.; Milne, F.J. Magnesium supplementation attenuates, but does not prevent, development of hypertension in spontaneously hypertensive rats. *Am. J. Hypertens.* **1999**, *12*, 757–765. [CrossRef]

102. Agus, M.S.D.; Agus, Z.S. Cardiovascular actions of magnesium. *Crit. Care Clin.* **2001**, *17*, 175–186. [CrossRef]

103. Mubagwa, K.; Gwanyanya, A.; Zakharov, S.; Macianskiene, R. Regulation of cation channels in cardiac and smooth muscle cells by intracellular magnesium. *Arch. Biochem. Biophys.* **2007**, *458*, 73–89. [CrossRef] [PubMed]

104. Johnson, C.J.; Peterson, D.R.; Smith, E.K. Myocardial tissue concentrations of magnesium and potassium in men dying suddenly from ischemic heart disease. *Am. J. Clin. Nutr.* **1979**, *32*, 967–970. [CrossRef] [PubMed]

105. Paravicini, T.M.; Chubanov, V.; Gudermann, T. TRPM7: A unique channel involved in magnesium homeostasis. *Int. J. Biochem. Cell Biol.* **2012**, *44*, 1381–1384. [CrossRef] [PubMed]

106. Touyz, R.M. Transient receptor potential melastatin 6 and 7 channels, magnesium transport, and vascular biology: Implications in hypertension. *Am. J. Physiol. Heart Circ. Physiol.* **2008**, *294*, H1103–H1118. [CrossRef] [PubMed]

107. Rodríguez-Ramírez, M.; Rodríguez-Morán, M.; Reyes-Romero, M.A.; Guerrero-Romero, F. Effect of oral magnesium supplementation on the transcription of TRPM6, TRPM7, and SLC41A1 in individuals newly diagnosed of pre-hypertension. A randomized, double-blind, placebo-controlled trial. *Magnes. Res.* **2017**, *30*, 80–87. [PubMed]

108. Kappeler, D.; Heimbeck, I.; Herpich, C.; Naue, N.; Höfler, J.; Timmer, W.; Michalke, B. Higher bioavailability of magnesium citrate as compared to magnesium oxide shown by evaluation of urinary excretion and serum levels after single-dose administration in a randomized cross-over study. *BMC Nutr.* **2017**, *3*, 7. [CrossRef]

109. Schuchardt, J.P.; Hahn, A. Intestinal Absorption and Factors Influencing Bioavailability of Magnesium—An Update. *Curr. Nutr. Food Sci.* **2017**, *13*, 260–278. [CrossRef] [PubMed]

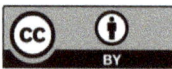

nutrients

MDPI

Article

Dietary Magnesium Intake and Hyperuricemia among US Adults

Yiying Zhang [1,2] **and Hongbin Qiu** [1,2,*]

[1]   Department of Epidemiology, School of Public Health, Harbin Medical University,
       Harbin 150081, China; yiyingzhang@hrbmu.edu.cn
[2]   School of Public Health, Jiamusi University, Jiamusi 154007, China
*   Correspondence: qiuhongbin@jmsu.edu.cn; Tel.: +86-139-0368-1456

Received: 23 January 2018; Accepted: 27 February 2018; Published: 2 March 2018

Abstract: To assess the association between dietary magnesium intake and hyperuricemia in United States (US) adults, we extracted 26,796 US adults aged 20–85 years from the National Health and Nutrition Examination Survey (NHANES) in 2001–2014. All dietary intake was measured through 24 h dietary recall method. Multivariable logistic regression analysis was performed to investigate the association between magnesium intake and hyperuricemia after adjusting for several important confounding variables. When compared to the lowest quintile (Q1), for male, adjusted odds ratios (ORs) of hyperuricemia in the second quintile (Q2) to the fifth quintile (Q5) of the magnesium intake were 0.83 (95% CI: 0.72–0.95), 0.74 (0.64–0.85), 0.78 (0.67–0.90), and 0.70 (0.58–0.84, p for trend = 0.0003), respectively. For female, OR was 0.75 (0.62–0.90) in the fourth quintile (Q4) (p for trend = 0.0242). As compared to Q4 of magnesium intake (contains recommended amount), the relative odds of hyperuricemia were increased by 1.29 times in Q1 (OR = 1.29, 1.11–1.50) in male. The ORs were 1.33 (1.11–1.61) in Q1, 1.27 (1.07–1.50) in Q2 in female. Our results indicated that increased magnesium intake was associated with decreased hyperuricemia risk. It also indicated the importance of recommended dietary allowance (RDA) of magnesium and the potential function of magnesium intake in the prevention of hyperuricemia.

Keywords: hyperuricemia; magnesium; NHANES; cross-sectional study

1. Introduction

Uric acid is the ultimate product of purine metabolism. When the level of serum uric acid transcends the normal level, hyperuricemia occurs. Previous studies indicated that hyperuricemia not only increased the risk of gout, but also had a close relationship with the development of hypertension, kidney disease, metabolic syndrome, obesity, cardiovascular disease [1–5], lipid metabolism disorders, and type 2 diabetes [6,7]. Nowadays, hyperuricemia is becoming a serious public health problem and epidemiological studies had shown a growing trend in the prevalence of hyperuricemia and gout. The reported prevalence of hyperuricemia ranged from 8.9% to 24.4% in diverse populations [8–11]. Nevertheless, the pathophysiology of hyperuricemia has not yet been completely illustrated.

Magnesium, which plays a significant role in prevention and treatment of several disorders, is a vital nutrient for human body. Recommended dietary allowance (RDA) of magnesium intake was developed by the Food and Nutrition Board (FNB) of the Institute of Medicine and was based on age and sex. For United States (US) adults, the RDAs for magnesium is 400 mg/day for male aged 19–30, 420 mg/day for male aged 30 and over; 310 mg/day for female aged 19 and 30, and 320 mg/day for female aged 30 and over. RDA is the average daily level of intake sufficient to meet the nutrient requirements of nearly all individuals in a life-stage and gender group [12]. Magnesium insufficiency can lead to many chronic diseases, including cardiovascular disease, type 2 diabetes, osteoporosis, pulmonary disease, depression, migraine headaches, inflammation, and tumors [13]. Many earlier studies proved that dietary magnesium intake is inversely correlated with serum C-reactive protein (CRP) which is an established biomarker of inflammation [14–18]. As hyperuricemia was positively connected with CRP [19–21], uric acid may also have a role in inflammation and subsequent inflammatory related diseases [22]. Although magnesium intake may represented an essential and potentially modifiable link to hyperuricemia certain extent, there were only two previous studies investigating the relationship between magnesium intake and hyperuricemia, one revealed a relationship between magnesium deficiency and increased serum uric acid level with 94 diabetic retinopathy patients [23], and another showed that dietary magnesium intake was inversely associated with hyperuricemia in Chinese male [24].

No known studies have explored the association between dietary magnesium intake and hyperuricemia using a nationally representative sample in US. Therefore, the purpose of this cross-sectional study is to assess this correlation in US population with a hypothesis that dietary magnesium intake is inversely correlated with hyperuricemia.

2. Materials and Methods

2.1. Study Populations

This cross-sectional study used data from the National Health and Nutrition Examination Survey (NHANES), which is a nationally representative survey managed by the Centers for Disease Control and Prevention (CDC) [25]. NHANES is a consecutive survey with every two years, representing one cycle of the US civilian noninstitutionalized population, using a stratified, multistage sampling design. The program covers clinical, physical, laboratory examinations, as well as interviews to get diet and health indicators. NHANES is a publicly available dataset, which resides in the public domain (available on the web at: http://www.cdc.gov/nchs/nhanes.htm). The NCHS Research Ethics Review Board at the National Center for Health Statistics approved the study protocols for NHANES 1999–2016 [26], and additional Institutional Review Board approval for the secondary analyses was not required [27].

A total of 37,215 individuals from 2001 to 2014 aged 20–85 years with uric acid value constituted the study sample. We excluded pregnant women (*n* = 1507) and those with missing essential information on demographic or total nutrient intakes dietary interview (*n* = 8912). After exclusion, 26,796 subjects (13,807 men and 12,989 women) were included in our study.

2.2. Study Variables

The major variables included concentrations of uric acid and the intake of magnesium. Serum concentrations of uric acid were detected on a Beckman UniCel® DxC800 Synchron or a Beckman Synchron LX20 (Beckman Coulter, Inc., Brea, CA, USA) after oxidation of uric acid by uricase to form allantoin and H_2O_2. Hyperuricemia was defined as serum uric acid ≥ 7.0 mg/dL in males and ≥ 6.0 mg/dL in females. The intake of magnesium, energy, and protein were collected from total nutrient intakes provided by the first 24 h dietary recall interview which was obtained in-person in the Mobile Examination Center (MEC). Using estimated amounts of foods, nutrient intakes were computed at the individual-level using a revised nutrient database that converted amounts of specific food intakes into amounts of various nutrients [28], detailed descriptions of the dietary interview methods are provided in the NHANES Dietary Interviewers Procedure Manuals [29]. In addition, factors that had been proved to be correlated with the intake of magnesium as well as hyperuricemia were included in regression models to control for potential confounding. The covariates included age, race/ethnicity, marital status, education background, smoking status, drinking status, body mass index (BMI), waist circumference, hypertension status, diabetes status, energy intake, protein intake, creatinine, gamma glutamyl transferase (GGT), total cholesterol, glucose, triglycerides, and high-density lipoprotein cholesterol (HDL-C). We categorized race/ethnicity as non-Hispanic white, non-Hispanic black, Mexican American, and others (other Hispanics and multi-racial participants). Education background was classified into above high school, high school graduation/General Educational Development (GED), and less than high school. Diabetes status was obtained from self-report. BMI (kg/m^2) was computed from weight and height. Hypertension was defined as systolic blood pressure ≥140 mm Hg or diastolic blood pressure ≥90 mm Hg.

2.3. Statistical Analyses

Respondents were grouped into five levels, according to the magnesium intake quintile: <176 (Q1), 176–234 (Q2), 235–298 (Q3), 299–387 (Q4), and ≥388 mg/day (Q5) for entire respondents; <200 (Q1), 200–265 (Q2), 266–334 (Q3), 335–432 (Q4), and ≥433 mg/day (Q5) for males; <158 (Q1), 158–207 (Q2), 208–260 (Q3), 261–336 (Q4), and ≥337 mg/day (Q5) for females. The continuous variable was presented as median and Inter-Quartile Range (skewed distributed data), and the categorical variable was expressed as percentage. Wilcoxon signed-rank test was used to compare the magnesium intake and the population RDAs (RDAs for magnesium were 400 mg/day for male aged 19–30, 420 mg/day for male aged 30 and over; 310 mg/day for female aged 19 and 30, 320 mg/day for female aged 30 and over [12]). Differences in continuous variable were assessed by the Wilcoxon rank sum test and Kruskal-Wallis H test (non-normally distributed data and heteroscedasticity). Differences in categorical variable were evaluated by the chi-square test and multiple comparisons based on Bonferroni correction. Multivariable logistic regression analysis was used to estimate the odds ratio (OR) and 95% confidence interval (CI) of hyperuricemia, according to the magnesium intake quintile for male and female separately, with the lowest quintile and the fourth quintile being considered as the references, respectively. Models 1 and 4 adjusted for age, race/ethnicity. Based on models 1 and 4, models 2 and 5 further adjusted for smoking status, drinking status, education background, marital status, hypertension status and diabetes status. Models 3 and 6 further adjusted for creatinine, GGT, energy intake, protein intake, total cholesterol, glucose, BMI, waist circumference, HDL-C, and triglycerides. The lowest quintile (Q1) was regarded as the reference in Models 1, 2 and 3. The fourth quintile (Q4 contains the recommended amount) was regarded as the reference in Models 4, 5 and 6. All of the p values were two-sided, $p < 0.05$ was regarded as statistically significant, and $p < 0.0125$ (0.05/4), $p < 0.0167$ (0.05/3), $p < 0.025$ (0.05/2) was considered as statistical significance after Bonferroni adjustment for multiple comparisons. All of the analyses were performed using SAS version 9.4 (SAS Institute Inc., Cary, NC, USA).

3. Results

The daily magnesium intake was 301 mg (215 mg–414 mg) for male aged 20–30 years, 299 mg (217 mg–400 mg) for male aged 31–85 years, 226 mg (164 mg–306.5 mg) for female aged 20–30 years, and 234 mg (173 mg–314 mg) for female aged 31–85 years, all significantly lower than their respective RDAs [12], as is shown in Table 1. The result of comparing the indicators between hyperuricemia and non-hyperuricemia for both sexes is shown in Table 2. For male, except for marital status ($p = 0.3895$), drinking status ($p = 0.1323$), and diabetes status ($p = 0.2630$), other indicators were all significantly different between hyperuricemia and non-hyperuricemia. Compared to the participants without hyperuricemia, those with hyperuricemia were more likely to be older, non-Hispanic black, former smoker, have hypertension, less likely to be Mexican American, currently smoking, have higher BMI, waist circumference, creatinine, GGT, total cholesterol, glucose, triglycerides, and have lower magnesium intake, energy intake, protein intake, HDL-C. For female, all of the indicators were significantly different between hyperuricemia and non-hyperuricemia. Participants with hyperuricemia were more likely to be older, non-Hispanic black, high school or GED, living alone, never drinking, former drinking, former smoking, have hypertension and diabetes, less likely to be Mexican American, above high school, married or living with partner, currently drinking, never smoking, have higher BMI, waist circumference, creatinine, GGT, total cholesterol, glucose, triglycerides, and have lower energy intake, protein intake, magnesium intake, and HDL-C than normal individuals. More detailed information is presented in Supplementary Table S1.

Table 1. Magnesium intake among United States (US) adults (>19 years) in NHANES 2001–2014.

Age (Years)	RDAs for Magnesium (mg/Day)	Magnesium Intake (mg/Day)	*p*
20–30 [a]	400.00	301.00 (215.00, 414.00)	<0.0001
31–85 [a]	420.00	299.00 (217.00, 400.00)	<0.0001
20–30 [b]	310.00	226.00 (164.00, 306.50)	<0.0001
31–85 [b]	320.00	234.00 (173.00, 314.00)	<0.0001

[a] Male; [b] Female.

A description of the characteristics of study participants according to the intake of magnesium is shown in Table 3. Significant differences were detected across all quintiles of magnesium intake for age, gender, race/ethnicity, marital status, education background, smoking status, drinking status, BMI, waist circumference, hypertension status, diabetes status, hyperuricemia, energy intake, protein intake, creatinine, GGT, glucose, triglycerides, and HDL-C. No significant relationship was found between magnesium intake and total cholesterol (*p* = 0.2454). More detailed information is presented in Supplementary Table S2. Participants with higher magnesium intake were more likely to be younger, male, and less likely to be hypertension, diabetes, and hyperuricemia.

The correlation between magnesium intake and hyperuricemia was examined by multivariable model, as is shown in Table 4. The results suggested a strong inverse relationship between magnesium intake and hyperuricemia in this cross-sectional study. Among all participants, the prevalence of hyperuricemia was 20.33%. For male, the prevalence of hyperuricemia was 22.66%, when compared to those consuming less than 200 mg magnesium daily, the relative odds of hyperuricemia were significantly decreased by 0.83 times among those that were consuming 200–265 mg magnesium daily (OR = 0.83, 95% CI: 0.72–0.95), 0.74 times among participants who consumed 266–334 mg daily (OR = 0.74, 95% CI: 0.64–0.85), 0.78 times among those consuming 335–432 mg daily (OR = 0.78, 95% CI: 0.67–0.90), and by 0.70 times among those consuming 433 mg or greater daily (OR = 0.70, 95% CI: 0.58 to 0.84), respectively, and *p* for trend was 0.0003. For female, the prevalence of hyperuricemia was 17.87%, the OR were decreased by 0.75 times among those consuming 261–336 mg magnesium daily (OR = 0.75, 95% CI: 0.62–0.90), when compared to those consuming less than 158 mg daily and *p* for trend was 0.0242. Furthermore, for male, compared to Q4 of magnesium intake (contains recommended amounts), the relative odds of hyperuricemia were increased by 1.29 times in those consuming less than 200 mg magnesium daily (OR = 1.29, 95% CI: 1.11–1.50). For female, the ORs were increased by 1.33 times (OR = 1.33, 95% CI: 1.11–1.61) in those consuming less than 158 mg daily, and by 1.27 times (OR = 1.27, 95% CI: 1.07–1.50) in those consuming 158 to 207 mg daily.

Table 2. Characteristics of participants with or without hyperuricemia.

Characteristic	Male			Female		
	Non-Hyperuricemia (n = 10,679)	Hyperuricemia (n = 3128)	p	Non-Hyperuricemia (n = 10,668)	Hyperuricemia (n = 2321)	p
Age (years)	48.00 (34.00, 63.00)	50.00 (35.00, 66.00)	<0.0001	47.00 (34.00, 62.00)	61.00 (48.00, 72.00)	<0.0001
Race/ethnicity (n, %)			<0.0001			<0.0001
Non-Hispanic white	5224 (48.92)	1603 (51.25)	0.1846 [c]	5190 (48.65)	1195 (51.49)	0.1506 [c]
Non-Hispanic black	1986 (18.60)	698 (22.31)	0.0002 [c]	1942 (18.20)	602 (25.94)	<0.0001 [c]
Mexican American	1984 (18.58)	399 (12.76)	<0.0001 [c]	1872 (17.55)	254 (10.94)	<0.0001 [c]
Others [a]	1485 (13.91)	428 (13.68)	0.7824 [c]	1664 (15.60)	270 (11.63)	<0.0001 [c]
Education background (n, %)			0.0120			<0.0001
>High School	5200 (48.69)	1597 (51.05)	0.1772 [d]	5709 (53.52)	1081 (46.57)	0.0006 [d]
High school or GED [b]	2571 (24.08)	760 (24.30)	0.8423 [d]	2352 (22.05)	613 (26.41)	0.0004 [d]
<High School	2908 (27.23)	771 (24.65)	0.0279 [d]	2607 (24.44)	627 (27.01)	0.0450 [d]
Marital status (n, %)			0.3895			<0.0001
Married or living with partner	7138 (66.84)	2065 (66.02)		5987 (56.12)	1118 (48.17)	0.0001 [e]
Living alone	3541 (33.16)	1063 (33.98)		4681 (43.88)	1203 (51.83)	<0.0001 [e]
Drinking status (n, %)			0.1323			<0.0001
Never	786 (7.36)	217 (6.94)		2032 (19.05)	522 (22.49)	0.0021 [d]
Current	8895 (83.29)	2651 (84.75)		6615 (62.01)	1291 (55.62)	0.0043 [d]
Former	998 (9.35)	260 (8.31)		2021 (18.94)	508 (21.89)	0.0082 [d]
Smoking status (n, %)			<0.0001			<0.0001
Never	4721 (44.21)	1371 (43.83)	0.8153 [d]	6656 (62.39)	1304 (56.18)	0.0058 [d]
Current	2823 (26.44)	661 (21.13)	<0.0001 [d]	2024 (18.97)	384 (16.54)	0.0228 [d]
Former	3135 (29.36)	1096 (35.04)	<0.0001 [d]	1988 (18.64)	633 (27.27)	<0.0001 [d]
Magnesium intake (mg/day)	305.00 (223.00, 408.00)	278.00 (199.00, 380.50)	<0.0001	237.00 (174.00, 317.00)	213.00 (158.00, 289.00)	<0.0001
BMI (kg/m^2)	27.10 (24.10, 30.44)	29.69 (26.59, 33.66)	<0.0001	27.11 (23.40, 31.91)	31.64 (27.42, 37.10)	<0.0001
Creatinine (mg/dL)	0.97 (0.86, 1.10)	1.04 (0.91, 1.20)	<0.0001	0.73 (0.65, 0.82)	0.90 (0.75, 1.08)	<0.0001
Hypertension status (n, %)	2245 (21.02)	877 (28.04)	<0.0001	2109 (19.77)	755 (32.53)	<0.0001
Diabetes status (n, %)	1183 (11.08)	369 (11.80)	0.2630	976 (9.15)	492 (21.20)	<0.0001

[a] Other Hispanics and other races including multi-racial participants; [b] General Educational Development; [c] Statistically significant after Bonferonni adjustment (0.05/4 = 0.0125); [d] Statistically significant after Bonferonni adjustment (0.05/3 = 0.0167); [e] Statistically significant after Bonferonni adjustment (0.05/2 = 0.025).

Table 3. Characteristics of the participants according to intake of magnesium.

Characteristic	Magnesium Intake (mg/Day)					*p*
	Q1 (<176) (*n* = 5406)	Q2 (176–234) (*n* = 5394)	Q3 (235–298) (*n* = 5335)	Q4 (299–387) (*n* = 5324)	Q5 (≥388) (*n* = 5337)	
Age (years)	51.00 (34.00, 67.00)	51.00 (36.00, 66.00)	50.00 (35.00, 65.00)	48.50 (35.00, 63.00)	45.00 (33.00, 59.00)	<0.0001
Male (*n*, %)	1935 (35.79)	2281 (42.29)	2654 (49.75)	3102 (58.26)	3835 (71.86)	<0.0001
Race/ethnicity (*n*, %)						<0.0001
Non-Hispanic white	2377 (43.97)	2612 (48.42)	2664 (49.93)	2774 (52.10)	2785 (52.18)	
Non-Hispanic black	1524 (28.19)	1165 (21.60)	957 (17.94)	835 (15.68)	747 (14.00)	
Mexican American	790 (14.61)	815 (15.11)	931 (17.45)	948 (17.81)	1025 (19.21)	
Others [a]	715 (13.23)	802 (14.87)	783 (14.68)	767 (14.41)	780 (14.61)	
Education background (*n*, %)						<0.0001
>High School	2113 (39.09)	2620 (48.57)	2737 (51.30)	2997 (56.29)	3120 (58.46)	
High school or GED [b]	1444 (26.71)	1338 (24.81)	1266 (23.73)	1145 (21.51)	1103 (20.67)	
<High School	1849 (34.20)	1436 (26.62)	1332 (24.97)	1182 (22.20)	1114 (20.87)	
Marital status (*n*, %)						<0.0001
Married or living with partner	2921 (54.03)	3177 (58.90)	3313 (62.10)	3432 (64.46)	3465 (64.92)	
Living alone	2485 (45.97)	2217 (41.10)	2022 (37.90)	1892 (35.54)	1872 (35.08)	
Drinking status (*n*, %)						<0.0001
Never	962 (17.80)	826 (15.31)	722 (13.53)	571 (10.73)	476 (8.92)	
Current	3411 (63.10)	3721 (68.98)	3858 (72.31)	4116 (77.31)	4346 (81.43)	
Former	1033 (19.11)	847 (15.70)	755 (14.15)	637 (11.96)	515 (9.65)	
Smoking status (*n*, %)						<0.0001
Never	2776 (51.35)	2909 (53.93)	2891 (54.19)	2797 (52.54)	2679 (50.20)	
Current	1417 (26.21)	1136 (21.06)	1057 (19.81)	1096 (20.59)	1186 (22.22)	
Former	1213 (22.44)	1349 (25.01)	1387 (26.00)	1431 (26.88)	1472 (27.58)	
Hypertension status (*n*, %)	1416 (26.19)	1305 (24.19)	1180 (22.12)	1134 (21.30)	951 (17.82)	<0.0001
Diabetes status (*n*, %)	770 (14.24)	669 (12.40)	566 (10.61)	563 (10.57)	452 (8.47)	<0.0001
Hyperuricemia (*n*, %)	1312 (24.27)	1176 (21.80)	1035 (19.40)	990 (18.60)	936 (17.54)	<0.0001

[a] Other Hispanics and other races including multi-racial participants; [b] General Educational Development.

Table 4. Adjusted odds ratios of hyperuricemia among participants associated with magnesium intake.

		Magnesium Intake (mg/Day)					p for Trend
		Q1 (<200) (n = 2771)	Q2 (200–265) (n = 2753)	Q3 (266–334) (n = 2761)	Q4 (335–432) (n = 2776)	Q5 (≥433) (n = 2746)	
Male (n = 13,807)	Model 1 [a,d]	Reference	0.80 (0.71, 0.90)	0.71 (0.62, 0.80)	0.73 (0.64, 0.82)	0.61 (0.53, 0.69)	<0.0001
	Model 2 [b,d]	Reference	0.78 (0.69, 0.88)	0.69 (0.61, 0.78)	0.70 (0.62, 0.80)	0.59 (0.51, 0.67)	<0.0001
	Model 3 [c,d]	Reference	0.83 (0.72, 0.95)	0.74 (0.64, 0.85)	0.78 (0.67, 0.90)	0.70 (0.58, 0.84)	0.0003
	Model 4 [a,e]	1.38 (1.22, 1.56)	1.10 (0.97, 1.25)	0.97 (0.85, 1.10)	Reference	0.84 (0.73, 0.95)	
	Model 5 [b,e]	1.43 (1.26, 1.62)	1.11 (0.98, 1.26)	0.98 (0.86, 1.11)	Reference	0.84 (0.73, 0.96)	
	Model 6 [c,e]	1.29 (1.11, 1.50)	1.07 (0.93, 1.23)	0.95 (0.83, 1.09)	Reference	0.91 (0.78, 1.05)	
		Q1 (<158) (n = 2631)	Q2 (158–207) (n = 2625)	Q3 (208–260) (n = 2542)	Q4 (261–336) (n = 2616)	Q5 (≥337) (n = 2575)	
Female (n = 12,989)	Model 1 [a,d]	Reference	0.92 (0.80, 1.06)	0.79 (0.68, 0.91)	0.66 (0.57, 0.76)	0.66 (0.57, 0.77)	<0.0001
	Model 2 [b,d]	Reference	0.93 (0.81, 1.06)	0.80 (0.70, 0.93)	0.68 (0.58, 0.79)	0.69 (0.59, 0.80)	<0.0001
	Model 3 [c,d]	Reference	0.95 (0.81, 1.11)	0.86 (0.73, 1.02)	0.75 (0.62, 0.90)	0.87 (0.70, 1.08)	0.0242
	Model 4 [a,e]	1.52 (1.31, 1.76)	1.40 (1.21, 1.62)	1.20 (1.03, 1.39)	Reference	1.01 (0.86, 1.18)	
	Model 5 [b,e]	1.48 (1.27, 1.72)	1.37 (1.18, 1.59)	1.19 (1.02, 1.39)	Reference	1.02 (0.87, 1.20)	
	Model 6 [c,e]	1.33 (1.11, 1.61)	1.27 (1.07, 1.50)	1.15 (0.97, 1.35)	Reference	1.16 (0.98, 1.39)	

[a] Adjusted for age, race/ethnicity; [b] adjusted for age, race/ethnicity, smoking status, drinking status, education background, marital status, hypertension status and diabetes status; [c] adjusted for age, race/ethnicity, smoking status, drinking status, education background, marital status, hypertension status, diabetes status, creatinine, gamma glutamyl transferase (GGT), energy intake, protein intake, total cholesterol, glucose, body mass index (BMI), waist circumference, high-density lipoprotein cholesterol (HDL-C) and triglycerides; [d] the lowest quintile (Q1) was regarded as the reference; [e] the fourth quintile (Q4) was regarded as the reference.

4. Discussion

In this cross-sectional study, we found that dietary magnesium intake was inversely associated with hyperuricemia in both male and female among US adults, after adjusting for major confounding factors, including age, race/ethnicity, smoking status, drinking status, education background, marital status, hypertension status, diabetes status, creatinine, GGT, energy intake, protein intake, total cholesterol, glucose, BMI, waist circumference, HDL-C, and triglycerides.

To the best of our knowledge, this is the first and the largest population-based study revealing the relationship between dietary magnesium intake and hyperuricemia in both male and female using a nationally representative sample of US adults. Our findings suggested that magnesium intake was inversely associated with the risk of hyperuricemia. Another similar research in the south India found an inverse correlation between the magnesium and the uric acid level among 94 diabetic retinopathy patients [23]. A cross-sectional study involving 5168 subjects aged 40 years old or above in China has shown a negative association between dietary magnesium intake and hyperuricemia valid for man merely [24], which is different from our result that the inverse association between hyperuricemia and dietary magnesium intake was observed in both men and women. Several factors may account for the difference. Firstly, when compared to previous studies, the sample of our study is the largest (26,796 American adults, including 13,807 men and 12,989 women). Secondly, the participants included women of all ages (20–85 years) and excluded pregnant women, while the subjects in the previous study in China were aged 40 years old or above and the effect of dietary magnesium intake on the exact magnesium level in bodies may be mitigated in middle aged and old women because of their lower serum estrogen level [30]. Thirdly, our study focused on American adults.

Previous studies showed that the dairy product consumption and vitamin C might be helpful in protection against hyperuricemia [31–34]. The intake of soy products are inversely associated with hyperuricemia [35], vegetable and dairy protein, nuts, legumes, fruits with less sugar, and whole grains would likely lower the risk of gout [36]. Thus, hyperuricemia may be related to dietary modification. Our findings showed that increased magnesium intake may decrease the risks of hyperuricemia. Similarly, magnesium is a component of chlorophyll and green leafy vegetables is an important source. Legumes, fruits, and white vegetables are good dietary sources of magnesium. Besides, nuts, seeds, whole grains, and fortified foods are all rich in magnesium [12,37,38]. In general, foods containing dietary fiber can provide magnesium. Fiber has been identified as being beneficial for intestinal motility and as having a potential act in binding uric acid in the gut for excretion. Therefore, adequate magnesium intake in the diet seems particularly effective in decreasing hyperuricemia risk.

Our results showed that the everyday intake of magnesium in US adults were lower than the recommended amounts, and indicated the importance of RDAs for magnesium: persons with lower intake of magnesium (less than 200 mg per day in male, less than 208 mg per day in female) may have a higher risk of hyperuricemia when compared to those following RDAs of magnesium intake. For males, the RDAs for magnesium ranges from as low as 400 mg/day (age of 19–30 years) to 420 mg/day (age of 30 and over). For females, the RDAs for magnesium ranges from 310 mg/day (age of 19–30 years) to 320 mg/day (age of 30 and over) [12]. Our findings suggested that adequate magnesium intake may have a potential function in the prevention of hyperuricemia, it is beneficial for individuals to keep sufficient magnesium intake, as suggested by RDAs through daily meals to prevent or decrease the risk of hyperuricemia.

The biological mechanism underlying the association between dietary magnesium intake and the prevalence of hyperuricemia was not completely understood, but may be related to the inflammatory mechanism. Laboratory studies have linked magnesium insufficiency to acute inflammatory response mediated by calcium, N-methyl-D-aspartate, interleukin-6 (IL-6), and tumor necrosis factor-alpha (TNF-α) [39]. Several epidemiological studies discovered that lower magnesium intake was inversely associated with higher CRP [18–22], which is a well-documented biomarker of inflammation in adults [40,41], children [15], and obese patients [42]. A meta-analysis and systematic review, which included seven cross-sectional studies approved that dietary magnesium intake was inversely correlated with CRP [14]. In addition, many studies reported that hyperuricemia was associated positively with TNF-α, IL-6 and CRP, which suggested that uric acid may have a role in inflammation and subsequent inflammatory related diseases [22,43–45]. Moreover, increasing the blood level of uric acid can produce inflammation in the joints and surrounding tissues when crystallized [46]. Further studies are required to investigate the biological mechanism between dietary magnesium intake and hyperuricemia.

In addition, previous studies have shown that growing age and BMI were related to increased hyperuricemia risk, and hypertension may play an independent role for hyperuricemia [10]. Hyperuricemia may also be linked to serum creatinine levels since uric acid had been confirmed to be an influence factor for renal failure [47]. Our study showed that participants with hyperuricemia were more likely to be older, have hypertension, and have higher BMI and creatinine than normal individuals. Previous studies reported that increasing the intake of magnesium in conjunction with taurine can lower blood pressure and improve blood lipid profiles and decrease cardiovascular diseases [48]. Magnesium intake was inversely associated with arterial calcification too, as has been proved in another study [49]. A meta-analysis found that the risk of diabetes decreased when increasing magnesium intake [50]. In our study, participants with higher magnesium intake were less likely to have hypertension and diabetes.

Our study has several strengths. Firstly, this is the first study to assess the relationship between the intake of magnesium and the risk of hyperuricemia among US adults, and use a large (26,796 participants) and nationally representative sample. Secondly, we adjusted for many important confounding variables. Thirdly, the use of trained staff following standardized protocols to measure the basic information of study subjects and conduct interviews improves the precision and efficacy of the data that is obtained.

Our study also has some limitations. First, our study was a cross-sectional study, which limited the definition of the causal correlations, further prospective longitudinal investigations would be important to prove those conclusions. Second, dietary intake levels were estimated from 24 h dietary recall, which may not exactly describe the long-term magnesium intake situation. However, when compared with food frequency questionnaires, 24 h recalls provide greater detail on the varieties and quantities of food eaten and decrease the risk of underestimating or overestimating the intake level of micronutrients. When compared with the blood concentration measurement, blood level may not completely show the nutritional situation, and serum magnesium level only represents less than 1% of the total body magnesium [13]. Finally, further studies are needed to investigate the mechanism of this association.

5. Conclusions

Our findings presented a negative correlation between dietary magnesium intake and hyperuricemia in both male and female among US adults after adjusting for major confounding factors. The intake of magnesium of American adults was significantly lower than their respective RDAs. The study indicated the importance of RDAs of magnesium and the potential function of magnesium intake in the prevention of hyperuricemia, and suggested that deficient magnesium intake may increase the risk of hyperuricemia.

Supplementary Materials: The following are available online at http://www.mdpi.com/2072-6643/10/3/296/s1, Table S1: Dietary and clinical characteristics of participants with and without hyperuricemia, Table S2: Dietary and clinical characteristics of the participants according to intake of magnesium.

Author Contributions: H.Q. and Y.Z. designed the study and wrote the manuscript. Y.Z. analyzed and interpreted the data. All authors read and approved the final manuscript.

Conflicts of Interest: The authors declare no conflict of interest.

References

1. Feig, D.I.; Kang, D.H.; Johnson, R.J. Uric acid and cardiovascular risk. *N. Engl. J. Med.* **2008**, *359*, 1811–1821. [CrossRef] [PubMed]
2. Borghi, C.; Rosei, E.A.; Bardin, T.; Dawson, J.; Dominiczak, A.; Kielstein, J.T.; Manolis, A.J.; Perez-Ruiz, F.; Mancia, G. Serum uric acid and the risk of cardiovascular and renal disease. *J. Hypertens* **2015**, *33*, 1729–1741. [CrossRef] [PubMed]
3. Fang, J.; Alderman, M.H. Serum uric acid and cardiovascular mortality the NHANES I epidemiologic follow-up study, 1971–1992. *JAMA* **2000**, *283*, 2404–2410. [CrossRef] [PubMed]
4. Xu, X.; Hu, J.; Song, N.; Chen, R.; Zhang, T.; Ding, X. Hyperuricemia increases the risk of acute kidney injury: A systematic review and meta-analysis. *BMC Nephrol.* **2017**, *18*, 27. [CrossRef] [PubMed]
5. Dai, X.; Yuan, J.; Yao, P.; Yang, B.; Gui, L.; Zhang, X.; Guo, H.; Wang, Y.; Chen, W.; Wei, S. Association between serum uric acid and the metabolic syndrome among a middle- and old-age Chinese population. *Eur. J. Epidemiol.* **2013**, *28*, 669–676. [CrossRef] [PubMed]
6. Keenan, T.; Blaha, M.J.; Nasir, K.; Silverman, M.G.; Tota-Maharaj, R.; Carvalho, J.A.; Conceicao, R.D.; Blumenthal, R.S.; Santos, R.D. Relation of uric acid to serum levels of high-sensitivity c-reactive protein, triglycerides, and high-density lipoprotein cholesterol and to hepatic steatosis. *Am. J. Cardiol.* **2012**, *110*, 1787–1792. [CrossRef] [PubMed]
7. Sluijs, I.; Beulens, J.W.; Dl, V.D.A.; Spijkerman, A.M.; Schulze, M.B.; Yt, V.D.S. Plasma uric acid is associated with increased risk of type 2 diabetes independent of diet and metabolic risk factors. *J. Nutr.* **2013**, *143*, 80–85. [CrossRef] [PubMed]
8. Wallace, K.L.; Riedel, A.A.; Josephridge, N.; Wortmann, R. Increasing prevalence of gout and hyperuricemia over 10 years among older adults in a managed care population. *J. Rheumatol.* **2004**, *31*, 1582–1587. [PubMed]
9. Liu, H.; Zhang, X.M.; Wang, Y.L.; Liu, B.C. Prevalence of hyperuricemia among Chinese adults: A national cross-sectional survey using multistage, stratified sampling. *J. Nephrol.* **2014**, *27*, 653–658. [CrossRef] [PubMed]
10. Zhu, Y.; Pandya, B.J.; Choi, H.K. Prevalence of gout and hyperuricemia in the US general population: The National Health and Nutrition Examination Survey 2007–2008. *Arthritis Rheum.* **2011**, *63*, 3136–3141. [CrossRef] [PubMed]
11. Uaratanawong, S.; Suraamornkul, S.; Angkeaw, S.; Uaratanawong, R. Prevalence of hyperuricemia in bangkok population. *Clin. Rheumatol.* **2011**, *30*, 887–893. [CrossRef] [PubMed]
12. Usa, I.O.M. *Dietary Reference Intakes for Calcium, Phosphorus, Magnesium, Vitamin D, Andfluoride*; National Academies Press: Washington, DC, USA, 1997.
13. De Baaij, J.H.; Hoenderop, J.G.; Bindels, R.J. Magnesium in man: Implications for health and disease. *Physiol. Rev.* **2015**, *95*, 1–46. [CrossRef] [PubMed]
14. Dibaba, D.T.; Xun, P.; He, K. Dietary magnesium intake is inversely associated with serum C-reactive protein levels: Meta-analysis and systematic review. *Eur. J. Clin. Nutr.* **2014**, *68*, 510–516. [CrossRef] [PubMed]
15. King, D.E.; Geesey, M.E.; Ellis, T. Magnesium intake and serum C-reactive protein levels in children. *Magnes. Res.* **2007**, *20*, 32–36. [PubMed]
16. Song, Y.; Li, T.Y.; Dam, R.M.V.; Manson, J.A.E.; Hu, F.B. Magnesium intake and plasma concentrations of markers of systemic inflammation and endothelial dysfunction in women. *Am. J. Clin. Nutr.* **2007**, *85*, 1068–1074. [CrossRef] [PubMed]
17. King, D.E.; Rd, M.A.; Geesey, M.E.; Woolson, R.F. Dietary magnesium and C-reactive protein levels. *J. Am. Coll. Nutr.* **2005**, *24*, 166–171. [CrossRef] [PubMed]
18. Song, Y.; Ridker, P.M.; Manson, J.E.; Cook, N.R.; Buring, J.E.; Liu, S. Magnesium intake, C-reactive protein, and the prevalence of metabolic syndrome in middle-aged and older US Women. *Diabetes Care* **2005**, *28*, 1438–1444. [CrossRef] [PubMed]
19. Saito, M.; Ishimitsu, T.; Minami, J.; Ono, H.; Ohrui, M.; Matsuoka, H. Relations of plasma high-sensitivity C-reactive protein to traditional cardiovascular risk factors. *Atherosclerosis* **2003**, *167*, 73–79. [CrossRef]
20. Fröhlich, M.; Imhof, A.; Berg, G.; Hutchinson, W.L.; Pepys, M.B.; Boeing, H.; Muche, R.; Brenner, H.; Koenig, W. Association between C-reactive protein and features of the metabolic syndrome: A population-based study. *Diabetes Care* **2000**, *23*, 1835–1839. [CrossRef] [PubMed]

21. Ruggiero, C.; Cherubini, A.; Ble, A.; Bos, A.J.G.; Maggio, M.; Dixit, V.D.; Lauretani, F.; Bandinelli, S.; Senin, U.; Ferrucci, L. Uric acid and inflammatory markers. *Eur. Heart J.* **2006**, *27*, 1174–1181. [CrossRef] [PubMed]

22. Lyngdoh, T.; Marquesvidal, P.; Paccaud, F.; Preisig, M.; Waeber, G.; Bochud, M.; Vollenweider, P. Elevated serum uric acid is associated with high circulating inflammatory cytokines in the population-based colaus study. *PLoS ONE* **2011**, *6*, e19901. [CrossRef] [PubMed]

23. Navin, S.; Krishnamurthy, N.; Ashakiran, S.; Dayanand, C.D. The association of hypomagnesaemia, high normal uricaemia and dyslipidaemia in the patients with diabetic retinopathy. *J. Clin. Diagn. Res.* **2013**, *7*, 1852–1854.

24. Wang, Y.; Zeng, C.; Wei, J.; Yang, T.; Li, H.; Deng, Z.; Yang, Y.; Zhang, Y.; Ding, X.; Xie, D. Association between dietary magnesium intake and hyperuricemia. *PLoS ONE* **2015**, *10*, e0141079. [CrossRef] [PubMed]

25. National Health and Nutrition Examination Survey Data. Centers for Disease Control and Prevention (CDC). Available online: http://www.cdc.gov/NCHS/nhanes.htm (accessed on 30 August 2017).

26. NCHS Research Ethics Review Board (ERB) Approval. Centers for Disease Control and Prevention (CDC). Available online: https://www.cdc.gov/nchs/nhanes/irba98.htm (accessed on 7 June 2017).

27. US Department of Health & Human Services. Office of Extramural Research. Available online: http://grants.nih.gov/grants/policy/hs/hs_policies.htm (accessed on 30 August 2017).

28. United States Department of Agriculture (USDA), Agriculture Research Service FSRG. Food and Nutrient Database for Dietary Studies, 5.0. Available online: http://www.ars.usda.gov/ba/bhnrc/fsrg (accessed on 30 August 2017).

29. National Health and Nutrition Examination Survey (NHANES). MEC In-Person Dietary Interviewers Procedures Manual. Available online: http://www.cdc.gov/nchs/data/nhanes/nhanes_05_06/dietary_mec.pdf (accessed on 30 August 2017).

30. Muneyyirci-Delale, O.; Nacharaju, V.L.; Dalloul, M.; Altura, B.M.; Altura, B.T. Serum ionized magnesium and calcium in women after menopause: Inverse relation of estrogen with ionized magnesium. *Fertil. Steril.* **1999**, *71*, 869–872. [CrossRef]

31. Huang, H.Y.; Appel, L.J.; Choi, M.J.; Gelber, A.C.; Charleston, J.; Norkus, E.P.; Miller, E.R. The effects of vitamin C supplementation on serum concentrations of uric acid: Results of a randomized controlled trial. *Arthritis Rheum.* **2005**, *52*, 1843–1847. [CrossRef] [PubMed]

32. Dalbeth, N.; Wong, S.; Gamble, G.D.; Horne, A.; Mason, B.; Pool, B.; Fairbanks, L.; Mcqueen, F.M.; Cornish, J.; Reid, I.R. Acute effect of milk on serum urate concentrations: A randomised controlled crossover trial. *Ann. Rheum. Dis.* **2010**, *69*, 1677–1682. [CrossRef] [PubMed]

33. Garrel, D.R.; Verdy, M.; Petitclerc, C.; Martin, C.; Brulé, D.; Hamet, P. Milk- and soy-protein ingestion: Acute effect on serum uric acid concentration. *Am. J. Clin. Nutr.* **1991**, *53*, 665–669. [CrossRef] [PubMed]

34. Ghadirian, P.; Shatenstein, B.; Verdy, M.; Hamet, P. The influence of dairy products on plasma uric acid in women. *Eur. J. Epidemiol.* **1995**, *11*, 275–281. [CrossRef] [PubMed]

35. Villegas, R.; Xiang, Y.B.; Elasy, T.; Xu, W.H.; Cai, H.; Cai, Q.; Linton, M.F.; Fazio, S.; Zheng, W.; Shu, X.O. Purine-rich foods, protein intake, and the prevalence of hyperuricemia: The Shanghai men's health study. *Nutr. Metab. Cardiovasc. Dis.* **2012**, *22*, 409–416. [CrossRef] [PubMed]

36. Choi, H.K. A prescription for lifestyle change in patients with hyperuricemia and gout. *Curr. Opin. Rheumatol.* **2010**, *22*, 165–172. [CrossRef] [PubMed]

37. National Institutes of Health Office of Dietary Supplements. Magnesium Fact Sheet for Health Professionals. Available online: https://ods.od.nih.gov/factsheets/Magnesium-HealthProfessional/ (accessed on 10 August 2017).

38. Freedman, M.R.; Keast, D.R. White potatoes, including French fries, contribute shortfall nutrients to children's and adolescents' diets. *Nutr. Res.* **2011**, *31*, 270–277. [CrossRef] [PubMed]

39. Nielsen, F.H. Magnesium, inflammation, and obesity in chronic disease. *Nutr. Rev.* **2010**, *68*, 333–340. [CrossRef] [PubMed]

40. King, D.E.; Mainous, A.G., III; Geesey, M.E.; Egan, B.M.; Rehman, S. Magnesium supplement intake and c-reactive protein levels in adults. *Nutr. Res.* **2006**, *26*, 193–196. [CrossRef]

41. Chacko, S.A.; Song, Y.; Nathan, L.; Tinker, L.; Boer, I.H.D.; Tylavsky, F.; Wallace, R.; Liu, S. Relations of dietary magnesium intake to biomarkers of inflammation and endothelial dysfunction in an ethnically diverse cohort of postmenopausal women. *Diabetes Care* **2010**, *33*, 304–310. [CrossRef] [PubMed]

42. Guerrero-Romero, F.; Rodríguez-Morán, M. Relationship between serum magnesium levels and C-reactive protein concentration, in non-diabetic, non-hypertensive obese subjects. *Int. J. Obes.* **2002**, *26*, 469. [CrossRef]

43. Leyva, F.; Anker, S.D.; Godsland, I.F.; Teixeira, M.; Hellewell, P.G.; Kox, W.J.; Poole-Wilson, P.A.; Coats, A.J. Uric acid in chronic heart failure: A marker of chronic inflammation. *Eur. Heart J.* **1998**, *19*, 1814–1822. [CrossRef] [PubMed]

44. Ruggiero, C.; Cherubini, A.; Edgar Miller, I.; Maggio, M.; Najjar, S.S.; Lauretani, F.; Bandinelli, S.; Senin, U.; Ferrucci, L. Usefulness of uric acid to predict changes in C-reactive protein and interleukin-6 in 3-year period in italians aged 21 to 98 years. *Am. J. Cardiol.* **2007**, *100*, 115–121. [CrossRef] [PubMed]

45. Kirilmaz, B.; Asgun, F.; Alioglu, E.; Ercan, E.; Tengiz, I.; Turk, U.; Saygi, S.; Özerkan, F. High inflammatory activity related to the number of metabolic syndrome components. *J. Clin. Hypertens.* **2010**, *12*, 136–144. [CrossRef] [PubMed]

46. Pluta, R.M.; Burke, A.E.; Glass, R.M. Jama patient page. *Gout. J. Am. Med. Assoc.* **2010**, *304*, 2314. [CrossRef] [PubMed]

47. Hunsicker, L.G.; Adler, S.; Caggiula, A.; England, B.K.; Greene, T.; Kusek, J.W.; Rogers, N.L.; Teschan, P.E. Predictors of the progression of renal disease in the modification of diet in renal disease study. *Kidney Int.* **1997**, *51*, 1908–1919. [CrossRef] [PubMed]

48. Yamori, Y.; Taguchi, T.; Mori, H.; Mori, M. Low cardiovascular risks in the middle aged males and females excreting greater 24-h urinary taurine and magnesium in 41 who-cardiac study populations in the world. *J. Biomed. Sci.* **2010**, *17*, 1–5. [CrossRef] [PubMed]

49. Hruby, A.; O'Donnell, C.J.; Jacques, P.F.; Meigs, J.B.; Hoffmann, U.; Mckeown, N.M. Magnesium intake is inversely associated with coronary artery calcification: The Framingham heart study. *JACC Cardiovasc. Imaging* **2014**, *7*, 59–69. [CrossRef] [PubMed]

50. Larsson, S.C.; Wolk, A. Magnesium intake and risk of type 2 diabetes: A meta-analysis. *J. Intern. Med.* **2007**, *262*, 208–214. [CrossRef] [PubMed]

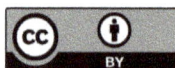

nutrients

MDPI

Article

Higher Dietary Magnesium Intake and Higher Magnesium Status Are Associated with Lower Prevalence of Coronary Heart Disease in Patients with Type 2 Diabetes

Christina M. Gant [1,2], Sabita S. Soedamah-Muthu [3,4], S. Heleen Binnenmars [2], Stephan J. L. Bakker [2], Gerjan Navis [2] and Gozewijn D. Laverman [1,*]

[1] Department of Internal Medicine/Nephrology, ZGT Hospital, 7609 PP Almelo, The Netherlands; c.gant@zgt.nl
[2] Department of Internal Medicine, Division of Nephrology, University of Groningen, University Medical Centre Groningen, 9713EZ Groningen, The Netherlands; s.h.binnenmars@umcg.nl (S.H.B.); s.j.l.bakker@umcg.nl (S.J.L.B.); g.j.navis@umcg.nl (G.N.)
[3] Centre of Research on Psychology in Somatic Diseases (CORPS), Department of Medical and Clinical Psychology, Tilburg University, 5037 AB Tilburg, The Netherlands; S.S.Soedamah@uvt.nl
[4] Institute for Food, Nutrition and Health, University of Reading, Reading RG1 5EX, UK
[*] Correspondence: g.laverman@zgt.nl; Tel.: +31-88-708-3079

Received: 23 January 2018; Accepted: 1 March 2018; Published: 5 March 2018

Abstract: In type 2 diabetes mellitus (T2D), the handling of magnesium is disturbed. Magnesium deficiency may be associated with a higher risk of coronary heart disease (CHD). We investigated the associations between (1) dietary magnesium intake; (2) 24 h urinary magnesium excretion; and (3) plasma magnesium concentration with prevalent CHD in T2D patients. This cross-sectional analysis was performed on baseline data from the DIAbetes and LifEstyle Cohort Twente-1 (DIALECT-1, $n = 450$, age 63 ± 9 years, 57% men, and diabetes duration of 11 (7–18) years). Prevalence ratios (95% CI) of CHD by sex-specific quartiles of magnesium indicators, as well as by magnesium intake per dietary source, were determined using multivariable Cox proportional hazard models. CHD was present in 100 (22%) subjects. Adjusted CHD prevalence ratios for the highest compared to the lowest quartiles were 0.40 (0.20, 0.79) for magnesium intake, 0.63 (0.32, 1.26) for 24 h urinary magnesium excretion, and 0.62 (0.32, 1.20) for plasma magnesium concentration. For every 10 mg increase of magnesium intake from vegetables, the prevalence of CHD was, statistically non-significantly, lower (0.75 (0.52, 1.08)). In this T2D cohort, higher magnesium intake, higher 24 h urinary magnesium excretion, and higher plasma magnesium concentration are associated with a lower prevalence of CHD.

Keywords: coronary heart disease; diabetes mellitus type 2; dietary magnesium intake; urinary magnesium excretion; plasma magnesium concentration

1. Introduction

Coronary heart disease (CHD) is one of the most prevalent and high-impact complications related to type 2 diabetes mellitus (T2D) [1,2]. In the general population, magnesium (Mg) deficiency might be associated with a greater risk of CHD; however, data on the inverse associations between Mg status and intake and CHD are inconsistent [3–9]. In T2D, the prevalence of hypomagnesemia is increased 14–48%, compared with 3–15% in those without T2D [10,11]. This could partly be due to increased urinary Mg excretion caused by insulin resistance, and partly due to poor dietary Mg intake [10–13].

However, surprisingly few studies report on the association between Mg and CHD in patients with established T2D [14,15].

In the DIAbetes and LifEstyle Cohort Twente (DIALECT), we collected extensive data on dietary Mg intake, 24 h urinary Mg excretion, and plasma Mg concentration. We aimed to study the association between the parameters of Mg (i.e., dietary Mg intake, 24 h urinary Mg excretion, and serum Mg concentration) and CHD. When we found that dietary Mg intake was inversely associated with CHD risk, we also explored whether there was an association between Mg intake from specific dietary sources (i.e., cereals, potatoes, etc.) and CHD risk.

2. Materials and Methods

2.1. Study Design

This was a cross-sectional analysis performed in the DIAbetes and LifEstyle Cohort Twente-1 (DIALECT-1). The study population and study procedures have been described previously [16]. The study has been approved by the relevant institutional review boards (METC-Twente, NL57219.044.16; METC-Groningen, 1009.68020), is registered in the Netherlands Trial Register (NTR trial code 5855), and is performed according to the guidelines of good clinical practice and the declaration of Helsinki.

2.2. Participants

All patients with T2D treated in the outpatient clinic of our hospital, aged 18+ years, were eligible for the study. Exclusion criteria were inability to understand the informed consent procedure, insufficient command of the Dutch language, or dialysis dependency. The inclusion flowchart has been described previously [16]. In total, 1082 patients were eligible for the study, of which 470 agreed to participate. The most important reasons for non-participation were no interest in the trial ($n = 123$), inability due to co-morbidity ($n = 62$), and no transport options ($n = 58$). After the baseline visit, 20 patients were excluded due to the fact that their diabetes diagnosis changed from type 2 diabetes to type 1 diabetes. Therefore, a total of 450 patients with type 2 diabetes were included in DIALECT-1. Missing values for specific variables are listed in Table 1.

2.3. Study Procedures

Eligible patients with type 2 diabetes were selected from the electronic patient file. At the clinic, sociodemographic characteristics, medical history, lifestyle behaviors, and current medications were recorded and anthropometric dimension were measured. Blood pressure was measured in a supine position by an automated device (Dinamap®; GE Medical systems, Milwaukee, WI, USA) for 15 min with a one-minute interval. The mean systolic and diastolic pressure of the final three measurements was used for further analysis. Physical activity was assessed using the Short QUestionnaire to ASses Health enhancing physical activity (SQUASH) questionnaire, which was previously validated and is commonly used in the Netherlands for population research [17].

Blood was drawn from venipuncture, for measurement of Mg and other variables relevant for diabetes. 24 h urine collections were performed as prescribed previously [16]. Samples of blood and urine were stored at −80 °C for later analysis.

Table 1. Baseline characteristics of patients with type 2 diabetes mellitus (T2D) by a breakup of prevalent coronary heart disease (CHD).

	n	Total Population $n = 450$	No CHD $n = 350$ (78%)	CHD $n = 100$ (22%)	p-Value
Patient characteristics					
Age, years	450	63 ± 9	62 ± 9	66 ± 7	<0.001
Male, n (%)	450	261 (58)	190 (54)	71 (71)	0.003
Diabetes duration, years	450	11 (7–18)	11 (7–17)	13 (7–20)	0.15
Systolic blood pressure, mmHg	449	136 ± 16	136 ± 16	136 ± 19	0.81
Diastolic blood pressure, mmHg	449	74 ± 9	75 ± 9	72 ± 10	0.01
Heart rate, beats/min	444	74 ± 13	75 ± 13	69 ± 11	<0.001
Body surface area, m^2	448	2.10 ± 0.22	2.10 ± 0.23	2.07 ± 0.19	0.27
Urinary creatinine excretion, μmol/24 h	446	13.8 ± 4.8	13.8 ± 5.0	13.8 ± 4.2	0.97
Complications					
Cerebrovascular disease, n (%)	450	47 (11)	87 (22)	13 (27)	0.44
Peripheral artery disease, n (%)	450	44 (10)	80 (20)	20 (44)	<0.001
Retinopathy, n (%)	447	106 (24)	78 (23)	32 (32)	0.05
Neuropathy, n (%)	450	157 (36)	116 (33)	46 (46)	0.02
Diabetic nephropathy, n (%)	446	183 (42)	131 (38)	58 (58)	<0.001
eGFR < 60 mL/min·1.73 m^2	450	101 (23)	74 (21)	30 (30)	0.06
Microalbuminuria, n (%)	445	131 (30)	92 (27)	44 (44)	0.001
Lifestyle					
Body mass index, kg/m^2	448	32.8 ± 6.2	33.1 ± 6.4	32.1 ± 5.6	0.15
Body mass index ≥ 30 kg/m^2, n (%)	448	290 (65)	233 (67)	57 (58)	0.12
Smoking, former or current, n (%)	450	306 (70)	235 (67)	78 (78)	0.04
Alcohol	424				
No alcohol, n (%)		148 (36)	123 (37)	32 (34)	0.80
0–13 units per week, n (%)		206 (50)	159 (48)	49 (52)	
≥14 units per week, n (%)		61 (15)	47 (14)	14 (15)	
Adherence guideline physical activity, n (%)	433	249 (59)	201 (60)	52 (54)	0.34
Pharmacological treatment					
Insulin use, n (%)	450	275 (63)	218 (62)	68 (68)	0.30
Statin use, n (%)	450	331 (76)	254 (73)	86 (86)	0.006
Beta blocker treatment, n (%)	450	202 (46)	131 (37)	77 (77)	<0.001
RAAS inhibition, n (%)	450	289 (66)	225 (64)	73 (73)	0.10
Calcium antagonists, n (%)	450	98 (22)	66 (19)	36 (36)	<0.001
Thiazide diuretics, n (%)	450	136 (31)	108 (31)	29 (29)	0.72
Loop diuretics, n (%)	450	75 (17)	48 (14)	33 (33)	<0.001
Number of antihypertensives	450	2 (1–3)	2 (1–3)	3 (2–4)	<0.001
Magnesium parameters					
Dietary magnesium intake *, mg/day	438	305 ± 46	309 ± 47	292 ± 40	0.001
Urinary magnesium excretion, mmol/24 h	402	3.94 ± 2.05	4.03 ± 2.05	3.66 ± 2.02	0.13
Plasma magnesium concentration, mmol/L	432	0.77 ± 0.09	0.78 ± 0.08	0.76 ± 0.09	0.06
Hypomagnesemia, n (%)	432	73 (17)	53 (16)	20 (20)	0.35
Serum values					
Total cholesterol, mmol/L	447	4.0 ± 0.9	4.1 ± 0.9	3.8 ± 1.1	0.04
HDL cholesterol, mmol/L	445	1.1 ± 0.3	1.2 ± 0.4	1.0 ± 0.3	<0.001
LDL cholesterol, mmol/L	428	2.0 ± 0.7	2.0 ± 0.7	1.9 ± 0.8	0.25
HbA1c, mmol/mol	448	57 ± 12	57 ± 12	58 ± 12	0.43
Dietary intake					
Total energy intake, kcal/day	438	1922 ± 629	1904 ± 649	1932 ± 630	0.71
Urinary sodium excretion, mmol/24 h	444	185 ± 79	183 ± 67	197 ± 84	0.14
Urinary potassium excretion, mmol/24 h	439	77 ± 25	78 ± 26	77 ± 21	0.87
Calcium intake, mg/day	438	969 ± 441	979 ± 467	905 ± 358	0.16
Fiber intake, g/day	438	20.9 ± 6.6	20.8 ± 7.0	20.4 ± 6.1	0.60
Cholesterol, g/day	438	194 ± 96	195 ± 101	188 ± 79	0.51
Total fat intake, g/day	438	79 ± 39	78 ± 34	81 ± 34	0.52
Total protein intake, g/day	438	79 ± 23	79 ± 24	76 ± 22	0.18
Total carbohydrate intake, g/day	438	207 ± 69	205 ± 72	209 ± 67	0.61

CHD: coronary heart disease, eGFR: estimated glomerular filtration rate (CKD-EPI), HDL: high density lipoprotein, LDL: low density lipoprotein, HbA1c: glycated hemoglobin. * Dietary magnesium intake was adjusted for total energy intake using the residual method.

2.4. Magnesium Measurements

We calculated dietary Mg intake using a semi-quantitative food frequency questionnaire (FFQ), inquiring about the intake of 177 items during the last month, taking seasonal variations into account [18]. The FFQ was developed and validated at the Wageningen University, and has been updated several times. For each food item, the frequency was recorded in times per day, week, or month. The number of servings was expressed in natural units (e.g., a slice of bread or a whole apple) or household measures (e.g., cup or spoon). Both questionnaires were self-administered and filled in at home. The filled-in questionnaires were checked for completeness by a trained researcher, and inconsistent answers were verified with the patients. If the patient could not remember an exact number, the trained researcher approximated the intake as closely as possible during the interview. Dietary data was converted into daily nutrient intake using the Dutch Food Composition Table of 2013 [19]. We calculated the average intake of Mg by multiplying the frequency of consumption of each food item by its Mg content in the Dutch Food Composition Table of 2013 [19], and summing the amount of Mg across all food items. We calculated Mg intake from different food categories by multiplying the frequency of consumption of each food item in that specific category by its Mg content, and summing across all food items in that category. Food items of the FFQ included in each category are listed in supplementary Table S1.

Plasma and urinary Mg were measured in stored plasma samples in routine laboratory measurements using the xylidyl blue method. Buffer/Ethylenediaminetetraacetic acid was added to mask calcium. After incubation, xylidyl blue was added to form a purple complex with Mg. Mg concentration was determined by the photometric measurement of xylidyl blue extinction. The detection range for plasma Mg was 0.1–5 mmol/L, and for 24 h urinary Mg the range was 0.5–25 mmol/L. There were no patients with values outside of the detection ranges. Hypomagnesemia was defined as serum Mg concentration <0.70 mmol/L.

2.5. Main Study Outcome

Coronary heart disease (CHD) is defined as physician-diagnosed unstable angina pectoris or myocardial infarction, percutaneous coronary intervention, or a coronary artery bypass graft in the medical history. Medical history was checked for CHD during the interview at the baseline visit, and was later reviewed in the hospital electronic patient files on three different occasions, by three different physician researchers, who were unaware of the magnesium data.

2.6. Statistics

All statistical analyses were performed using the Statistical Package for the Social Sciences (SPSS), version 23.0. Normally-distributed data are presented as mean ± standard deviation. Skewed variables are expressed as median (interquartile range). Dichotomous variables are presented in number and percentage. Dietary intake of Mg was adjusted for energy intake by the residual method [20].

Differences between T2D patients with and without CHD were determined using the Student *t* (normal distribution), Mann–Whitney U (skewed distribution), or Chi-Square (categorical variables) test. In order to examine parameters associated with magnesium intake, we divided the population into sex-specific quartiles of adjusted magnesium intake. Differences between the quartiles were assessed using one-way ANOVA (normal distribution), Kruskal–Wallis (skewed distribution), or Chi-Square (categorical variables) analysis.

Correlations between Mg parameters were assessed using Pearson's correlation coefficient.

We calculated the prevalence ratio (95% CI) of CHD by sex-specific quartiles of (1) dietary Mg intake; (2) 24 h urinary Mg excretion; and (3) plasma Mg concentration, using multivariable Cox proportional hazard models, with the time to event set at 1 for all patients. The models were adjusted for the potential confounding of lifestyle parameters (BMI, smoking, alcohol, and physical activity) and nutritional intake (24 h urinary sodium excretion and 24 h urinary potassium excretion) [3,21].

There was a strong correlation between dietary calcium and Mg intake (R = 0.70), therefore we did not adjust for calcium intake in the final model. Effect modification was checked for gender, BMI, smoking, and alcohol, and no significant effect modification was found ($p > 0.20$ for all interaction terms). Sensitivity analyses were performed by excluding patients with diabetic kidney disease, and prevalence ratios were similar as in the primary analyses.

Additionally, we performed multivariable Cox proportional hazard models, and calculated the prevalence ratios of CHD for each 10 mg increment of dietary Mg intake from different sources (cereals, dairy, coffee, potatoes, meat, legumes and nuts, fruit, vegetables, and other). The models were adjusted for potential confounding of lifestyle parameters (age, BMI, smoking, alcohol, and physical activity) and Mg intake from the miscellaneous sources.

3. Results

In total, 450 patients with T2D were included in DIALECT-1. Baseline characteristics are shown in Table 1. In short, patients were 63 ± 9 years old, and the majority of the population was male (57%). The population represents T2D in secondary health care, with a median diabetes duration of 11 (7–18) years, and a high prevalence of diabetic nephropathy (42%).

There were 100 (22%) CHD cases diagnosed in our population (Table 1). T2D patients with CHD were older (66 ± 7 vs. 62 ± 9 years, $p < 0.001$), were more often men (71% vs. 54%, $p = 0.003$), and more often had peripheral artery disease (44% vs. 20%, $p < 0.001$), and nephropathy (58% vs. 38%, $p < 0.001$) than patients without CHD. There were no differences in lifestyle parameters between those with and without CHD. Regarding pharmacological treatment, those with CHD more often used beta-blockers (77% vs. 37%, $p < 0.001$), and loop diuretics (33% vs. 14%, $p < 0.001$) than those without CHD. This was paralleled by a lower diastolic blood pressure (72 ± 10 mmHg vs. 75 ± 9 mmHg, $p = 0.01$) and heart rate (69 ± 11 beats/min vs. 75 ± 13 beats/min, $p < 0.001$) in patients with CHD. Systolic blood pressure was 136 ± 16 mmHg, and did not differ between the groups. Although patients with CHD more often used statins (86% vs. 73%, $p = 0.006$), serum LDL was similar in the groups (2.0 ± 0.7 mmol/L), and serum HDL cholesterol was lower in those with CHD (1.0 ± 0.3 mmol/L vs. 1.2 ± 0.4 mmol/L, $p < 0.001$) compared to those without CHD.

Mean energy-adjusted dietary Mg intake was 305 ± 46 mg/day, and was lower in those with CHD (adjusted standardized beta = -0.14, $p = 0.003$). Mean 24 h urinary Mg excretion was 3.94 ± 2.05 mmol/24 h, and mean plasma Mg concentration was 0.77 ± 0.09 mmol/L; neither differed statistically significantly between those with and without CHD (Table 1). Hypomagnesemia (plasma Mg < 0.7 mmol/L) was present in 73 patients (17%), of which 11 patients (3%) had a plasma Mg of <0.6 mmol/L.

Dietary Mg intake was significantly correlated with 24 h urinary Mg excretion (Pearson R = 0.24, $p < 0.001$), but not with plasma Mg (R = 0.02, $p = 0.64$). 24 h urinary Mg excretion was significantly correlated with plasma Mg (R = 0.13, $p < 0.008$).

Systolic blood pressure was lowest in the highest gender-specific quartile of energy-adjusted magnesium intake (4th quartile 133 ± 13 vs. 1st quartile 137 ± 17 mmHg; Supplementary Table S2), and the number of antihypertensive drugs used was lowest in this quartile as well (4th quartile 2 (0–3) vs. 2 (1–3) in other quartiles, $p = 0.008$). Serum HbA1c and cholesterol levels were similar in all Mg intake quartiles. There was a trend towards higher urinary potassium excretion, dietary calcium, fiber, protein, and carbohydrate intake, as well as a lower dietary intake of fat in each of the higher quartiles of magnesium intake.

3.1. Association between Dietary Magnesium Intake, 24 h Urinary Magnesium Excretion, Plasma Magnesium Concentration, and the Prevalence of Coronary Heart Disease

The highest quartile of Mg intake was significantly associated with a lower prevalence ratio (PR) of CHD than the lowest quartile of Mg intake (0.40 (0.20, 0.77); Table 2). When adjusting for age and lifestyle parameters (BMI, smoking, alcohol, and physical activity), the PR remained largely unchanged

(0.42 (0.22, 0.82)). After adjustment for dietary intake of other micronutrients (total energy intake, sodium, and potassium), the PR became (0.40 (0.20, 0.79)), and the *p*-trend was 0.01.

There was a similar trend towards a lower prevalence of CHD in the highest quartile of 24 h urinary Mg excretion, which was not statistically significant (PR 0.63 (0.33, 1.19)). After adjustment for lifestyle and nutritional factors, the PR remained similar (0.63 (0.32, 1.26)). Also, the highest quartile of plasma Mg concentration had a non-significant trend towards a lower prevalence of CHD (unadjusted PR 0.60 (0.31, 1.14), adjusted PR 0.62 (0.32, 1.20)). The PR ratios for dietary Mg intake, urinary Mg excretion and plasma Mg concentration did not change after further adjustment for other classic CHD risk factors, namely systolic blood pressure and LDL cholesterol (data not shown).

Table 2. Prevalence ratios (95% CI) for associations between dietary, urinary and plasma Magnesium and coronary heart disease in type 2 diabetes from the DIAbetes and LifEstyle Cohort Twente (DIALECT) (*n* = 450).

	Quartile 1	Quartile 2	Quartile 3	Quartile 4	*p*-Trend
Dietary Mg intake *, mg/day	254 ± 25	291 ± 7	315 ± 8	361 ± 39	
n cases/*n* total	33/109	25/110	23/110	13/109	
Model 1 [a]	1.00	0.71 (0.42, 1.22)	0.64 (0.37, 1.10)	0.40 (0.20, 0.77)	0.005
Model 2 [b]	1.00	0.72 (0.42, 1.23)	0.69 (0.40, 1.21)	0.42 (0.22, 0.82)	0.01
Model 3 [c]	1.00	0.71 (0.41, 1.23)	0.72 (0.41, 1.27)	0.40 (0.20, 0.79)	0.01
Urinary Mg excretion, mmol/24 h	1.81 ± 0.63	3.05 ± 0.32	4.32 ± 0.57	6.64 ± 1.75	
n cases/*n* total	24/101	24/100	19/101	15/100	
Model 1 [a]	1.00	0.95 (0.54, 1.67)	0.73 (0.39, 1.35)	0.63 (0.33, 1.19)	0.24
Model 2 [b]	1.00	1.28 (0.71, 2.30)	0.96 (0.51, 1.82)	0.74 (0.39, 1.42)	0.33
Model 3 [c]	1.00	1.27 (0.70, 2.30)	0.85 (0.44, 1.65)	0.63 (0.32, 1.26)	0.13
Plasma Mg concentration, mmol/L	0.67 ± 0.06	0.75 ± 0.02	0.80 ± 0.02	0.88 ± 0.04	
n cases/*n* total	29/113	22/106	27/111	16/102	
Model 1 [a]	1.00	0.91 (0.52, 1.60)	1.03 (0.60, 1.77)	0.60 (0.31, 1.14)	0.15
Model 2 [b]	1.00	0.91 (0.51, 1.62)	1.09 (0.63, 1.89)	0.58 (0.30, 1.12)	0.17
Model 3 [c]	1.00	0.91 (0.51, 1.63)	1.12 (0.65, 1.94)	0.62 (0.32, 1.20)	0.26

[a] Model 1: Crude model [b] Model 2: Adjusted for age (years), BMI (kg/m^2), smoking (never, former or current), alcohol consumption (none, 1–13 units per week, ≥14 units per week), physical activity (not adherent to guideline, adherent to guideline).[c] Model 3: Model 2 + Total energy intake (kcal), 24 h urinary sodium excretion (mmol/24 h) and 24 h urinary potassium excretion (mmol/24 h).* Dietary magnesium intake was adjusted for total energy intake using the residual method.

3.2. Analysis on Source of Magnesium Intake and Prevalence of CHD

We performed an explorative analysis whether there was an association between Mg intake from specific dietary sources and CHD. The largest dietary contributors to total dietary Mg intake for patients with T2D (Figure 1) were cereals at 22% (16–26%), dairy at 14% (10–20%), coffee at 9% (6–13%), potatoes at 7% (4–10%), meat at 6% (5–8%), legumes and nuts at 6% (4–11%), fruit at 5% (3–8%), and vegetables with 3% (2–5%). We found no statistically significant association between Mg intake from specific food groups and CHD (Table 3). However, there was a non-significant trend towards a lower prevalence of CHD for every 10 mg increase of dietary Mg intake derived from vegetables (PR 0.75 (0.52, 1.08)).

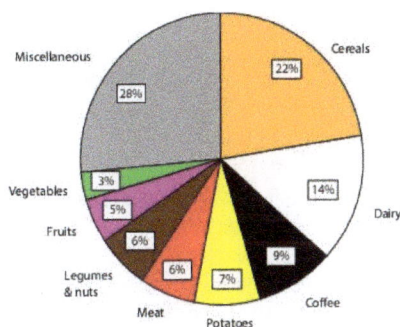

Figure 1. Sources of magnesium intake from different food product categories in patients with T2D.

Table 3. Prevalence ratios (95% CI) for associations between magnesium intake from different food sources in type 2 diabetes patients from the DIALECT cohort (*n* = 450).

	Model 1 [a]	Model 2 [b]	Model 3 [c]
Source of magnesium intake	PR (95% CI)	PR (95% CI)	PR (95% CI)
Magnesium intake from cereals *, 10 mg/day	1.02 (0.94, 1.10)	1.02 (0.94, 1.10)	0.95 (0.86, 1.05)
Magnesium intake from dairy *, 10 mg/day	0.95 (0.87, 1.03)	0.95 (0.87, 1.03)	0.92 (0.84, 1.01)
Magnesium intake from coffee *, 10 mg/day	0.95 (0.83, 1.06)	0.95 (0.83, 1.08)	0.96 (0.84, 1.10)
Magnesium intake from potatoes *, 10 mg/day	1.03 (0.87, 1.22)	1.02 (0.86, 1.21)	0.97 (0.80, 1.16)
Magnesium intake from meat *, 10 mg/day	0.91 (0.70, 1.20)	0.91 (0.69, 1.19)	0.80 (0.59, 1.09)
Magnesium intake from legumes & nuts *, 10 mg/day	0.96 (0.89, 1.05)	0.96 (0.88, 1.06)	0.95 (0.86, 1.05)
Magnesium intake from fruit *, 10 mg/day	1.00 (0.81, 1.23)	0.98 (0.79, 1.20)	0.96 (0.78, 1.19)
Magnesium intake from vegetables *, 10 mg/day	0.71 (0.51, 1.01)	0.71 (0.50, 1.01)	0.75 (0.52, 1.08)
Magnesium intake from miscellaneous sources *, 10 mg/day	0.95 (0.89, 1.02)	0.95 (0.89, 1.03)	0.90 (0.82, 0.99)

[a] Model 1: Crude model [b] Model 2: Adjusted for age (years), BMI (kg/m^2), smoking (never, former/current), alcohol consumption (none, 1–13 units per week, ≥14 units per week), physical activity (not adherent to guideline, adherent to guideline).[c] Model 3: Model 2 + Total energy intake (kcal), magnesium intake from the other sources (cereals (mg/day), dairy (mg/day), coffee (mg/day), potatoes (mg/day), meat (mg/day), legumes and nuts (mg/day), fruit (mg/day), vegetables (mg/day), and other (mg/day)). * Magnesium intake from food sources was adjusted for total energy intake using the residual method. An increment of 10 mg magnesium intake per day was used to calculate PR.PR, prevalence ratio; CI, confidence interval.

4. Discussion

We found inverse associations for dietary Mg intake, 24 h urinary Mg excretion, and plasma Mg concentration with the prevalence of CHD in patients with T2D. As far as we know, this is the first study in T2D patients which simultaneously reports on these three Mg parameters in relation to CHD. The inverse association between dietary Mg intake and the prevalence of CHD we found was strongest for Mg intake derived from vegetables, albeit not statistically significant.

The mean dietary Mg intake we report (305 ± 46 mg/day) was somewhat lower than the median Mg intake in the general Dutch population, which is around 350 mg/day [22], but was comparable to median Mg intake of population studies in the U.S. (308 mg/day) [4]. We found that in the Dutch population, cereals, dairy, and coffee intake were the largest contributors to total Mg intake, at 22%, 14%, and 9% respectively. This was somewhat different from the U.K. population, where cereals (34%), meat (19%), and dairy (18%) intake were the most important contributors [23]. In contrast, in the U.S. population the most important food groups were vegetables (13%), milk (8%), and meat (7%) [24]. It should be noted that different groupings of food products renders a head-to-head comparison between these percentages difficult. The 24 h urinary Mg excretion we report (4.0 ± 2.1 mmol/24 h) was in line with the general population the Netherlands (4.2 ± 1.7 mmol/24 h for men and 3.5 ± 1.4 mmol/24 h for women) [5]. Plasma Mg concentration (0.77 ± 0.09 mmol/L) was similar to an earlier report about Dutch diabetes patients (0.74 ± 0.10 mmol/L) [25]. The prevalence of hypomagnesemia we found (17%) was in the range of the reported prevalence of hypomagnesemia in patients with T2D, between 14% and 48% [10,11], and emphasizes that clinical vigilance for hypomagnesemia is warranted in T2D, because it is associated with increased insulin resistance and faster renal function decline [26].

We are the first to report an inverse association between dietary Mg intake and the prevalence of CHD in T2D. In contrast, a large meta-analysis in non-T2D patients demonstrated no association between dietary Mg intake and incident CHD [9]. However, low dietary Mg intake was associated with a higher risk of stroke, heart failure, new-onset diabetes, and all-cause mortality [9]. It is known that in T2D renal wasting of Mg occurs [27]. Additionally, Mg supplementation in T2D can improve insulin sensitivity and metabolic control [28]. Possibly, an adequate Mg intake in patients with T2D is even more important than in those without T2D, in order to maintain an adequate Mg status and prevent diabetes-related complications. These data fuel the hypothesis that magnesium intake is beneficial in T2D patients.

In addition, when investigating Mg intake from specific food sources, we found the strongest inverse association between Mg derived from vegetables and CHD, albeit not quite reaching statistical significance. To our knowledge, the association with vegetable-derived Mg intake and CHD has not been described before. When studying Mg intake and Mg status, it is important to consider bioavailability of ingested Mg for intestinal uptake, as this might vary considerably depending on the source of Mg intake [29]. Possibly, bioavailability from Mg in vegetables is greater than from other food sources; however, this issue would have to be addressed an in-depth mechanistic study. Nevertheless, our data illustrate that when studying the association between micronutrients and outcomes, intake of different food groups is also important. As vegetable intake in our population was low [30], and vegetable intake only accounted for 3% of total Mg intake in this population, increasing vegetable intake is a good opportunity to not only increase Mg intake, but also to improve overall diet quality. It should be noted that in our study, it is difficult to distinguish between the protective effects of overall vegetable intake and those from vegetable-derived Mg intake. Other vegetable-derived components like antioxidants, but also potassium and vitamin K, might contribute to or interact with Mg in the eventual association with CHD [31–34]. Maybe the possible cohort effect from these micronutrients and Mg could amplify such protection. Since such an analysis is beyond the scope and available data of the current study, future studies are necessary to further investigate mechanisms behind vegetable intake and risk of coronary heart disease.

Additionally, we found that lower 24 h urinary Mg excretion was associated with more prevalent CHD. In line with this finding, in the general population an inverse association between Mg excretion and CHD was reported [5]. Potential renal Mg wasting in T2D renders the interpretation of urinary Mg excretion difficult. High urinary Mg excretion could, on the one hand, reflect a high dietary Mg intake; on the other hand, though, it could reflect the hypermagnesuria found in T2D [10,11]. This could explain why, in our cohort, dietary Mg intake is more strongly associated with CHD than 24 h urinary excretion.

In parallel, lower plasma Mg concentration was also associated with prevalent CHD. In T2D, the association between plasma Mg concentration and CHD was investigated previously, and conflicting results were reported [14,15]. In non-T2D subjects, conflicting results on the association between plasma Mg have been reported as well; however, a meta-analysis demonstrated an inverse association between plasma Mg and incident CHD [8]. As Mg is mainly an intracellular cation, and therefore plasma Mg only reflects 1% of bodily Mg stores, the validity of using plasma Mg as a marker for Mg status has been questioned; Mg deficiency has been reported in patients without overt hypomagnesemia [11,35].

Our paper was not designed to unravel mechanisms behind the inverse associations between Mg intake, Mg status, and CHD. However, several mechanisms have been proposed that could underlie this association. First, animal studies have consistently shown that higher Mg status inhibits vascular calcification [36,37]. In human subjects, serum Mg and dietary Mg intake were inversely associated with the degree of coronary calcification [4,6]. Second, low Mg status might be associated with cardiac arrhythmias [38]. Lastly, increased CHD risk might be mediated through the association between low

Mg status or intake and increased traditional CHD risk factors, such as blood pressure [39] and insulin resistance [12].

Our paper is the first to simultaneously report the association between dietary Mg intake, factors of Mg status (24 h urinary Mg excretion and plasma Mg), and CHD in patients with established T2D. The robustness of our findings is established through the fact that all three Mg parameters were inversely associated with CHD. The main limitation of our paper is the cross-sectional design, which only allowed us to study associations and not causality, and therefore there is a risk of reverse causality bias. Another limitation is that the FFQ we used in our study was not validated to estimate magnesium intake. However, because there was a moderate correlation between dietary Mg intake and urinary Mg excretion, we deemed the results sufficiently valid.

Our study has several clinical implications. First, we show that Mg intake is of the utmost importance with relation to T2D. Patients with T2D are at risk of developing hypomagnesemia, as Mg intake in our population was somewhat lower in comparison to the general population. Additionally, patients with T2D have increased renal Mg excretion [27]. We show that Mg intake and Mg status is reduced in those with CHD, possibly indicating that higher Mg intake is associated with a lower risk of CHD. The best opportunity to increase Mg intake is to increase intake of Mg-rich vegetables. As Mg intake in the highest quartile is approximately 100 mg/day higher than in the lowest quartile, in clinical practice this could correspond with increasing vegetable intake by, for example, 200 g spinach, or 100 g rucola lettuce and two avocados per day. Alternatively, previous research has shown that several dietary patterns might reduce CHD risk or improve cardiac function, such as the Mediterranean diet; the Dietary Approaches to Stop Hypertension diet; or a high-protein, intermittent fasting, low-calorie diet [40–42]. We add to these findings by illustrating that Mg is an important component in such diets. For future studies, it would be of interest to investigate how Mg and other beneficial nutritional approaches could reinforce each other in the pursuit of the reduction of CHD in diabetes patients. Additionally, future mechanistic studies should be done to investigate how vegetable-derived nutrients, particularly Mg, might reduce CHD risk.

5. Conclusions

In a cohort of patients with established T2D, dietary magnesium intake, 24 h urinary magnesium excretion, and plasma magnesium concentration were inversely associated with the prevalence of coronary heart disease. Increasing dietary magnesium intake, especially through increasing vegetable intake, may reduce the risk of CHD in patients with established T2D.

Supplementary Materials: The following are available online at www.mdpi.com/2072-6643/10/3/307/s1, Table S1: Overview of food items included in each food category, Table S2: Baseline characteristics of patients with T2D by a breakup of dietary magnesium intake.

Acknowledgments: We thank Else van den Berg, Willeke van Kampen, Sanne van Huizen, Anne Davina, Manon Harmelink and Jolien Jaspers for their contribution to patient inclusion. We thank Jelle Sanderman for supervising laboratory measurements. This work was performed without external financial support.

Author Contributions: S.H.B., G.N., S.S.S.-M. and G.D.L. conceived and designed the study; C.M.G. and S.H.B. included patients; C.M.G. and S.S.S.-M. analyzed the data; S.J.L.B., G.N. and G.D.L. contributed reagents/materials/analysis tools; C.G. wrote the paper.

Conflicts of Interest: The authors declare no conflict of interest.

References

1. Rana, J.S.; Liu, J.Y.; Moffet, H.H.; Jaffe, M.; Karter, A.J. Diabetes and Prior Coronary Heart Disease are Not Necessarily Risk Equivalent for Future Coronary Heart Disease Events. *J. Gen. Intern. Med.* **2016**, *31*, 387–393. [CrossRef] [PubMed]
2. Emerging Risk Factors Collaboration; Sarwar, N.; Gao, P.; Seshasai, S.R.; Gobin, R.; Kaptoge, S.; Di Angelantonio, E.; Ingelsson, E.; Lawlor, D.A.; Selvin, E.; et al. Diabetes Mellitus, Fasting Blood Glucose Concentration, and Risk of Vascular Disease: A Collaborative Meta-Analysis of 102 Prospective Studies. *Lancet* **2010**, *375*, 2215–2222. [PubMed]

3. Chiuve, S.E.; Sun, Q.; Curhan, G.C.; Taylor, E.N.; Spiegelman, D.; Willett, W.C.; Manson, J.E.; Rexrode, K.M.; Albert, C.M. Dietary and Plasma Magnesium and Risk of Coronary Heart Disease among Women. *J. Am. Heart Assoc.* **2013**, *2*, e000114. [CrossRef] [PubMed]

4. Hruby, A.; O'Donnell, C.J.; Jacques, P.F.; Meigs, J.B.; Hoffmann, U.; McKeown, N.M. Magnesium Intake is Inversely Associated with Coronary Artery Calcification: The Framingham Heart Study. *JACC Cardiovasc. Imaging* **2014**, *7*, 59–69. [CrossRef] [PubMed]

5. Joosten, M.M.; Gansevoort, R.T.; Mukamal, K.J.; van der Harst, P.; Geleijnse, J.M.; Feskens, E.J.; Navis, G.; Bakker, S.J.; PREVEND Study Group. Urinary and Plasma Magnesium and Risk of Ischemic Heart Disease. *Am. J. Clin. Nutr.* **2013**, *97*, 1299–1306. [CrossRef] [PubMed]

6. Posadas-Sanchez, R.; Posadas-Romero, C.; Cardoso-Saldana, G.; Vargas-Alarcon, G.; Villarreal-Molina, M.T.; Perez-Hernandez, N.; Rodriguez-Perez, J.M.; Medina-Urrutia, A.; Jorge-Galarza, E.; Juarez-Rojas, J.G.; et al. Serum Magnesium is Inversely Associated with Coronary Artery Calcification in the Genetics of Atherosclerotic Disease (GEA) Study. *Nutr. J.* **2016**, *15*, 22. [CrossRef] [PubMed]

7. Sakaguchi, Y.; Hamano, T.; Nakano, C.; Obi, Y.; Matsui, I.; Kusunoki, Y.; Mori, D.; Oka, T.; Hashimoto, N.; Takabatake, Y.; et al. Association between Density of Coronary Artery Calcification and Serum Magnesium Levels among Patients with Chronic Kidney Disease. *PLoS ONE* **2016**, *11*, e0163673. [CrossRef] [PubMed]

8. Wu, J.; Xun, P.; Tang, Q.; Cai, W.; He, K. Circulating Magnesium Levels and Incidence of Coronary Heart Diseases, Hypertension, and Type 2 Diabetes Mellitus: A Meta-Analysis of Prospective Cohort Studies. *Nutr. J.* **2017**, *16*, 60. [CrossRef] [PubMed]

9. Fang, X.; Wang, K.; Han, D.; He, X.; Wei, J.; Zhao, L.; Imam, M.U.; Ping, Z.; Li, Y.; Xu, Y.; et al. Dietary Magnesium Intake and the Risk of Cardiovascular Disease, Type 2 Diabetes, and all-Cause Mortality: A Dose-Response Meta-Analysis of Prospective Cohort Studies. *BMC Med.* **2016**, *14*, 210. [CrossRef] [PubMed]

10. Gommers, L.M.; Hoenderop, J.G.; Bindels, R.J.; de Baaij, J.H. Hypomagnesemia in Type 2 Diabetes: A Vicious Circle? *Diabetes* **2016**, *65*, 3–13. [CrossRef] [PubMed]

11. Pham, P.C.; Pham, P.M.; Pham, S.V.; Miller, J.M.; Pham, P.T. Hypomagnesemia in Patients with Type 2 Diabetes. *Clin. J. Am. Soc. Nephrol.* **2007**, *2*, 366–373. [CrossRef] [PubMed]

12. Fang, X.; Han, H.; Li, M.; Liang, C.; Fan, Z.; Aaseth, J.; He, J.; Montgomery, S.; Cao, Y. Dose-Response Relationship between Dietary Magnesium Intake and Risk of Type 2 Diabetes Mellitus: A Systematic Review and Meta-Regression Analysis of Prospective Cohort Studies. *Nutrients* **2016**, *8*, 739. [CrossRef] [PubMed]

13. Hruby, A.; Meigs, J.B.; O'Donnell, C.J.; Jacques, P.F.; McKeown, N.M. Higher Magnesium Intake Reduces Risk of Impaired Glucose and Insulin Metabolism and Progression from Prediabetes to Diabetes in Middle-Aged Americans. *Diabetes Care* **2014**, *37*, 419–427. [CrossRef] [PubMed]

14. Liao, F.; Folsom, A.R.; Brancati, F.L. Is Low Magnesium Concentration a Risk Factor for Coronary Heart Disease? The Atherosclerosis Risk in Communities (ARIC) Study. *Am. Heart J.* **1998**, *136*, 480–490. [CrossRef]

15. Peters, K.E.; Chubb, S.A.; Davis, W.A.; Davis, T.M. The Relationship between Hypomagnesemia, Metformin Therapy and Cardiovascular Disease Complicating Type 2 Diabetes: The Fremantle Diabetes Study. *PLoS ONE* **2013**, *8*, e74355. [CrossRef] [PubMed]

16. Gant, C.M.; Binnenmars, S.H.; Berg, E.V.D.; Bakker, S.J.L.; Navis, G.; Laverman, G.D. Integrated Assessment of Pharmacological and Nutritional Cardiovascular Risk Management: Blood Pressure Control in the DIAbetes and LifEstyle Cohort Twente (DIALECT). *Nutrients* **2017**, *9*, 709. [CrossRef] [PubMed]

17. Wendel-Vos, G.C.; Schuit, A.J.; Saris, W.H.; Kromhout, D. Reproducibility and Relative Validity of the Short Questionnaire to Assess Health-Enhancing Physical Activity. *J. Clin. Epidemiol.* **2003**, *56*, 1163–1169. [CrossRef]

18. Feunekes, G.I.; Van Staveren, W.A.; De Vries, J.H.; Burema, J.; Hautvast, J.G. Relative and Biomarker-Based Validity of a Food-Frequency Questionnaire Estimating Intake of Fats and Cholesterol. *Am. J. Clin. Nutr.* **1993**, *58*, 489–496. [CrossRef] [PubMed]

19. Rijksinstituut voor Volksgezondheid en Milieu. *NEVO-Tabel (Dutch Food Composition Table): Nederlands Voedingsstoffenbestand, version 4.0*; Rijksinstituut voor Volksgezondheid en Milieu: Bilthoven, The Netherlands, 2013.

20. Willett, W.C.; Stampfer, M. Implications of total energy intake for epidemiologic analyses. In *Nutritional Epidemiology*; Willett, W.C., Ed.; Oxford University Press: New York, NY, USA, 1998; pp. 273–301.

21. Zhang, W.; Iso, H.; Ohira, T.; Date, C.; Tamakoshi, A.; JACC Study Group. Associations of Dietary Magnesium Intake with Mortality from Cardiovascular Disease: The JACC Study. *Atherosclerosis* **2012**, *221*, 587–595. [CrossRef] [PubMed]

22. Van Rossum, C.; Fransen, H.; Verkaik-Kloosterman, J.; Buurma-Rethans, E.; Ocke, M. *Dutch National Food Consumption Survey 2007–2010: Diet of Children and Adults Aged 7 to 69 Years*; National Institute for Public Health and the Environment: Bilthoven, The Netherlands, 2011.

23. Davies, B.E. The UK Geochemical Environment and Cardiovascular Diseases: Magnesium in Food and Water. *Environ. Geochem. Health* **2015**, *37*, 411–427. [CrossRef] [PubMed]

24. Ford, E.S.; Mokdad, A.H. Dietary Magnesium Intake in a National Sample of US Adults. *J. Nutr.* **2003**, *133*, 2879–2882. [CrossRef] [PubMed]

25. Kurstjens, S.; de Baaij, J.H.; Bouras, H.; Bindels, R.J.; Tack, C.J.; Hoenderop, J.G. Determinants of Hypomagnesemia in Patients with Type 2 Diabetes Mellitus. *Eur. J. Endocrinol.* **2017**, *176*, 11–19. [CrossRef] [PubMed]

26. Grober, U.; Schmidt, J.; Kisters, K. Magnesium in Prevention and Therapy. *Nutrients* **2015**, *7*, 8199–8226. [CrossRef] [PubMed]

27. McNair, P.; Christensen, M.S.; Christiansen, C.; Madsbad, S.; Transbol, I. Renal Hypomagnesaemia in Human Diabetes Mellitus: Its Relation to Glucose Homeostasis. *Eur. J. Clin. Investig.* **1982**, *12*, 81–85. [CrossRef]

28. Rodriguez-Moran, M.; Guerrero-Romero, F. Oral Magnesium Supplementation Improves Insulin Sensitivity and Metabolic Control in Type 2 Diabetic Subjects: A Randomized Double-Blind Controlled Trial. *Diabetes Care* **2003**, *26*, 1147–1152. [CrossRef] [PubMed]

29. Schuchardt, J.P.; Hahn, A. Intestinal Absorption and Factors Influencing Bioavailability of Magnesium-an Update. *Curr. Nutr. Food Sci.* **2017**, *13*, 260–278. [CrossRef] [PubMed]

30. Gant, C.M.; Binnenmars, S.H.; Harmelink, M.; Soedamah-Muthu, S.S.; Bakker, S.J.L.; Navis, G.J.; Laverman, G.D. Real-Life Achievement of Lipid-Lowering Treatment Targets in the DIAbetes and LifEstyle Cohort Twente: Systemic Assessment of Pharmacological and Nutritional Factors. *Nutr. Diabetes* **2018**, in press.

31. Zhu, X.; Zuo, L. Characterization of Oxygen Radical Formation Mechanism at Early Cardiac Ischemia. *Cell Death Dis.* **2013**, *4*, e787. [CrossRef] [PubMed]

32. Keyzer, C.A.; Vermeer, C.; Joosten, M.M.; Knapen, M.H.; Drummen, N.E.; Navis, G.; Bakker, S.J.; de Borst, M.H. Vitamin K Status and Mortality After Kidney Transplantation: A Cohort Study. *Am. J. Kidney Dis.* **2015**, *65*, 474–483. [CrossRef] [PubMed]

33. Riphagen, I.J.; Keyzer, C.A.; Drummen, N.E.A.; de Borst, M.H.; Beulens, J.W.J.; Gansevoort, R.T.; Geleijnse, J.M.; Muskiet, F.A.J.; Navis, G.; Visser, S.T.; et al. Prevalence and Effects of Functional Vitamin K Insufficiency: The PREVEND Study. *Nutrients* **2017**, *9*, 1334. [CrossRef] [PubMed]

34. Kieneker, L.M.; Gansevoort, R.T.; Mukamal, K.J.; de Boer, R.A.; Navis, G.; Bakker, S.J.; Joosten, M.M. Urinary Potassium Excretion and Risk of Developing Hypertension: The Prevention of Renal and Vascular End-Stage Disease Study. *Hypertension* **2014**, *64*, 769–776. [CrossRef] [PubMed]

35. Barbagallo, M.; Di Bella, G.; Brucato, V.; D'Angelo, D.; Damiani, P.; Monteverde, A.; Belvedere, M.; Dominguez, L.J. Serum Ionized Magnesium in Diabetic Older Persons. *Metabolism* **2014**, *63*, 502–509. [CrossRef] [PubMed]

36. Alesutan, I.; Tuffaha, R.; Auer, T.; Feger, M.; Pieske, B.; Lang, F.; Voelkl, J. Inhibition of Osteo/Chondrogenic Transformation of Vascular Smooth Muscle Cells by $MgCl_2$ Via Calcium-Sensing Receptor. *J. Hypertens.* **2017**, *35*, 523–532. [CrossRef] [PubMed]

37. Kircelli, F.; Peter, M.E.; Sevinc Ok, E.; Celenk, F.G.; Yilmaz, M.; Steppan, S.; Asci, G.; Ok, E.; Passlick-Deetjen, J. Magnesium Reduces Calcification in Bovine Vascular Smooth Muscle Cells in a Dose-Dependent Manner. *Nephrol. Dial. Transplant.* **2012**, *27*, 514–521. [CrossRef] [PubMed]

38. Verduyn, S.C.; Vos, M.A.; van der Zande, J.; van der Hulst, F.F.; Wellens, H.J. Role of Interventricular Dispersion of Repolarization in Acquired Torsade-De-Pointes Arrhythmias: Reversal by Magnesium. *Cardiovasc. Res.* **1997**, *34*, 453–463. [CrossRef]

39. Dibaba, D.T.; Xun, P.; Song, Y.; Rosanoff, A.; Shechter, M.; He, K. The Effect of Magnesium Supplementation on Blood Pressure in Individuals with Insulin Resistance, Prediabetes, or Noncommunicable Chronic Diseases: A Meta-Analysis of Randomized Controlled Trials. *Am. J. Clin. Nutr.* **2017**, *106*, 921–929. [CrossRef] [PubMed]

40. Rosato, V.; Temple, N.J.; La Vecchia, C.; Castellan, G.; Tavani, A.; Guercio, V. Mediterranean Diet and Cardiovascular Disease: A Systematic Review and Meta-Analysis of Observational Studies. *Eur. J. Nutr.* **2017**. [CrossRef] [PubMed]

41. Fung, T.T.; Chiuve, S.E.; McCullough, M.L.; Rexrode, K.M.; Logroscino, G.; Hu, F.B. Adherence to a DASH-Style Diet and Risk of Coronary Heart Disease and Stroke in Women. *Arch. Intern. Med.* **2008**, *168*, 713–720. [CrossRef] [PubMed]

42. Zuo, L.; He, F.; Tinsley, G.M.; Pannell, B.K.; Ward, E.; Arciero, P.J. Comparison of High-Protein, Intermittent Fasting Low-Calorie Diet and Heart Healthy Diet for Vascular Health of the Obese. *Front. Physiol.* **2016**, *7*, 350. [CrossRef] [PubMed]

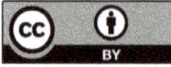

nutrients

MDPI

Article

Dietary Intake of Magnesium or Calcium and Chemotherapy-Induced Peripheral Neuropathy in Colorectal Cancer Patients

Evertine Wesselink [1], Renate M. Winkels [1], Harm van Baar [1], Anne J. M. R. Geijsen [1], Moniek van Zutphen [1], Henk K. van Halteren [2], Bibi M. E. Hansson [3], Sandra A. Radema [4], Johannes H. W. de Wilt [5], Ellen Kampman [1] and Dieuwertje E. G. Kok [1],*

[1] Division of Human Nutrition, Wageningen University & Research, Stippeneng 4, 6708 WE Wageningen, The Netherlands; vera.wesselink@wur.nl (E.W.); renate.winkels@wur.nl (R.M.W.); harm.vanbaar@wur.nl (H.v.B.); anne.geijsen@wur.nl (A.J.M.R.G.); moniek.vanzutphen@wur.nl (M.v.Z.); ellen.kampman@wur.nl (E.K.)
[2] Department of Internal Medicine, Admiraal de Ruyter Ziekenhuis, 's-Gravenpolderseweg 114, 4462 RA Goes, The Netherlands; h.vanhalteren@adrz.nl
[3] Department of Surgery, Canisius Wilhelmina Ziekenhuis, Weg door het Jonkerbos 100, 6532 SZ Nijmegen, The Netherlands; b.hansson@cwz.nl
[4] Department of Medical Oncology, Radboud University Medical Centre, Geert Grooteplein-Zuid 22, 6525 GA Nijmegen, The Netherlands; sandra.radema@radboudumc.nl
[5] Department of Surgery, Radboud University Medical Centre, Geert Grooteplein-Zuid 22, 6525 GA Nijmegen, The Netherlands; Hans.deWilt@radboudumc.nl
* Correspondence: dieuwertje.kok@wur.nl; Tel.: +31-317-485-901

Received: 15 February 2018; Accepted: 21 March 2018; Published: 23 March 2018

Abstract: Chemotherapy-induced peripheral neuropathy (CIPN) is a common and severe side-effect in colorectal cancer (CRC) patients. This study assessed the association between habitual dietary intake of magnesium or calcium and prevalence and severity of chronic CIPN in CRC patients receiving adjuvant chemotherapy. For this prospective cohort study, 196 CRC patients were considered. Magnesium and calcium intake was determined using a food frequency questionnaire at diagnosis, during and after chemotherapy. Chronic CIPN was assessed 12 months after diagnosis using the quality of life questionnaire CIPN20. Prevalence ratios were calculated to assess the association between magnesium or calcium intake and the prevalence of CIPN. Multivariable linear regression analysis was used to assess the association between magnesium or calcium intake and severity of CIPN. CIPN was reported by 160 (82%) patients. Magnesium intake during chemotherapy was statistically significantly associated with lower prevalence of CIPN (prevalence ratio (PR) 0.53, 95% confidence interval (CI) 0.32, 0.92). Furthermore, higher dietary intake of magnesium during (β -1.08, 95% CI -1.95, -0.22) and after chemotherapy (β -0.93, 95% CI -1.81, -0.06) was associated with less severe CIPN. No associations were found for calcium intake and the prevalence and severity of CIPN. To conclude, we observed an association between higher dietary magnesium intake and lower prevalence and severity of CIPN in CRC patients.

Keywords: calcium; chemotherapy; colorectal cancer; magnesium; neuropathy; oxaliplatin

---

1. Introduction

Chemotherapy-induced peripheral neuropathy (CIPN) is a common side-effect in colorectal cancer (CRC) patients treated with oxaliplatin [1]. Oxaliplatin can cause both acute and chronic CIPN. Symptoms of chronic CIPN include distal paresthesia, tingling sensations and numbness. Chronic CIPN predominantly affects sensory nerves and can lead to long-term disability [1]. Occurrence and severity of chronic CIPN are related to the cumulative dose and dose-intensity of the treatment [1–3].

Six to eight months after the end of oxaliplatin treatment, 40–60% of the patients still suffer from CIPN [4–7]. In order to minimize the detrimental effects in CRC patients, it is important to understand which factors can influence the development and severity of CIPN.

Magnesium and calcium are proposed to be important in the etiology of CIPN, because they are both involved in electric excitability of neurons and muscle contraction [8]. Low circulating levels of magnesium, but not calcium, before treatment have been associated with more severe CIPN in CRC patients [3]. Besides circulating levels of magnesium and calcium, several studies focused on intravenous administration of magnesium and calcium and the severity of CIPN [9–16]. The clinical observational study of Gamelin et al. found a lower occurrence and severity of CIPN in CRC patients who received magnesium and calcium in comparison to patients who did not receive magnesium and calcium for several reasons [9]. Other observational studies in CRC patients did not find an association between intravenous magnesium and calcium infusions and CIPN [10,11].

Several randomized-controlled trials (RCTs) [11–15] studied the effect of intravenous magnesium and calcium infusions on CIPN, but results are inconclusive. Grothey et al. reported a protective effect of magnesium and calcium on the prevalence of CIPN in 102 colon cancer patients [12]. The prevalence of CIPN was 22% in the magnesium and calcium group compared to 41% in the placebo group ($p = 0.04$) [12]. On the contrary, four other RCTs conducted among 27–353 CRC patients, did not find a protective effect of magnesium and calcium infusions on CIPN [13–16]. So far, no consensus about the use of magnesium and calcium infusions to reduce or prevent CIPN has been reached [17].

Most studies conducted so far focused on acute CIPN during and directly after treatment. It has been shown that further progression of CIPN can occur months after the end of treatment [1]. Moreover, the associations between dietary magnesium or calcium intake and the prevalence and severity of chronic CIPN have not been described so far. Dietary intake in relation to CIPN is important as dietary magnesium intake is the main contributor to the magnesium status. Further insights into the relation between diet and CIPN may provide feasible opportunities for dietary strategies directed against CIPN in cancer patients. In this prospective cohort study, we assessed the association between habitual dietary intake of magnesium or calcium and the prevalence and severity of CIPN approximately six months after chemotherapy, i.e., 12 months after diagnosis, in CRC patients receiving adjuvant chemotherapy.

2. Materials and Methods

2.1. Patients

This study is embedded in the longitudinal observational study on nutritional and lifestyle factors (COLON study), which is a prospective cohort study focusing on nutritional and lifestyle factors in relation to clinical outcomes and quality of life of CRC patients in the Netherlands [18]. The design and recruitment of the COLON study has been described in detail previously [18]. In short, newly diagnosed CRC patients were recruited directly after diagnosis in 12 hospitals in the Netherlands and were followed up during and after treatment. Men and women of all ages, who were in any stage of the disease were eligible for the study. Non-Dutch speaking patients, or patients with a history of CRC or (partial) bowel resection, chronic inflammatory bowel disease, hereditary CRC syndromes (e.g., Lynch syndrome, Familial Adenomatous Polyposis, Peutz-Jegher), dementia or another mental condition that made it impossible to fill out a questionnaire correctly, were excluded from the study. Participants of the COLON study who were included between April 2012 and December 2015 and who received adjuvant chemotherapy were eligible for the current study ($n = 293$). Patients who also received neoadjuvant chemotherapy ($n = 8$), who did not start with chemotherapy ($n = 22$), or did not fill out the questionnaire on CIPN ($n = 67$) were excluded, resulting in a total of 196 newly diagnosed CRC patients eligible for the current study (Figure 1). Hospital records and linkage with the Dutch ColoRectal Audit (DCRA) [19] were used to obtain data regarding cancer type, cancer stage and type of chemotherapy. All patients provided written informed consent. All procedures followed were in accordance with the ethical standards of the institution and the COLON study was approved by the Committee on Research involving Human Subjects, region Arnhem-Nijmegen, the Netherlands (file 2009-349).

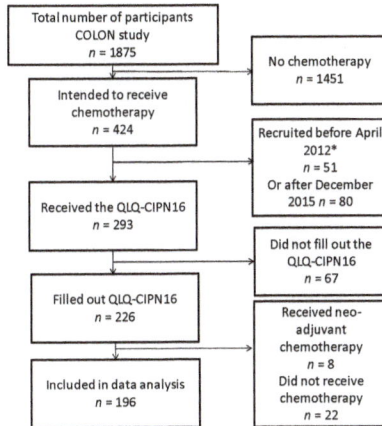

Figure 1. Flowchart representing patient selection for the current study. Colorectal cancer patients participating in the longitudinal observational study on nutritional and lifestyle factors (the COLON study) and who received adjuvant chemotherapy and filled out the quality of life questionnaire to assess chemotherapy-induced peripheral neuropathy (QLQ-CIPN16) were included in the present study. * Patients who were recruited before April 2012 were not included in this study, because the QLQ-CIPN16 questionnaire was implemented from April 2012 onwards.

2.2. Magnesium and Calcium Intake

A 204-item semi-quantitative food frequency questionnaire (FFQ) developed by the Division of Human Nutrition of Wageningen University and Research, the Netherlands, was used to assess habitual intake of magnesium and calcium from the diet during the previous month. The magnesium or calcium content of a product was determined based on data from the Dutch food composition table of 2011 [20]. Dietary intake of magnesium and calcium was calculated for each food item based on frequency of intake, number of portions and portion size, as well as the type of product (e.g., whole grain bread or brown bread). The total amount of the nutrients consumed per day was calculated by adding all items containing the respective nutrient. The dietary intake of magnesium and calcium was adjusted for total energy intake using the residual method [21]. Dietary supplement use was assessed by a dietary supplement questionnaire developed by the Division of Human Nutrition of Wageningen University and Research [18]. Intake of magnesium and calcium from dietary supplements was not considered for the current study, due to the relatively low number of supplement users and the lack of details on exact dosages, frequency and compliance. However, we performed sensitivity analyses excluding patients who reported use of dietary supplements containing magnesium or calcium. The FFQs and dietary supplement questionnaires were filled out at diagnosis and six and 12 months after diagnosis. These three time points represent the usual dietary intake before surgery, during chemotherapy and six months after chemotherapy, respectively.

2.3. Chemotherapy-Induced Peripheral Neuropathy

Prevalence and severity of chronic CIPN were assessed using the 'European Organization for Research and Treatment of Cancer Quality of Life Questionnaire to assess Chemotherapy Induced Peripheral Neuropathy' (EORTC QLQ-CIPN16). This is an abbreviated version of the QLQ-CIPN20 [22], which is used in the COLON study. This questionnaire was filled out 12 months after diagnosis, representing approximately six months after the end of chemotherapy. The QLQ-CIPN16 consists of 16 questions of which eight assessing sensory symptoms and eight assessing motor symptoms. These questions were shown to be valid and reliable to assess patient-reported CIPN [22]. Patients reported the degree to which they have experienced sensory and motor symptoms during the past week using a 4-point Likert scale. Sensory and motor scale scores from the QLQ-CIPN16 ranged from 1–32. The scores of the QLQ-CIPN16 were linear transformed to a 0–100 scale. Based on mean scores of CIPN in the general Dutch population, the presence of CIPN was defined as >3.6 for the total CIPN16 score, >3.2 for the sensory sub-score and >3.8 for the motor sub-score [23]. Furthermore, we have evaluated severity of CIPN-related symptoms by specifically focusing on the CIPN scores, with higher scores indicating more severe CIPN. Missing values were handled by the mean-person imputation method [24], however, participants were excluded from analyses when more than two items in the QLQ-CIPN16 were missing.

2.4. Data Analysis

To study the association between magnesium and calcium and the prevalence of CIPN, prevalence ratios (PR) were calculated using a Cox proportional hazards regression model, with a fixed time variable. PRs were used, since odds ratios tend to overestimate the size of the association when the outcome is common [25]. Subsequently, among patients suffering from CIPN, the association between magnesium or calcium intake and the severity of CIPN was assessed by using multivariable linear regression analysis.

The Shapiro-Wilk test was used to determine whether data were normally distributed. Dietary intake of magnesium, calcium, vitamin D, total energy, as well as CIPN scores were natural-log transformed. To adjust for potential confounding, the models were adjusted for age, gender as well as energy adjusted dietary calcium or magnesium and vitamin D intake. When a variable changed the regression coefficient of the independent variable with 10% or more, the variable was considered to be a confounder and was added as a covariate to the model. Self-reported magnesium or calcium supplement use, diabetes mellitus, physical activity, smoking, as well as B vitamins and alcohol intake did not influence the observed associations. There was a strong correlation between protein and magnesium intake ($r = 0.81$), as well as between protein and calcium intake ($r = 0.80$), therefore we did not adjust for protein intake in the final model. Sensitivity analyses were performed for oxaliplatin-containing chemotherapy (OX), patients with colon cancer and non-supplement users. Stratified analysis was done for age (<65 and ≥65 years of age) to assess possible age differences.

Statistical analyses were performed in SAS 9.4 (SAS Institute, Cary, NC, USA). Ninety-five percent confidence intervals (95% CIs), not containing 1 for the Cox regression analyses and not containing 0 for the multivariable regression analyses, represent statistically significant associations [26].

3. Results

3.1. Patients Characteristics

In total, 196 CRC patients from 12 hospitals in the Netherlands were included in this study. The majority of the patients started with OX ($n = 166$, 85%), while 23 (11%) patients received capecitabine monotherapy (Table 1). In our study population, 160 patients (82%) reported CIPN 12 months after diagnosis. Among these patients, both sensory as well as motor CIPN symptoms were commonly reported (81% and 76%, respectively). Common sensory symptoms included tingling and numbness in fingers and toes, whereas difficulty with manipulating small objects and opening jars or bottles were commonly reported motor symptoms. The severity of sensory symptoms was higher than the severity of motor symptoms (mean score 20.8 and 12.5, respectively).

The median intake of magnesium was 317 mg/day and for calcium this was 851 g/day. The most important food sources of magnesium in our population were whole grain bread and nuts. Also, coffee, dairy products, dark chocolate, banana and legumes were common sources of magnesium.

For calcium the most important food source was dairy products, especially cheese, yoghurt and milk. The intake of magnesium was below the estimated average requirement of 350 mg/day for men and 265 mg/day for women [27] in 48% of our study population at the time of diagnosis. During and after chemotherapy, 65% and 57% of the patients had an intake below the estimated average requirement, respectively. The intake of calcium was below the estimated average requirement of 800 mg/day for man <70 years and 1000 mg/day for man >70 years and 1000 mg for women [28] in 58% of our population at the time of diagnosis, 59% during treatment and 65% after treatment.

Table 1. Characteristics of colorectal cancer patients who received adjuvant chemotherapy by prevalence of chemotherapy-induced peripheral chemotherapy (CIPN).

		CIPN	
	Total Population *n* = 196	CIPN No *n* = 36 (18%)	Yes [1] *n* = 160 (82%)
Gender, women	71 (36%)	12 (33%)	59 (37%)
Age (years)	64.0 (59.8–68.1)	65.4 (59.0–68.2)	63.7 (59.9–68.0)
Diabetes mellitus (yes) [2]	15 (8%)	3 (8%)	12 (8%)
Physical activity (meeting norm) [3]	143 (73%)	25 (69%)	118 (74%)
Tumor stage			
Stage II	15 (8%)	2 (6%)	13 (8%)
Stage III	145 (74%)	28 (76%)	117 (73%)
Stage IV	21 (10%)	3 (9%)	18 (11%)
Missing	15 (8%)	3 (9%)	12 (8%)
Cancer site			
Colon	181 (93%)	33 (92%)	148 (93%)
Rectum	14 (7%)	3 (8%)	11 (7%)
Missing	1 (0%)	0 (0%)	1 (0%)
Type of chemotherapy			
Oxaliplatin-containing (OX)	166 (85%)	27 (75%)	139 (87%)
Capecitabine monotherapy	23 (12%)	9 (25%)	14 (9%)
Other	2 (1%)	0 (0%)	2 (1%)
Missing	5 (2%)	0 (0%)	5 (3%)
Dietary factors			
Magnesium intake from diet (mg/day) [2,4]	317 (261–383)	325 (261–396)	313 (261–380)
Use of magnesium supplements (yes)	36 (18%)	6 (17%)	30 (18%)
Calcium intake from diet (mg/day) [2,4]	851 (621–1143)	789 (597–1155)	861 (631–1123)
Use of calcium supplements (yes)	35 (18%)	6 (17%)	29 (18%)
Vitamin D intake from diet (mg/day) [2,4]	3.1 (2.4–4.1)	2.8 (2.2–3.7)	3.2 (2.4–4.2)
Total energy intake (kcal/day) [2,4]	1893 (1534–2265)	1898 (1547–2230)	1893 (1534–2285)
CIPN [5]			
Total score [6]	14.6 (6.3–26.4)	0.0 (0–2.1)	16.7 (10.4–29.2)
Sensory score [7]	16.7 (4.2–37.5)	0.0 (0–0)	20.8 (12.5–37.5)
Motor score [8]	8.3 (4.2–20.8)	0.0 (0–0)	12.5 (8.3–20.8)

Values presented are median (quartile 1–quartile 3) or number (percentage). [1] Cut-off point for CIPN total score: 3.6, [2] Assessed at diagnosis. [3] Meeting the Dutch physical activity guideline of 150 min per week of moderate intensive exercise at baseline, [4] Intake is missing for two patients, [5] Assessed 12 months after diagnosis. [6] Data for one patient missing. [7] Data for two patients missing. [8] Data for five patients missing.

3.2. Dietary Magnesium or Calcium Intake and CIPN

Dietary intake of magnesium during chemotherapy was associated with the prevalence of chronic CIPN (PR 0.53, 95% CI 0.32, 0.90) (Table 2). Among patients suffering from CIPN, a higher dietary intake of magnesium was associated with less severe symptoms of CIPN (β −1.08, 95% CI −1.95, −0.22 for the intake during chemotherapy and β −0.93, 95% CI −1.81, −0.06 for the intake after chemotherapy) (Table 3). Dietary intake of calcium was not associated with the prevalence (Table 2) and severity (Table 3) of CIPN.

Sensitivity analyses including only patients receiving OX (*n* = 166) or only patients with colon cancer (*n* = 181) or only non-supplement users (*n* = 160–171) showed similar results (Table 4).

Table 2. Association between dietary magnesium or calcium intake and the prevalence of chronic chemotherapy-induced neuropathy in colorectal cancer patients receiving adjuvant chemotherapy.

	n/Events	Prevalence Ratio (95% CI) Total Score CIPN16[1]	n/Events	Sensory Symptoms[1]	n/Events	Motor Symptoms[1]
Magnesium intake						
Crude model						
At diagnosis	194/158	0.81 (0.51, 1.29)	194/157	0.98 (0.64, 1.52)	194/147	0.95 (0.54, 1.67)
During chemotherapy	192/156	**0.57 (0.35, 0.92)**	192/156	0.70 (0.44, 1.12)	192/145	0.59 (0.33, 1.05)
After chemotherapy	181/147	0.67 (0.43, 1.05)	181/146	0.86 (0.57, 1.31)	181/136	0.61 (0.36, 1.03)
Full model						
At diagnosis	194/158	0.69 (0.42, 1.13)	194/157	0.84 (0.51, 1.39)	194/147	0.81 (0.43, 1.52)
During chemotherapy	192/156	**0.53 (0.32, 0.90)**	192/156	0.67 (0.40, 1.10)	192/145	0.57 (0.30, 1.09)
After chemotherapy	181/147	0.61 (0.37, 1.03)	181/146	0.84 (0.51, 1.37)	181/136	**0.51 (0.28, 0.93)**
Calcium intake						
Crude model						
At diagnosis	194/158	1.15 (0.93, 1.41)	194/157	1.20 (0.98, 1.46)	194/147	1.12 (0.89, 1.41)
During chemotherapy	192/156	0.97 (0.83, 1.13)	192/156	1.02 (0.87, 1.19)	192/145	0.89 (0.73, 1.09)
After Chemotherapy	181/147	1.03 (0.86, 1.23)	181/146	1.08 (0.90, 1.30)	181/136	0.96 (0.78, 1.17)
Full model						
At diagnosis	194/158	1.21 (0.95, 1.56)	194/157	1.24 (0.97, 1.58)	194/147	1.15 (0.88, 1.50)
During chemotherapy	192/156	1.03 (0.86, 1.23)	192/156	1.06 (0.89, 1.28)	192/145	0.92 (0.73, 1.16)
After Chemotherapy	181/147	1.08 (0.89, 1.32)	181/146	1.10 (0.89, 1.35)	181/136	0.99 (0.79, 1.24)

Analyses were performed using a Cox proportional hazard regression model, with a fixed time variable. Crude models: energy-adjusted intake of magnesium or calcium. Full model for magnesium was adjusted for, energy-adjusted dietary calcium and vitamin D intake as well as age and gender. Full model for calcium was adjusted for, energy-adjusted dietary magnesium and vitamin D intake as well as age and gender. [1] CIPN was defined as a score >3.6 for the total CIPN16 score, >3.2 for the sensory sub-score and >3.8 for the motor sub-score.

Table 3. Associations between dietary magnesium or calcium intake and severity of chronic chemotherapy-induced neuropathy in colorectal cancer patients receiving adjuvant chemotherapy.

		Beta (95% CI)				
	n	Total Score CIPN16	n	Sensory Symptoms	n	Motor Symptoms
Magnesium intake						
Crude model						
At diagnosis	158	−0.68 (−1.45, 0.08)	157	−1.09 (−1.90 −0.27)	147	−0.45 (−1.33, 0.43)
During chemotherapy	156	−1.21 (−2.01, −0.41)	156	−1.43 (−2.30, −0.57)	145	−1.25 (−2.16, −0.35)
After chemotherapy	147	−0.81 (−1.59, −0.04)	146	−1.05 (−1.87, −0.22)	136	−0.64 (−1.48, 0.21)
Full model						
At diagnosis	158	−0.65 (−1.52, 0.20)	157	−1.10 (−2.01, −0.18)	147	−0.36 (−1.36, 0.63)
During chemotherapy	156	−1.08 (−1.95, −0.22)	156	−1.24 (−2.17, −0.32)	145	−1.25 (−2.24, −0.27)
After chemotherapy	147	−0.93 (−1.81, −0.06)	146	−1.11 (−2.04, −0.19)	136	−0.76 (−1.73, 0.21)
Calcium intake						
Crude model						
At diagnosis	158	−0.20 (−0.55, 0.14)	157	−0.31 (−0.68, 0.06)	147	−0.19 (−0.56, 0.18)
During chemotherapy	156	−0.31 (−0.62, 0.00)	156	−0.39 (−0.74, −0.04)	145	−0.31 (−0.66, 0.04)
After chemotherapy	147	−0.19 (−0.55, 0.17)	146	−0.36 (−0.75, 0.03)	136	−0.04 (−0.42, 0.35)
Full model						
At diagnosis	158	−0.05 (−0.45, 0.35)	157	0.03 (−0.40, 0.45)	147	−0.19 (−0.61, 0.23)
During chemotherapy	156	−0.16 (−0.51, 0.19)	156	−0.14 (−0.52, 0.23)	145	−0.19 (−0.57, 0.19)
After chemotherapy	147	−0.03 (−0.42, 0.35)	146	−0.10 (−0.52, 0.32)	136	0.01 (−0.40, 0.43)

Analyses were performed using multivariable linear regression analyses. Crude models: energy-adjusted intake of magnesium or calcium. Full model for magnesium was adjusted for energy-adjusted dietary calcium and vitamin D intake as well as age and gender. Full model for calcium was adjusted for energy-adjusted dietary magnesium and vitamin D intake as well as age and gender.

Table 4. Sensitivity analyses for the associations between dietary magnesium or calcium intake and severity of chronic chemotherapy-induced neuropathy.

		Beta (95% CI)				
	n	Total Score CIPN16	n	Sensory Symptoms	n	Motor Symptoms
Patients receiving oxaliplatin-containing chemotherapy						
Magnesium						
At diagnosis	137	−0.68 (−1.58, 0.22)	138	−1.01 (−1.97, −0.05)	126	−0.48 (−0.53, 0.57)
During chemotherapy	136	−0.90 (−1.80, −0.00)	137	−1.10 (−2.06, −0.14)	125	−1.28 (−2.33, −0.24)
After chemotherapy	132	−0.94 (−1.85, −0.02)	133	−1.10 (−2.07, −0.12)	121	−0.94 (−1.98, 0.10)
Calcium						
At diagnosis	137	0.00 (−0.42, 0.42)	138	0.08 (−0.36, 0.53)	132	−0.19 (−0.63, 0.26)
During chemotherapy	136	−0.18 (−0.54; 0.18)	137	−0.11 (−0.51; 0.28)	125	−0.28 (−0.69; 0.13)
After chemotherapy	132	0.00 (−0.39, 0.41)	133	−0.06 (−0.49, 0.38)	121	0.01 (−0.43, 0.45)
Not supplement users						
Magnesium						
At diagnosis	128	−0.80 (−1.80, 0.20)	126	−0.99 (−2.08, 0.10)	119	−0.68 (−1.83, 0.48)
During chemotherapy	136	−1.24 (−2.21, −0.27)	134	−1.20 (−2.27, −0.13)	128	−1.81 (−2.90, −0.71)
After chemotherapy	129	−1.34 (−2.30, −0.37)	126	−1.29 (−2.37, −0.21)	119	−1.38 (−2.44, −0.32)
Calcium						
At diagnosis	127	−0.06 (−0.50, 0.37)	127	0.06 (−0.41, 0.53)	119	−0.08 (−0.56, 0.38)
During chemotherapy	140	−0.12 (−0.48, 0.23)	138	−0.07 (−0.45, 0.32)	132	−0.20 (−0.60, 0.20)
After chemotherapy	127	−0.00 (−0.41, 0.42)	130	−0.09 (−0.54, 0.36)	119	0.09 (−0.35, 0.53)
Colon cancer patients						
Magnesium						
At diagnosis	146	−0.66 (−1.54, 0.22)	145	−1.11 (−2.04, −0.18)	135	−0.34 (−1.37, 0.68)
During chemotherapy	145	−1.13 (−2.03, −0.23)	145	−1.34 (−2.30, −0.38)	134	−1.30 (−2.33, −0.26)
After chemotherapy	139	−0.80 (−1.71, 0.11)	137	−0.98 (−1.95, −0.02)	128	−0.66 (−1.67, 0.36)
Calcium						
At diagnosis	146	−0.00 (−0.42, 0.41)	145	0.07 (−0.37, 0.51)	135	−0.15 (−0.58, 0.28)
During chemotherapy	145	−0.11 (−0.48, 0.25)	145	−0.07 (−0.47, 0.35)	134	−0.16 (−0.57, 0.26)
After chemotherapy	139	−0.03 (−0.45, 0.39)	137	−0.11 (−0.56, 0.34)	128	0.04 (−0.41, 0.50)

Analyses were performed using multivariable linear regression analyses. Models for magnesium was adjusted for energy-adjusted dietary calcium and vitamin D intake as well as age and gender. Models for calcium was adjusted for energy-adjusted dietary magnesium and vitamin D intake as well as age and gender.

Stratified analyses for age showed statistically significant associations between magnesium intake at all three time points and the severity of CIPN for patients aged 65 and older ($n = 88$), but not for patients younger than 65 years ($n = 108$) (data not shown).

4. Discussion

The aim of this study was to assess the association between magnesium and calcium intake and CIPN in a prospective cohort of CRC patients. Dietary intake of magnesium during chemotherapy was associated with a lower prevalence of CIPN. A higher dietary intake of magnesium, but not calcium, during and after chemotherapy was associated with a lower severity of total CIPN symptoms.

The prevalence of CIPN approximately six months after chemotherapy, i.e., 12 months after diagnosis, was higher than expected (81%) in our study population consisting of 196 CRC patients treated with adjuvant chemotherapy. Argyriou et al. reported a prevalence of 40% for CIPN in CRC patients six to eight months after finalizing their treatment containing OX [1]. CIPN is related to various risk factors, including treatment schedule, dose per course, cumulative dose, time of infusion and pre-existing peripheral neuropathy [1]. These factors likely vary between studies and countries. Furthermore, difference in the prevalence of CIPN may be explained by different methods to assess CIPN. Most previous studies used criteria of the National Cancer Institute (NCI-CTCAE) or the total neuropathy score (TNSc) to assess CIPN [4–7]. These methods are based on clinical examination, while the QLQ-CIPN16 is a patient-reported assessment of CIPN. The use of the QLQ-CIPN16 is inherent to the large-scale setting of the COLON cohort study. Recent studies compared several commonly used methods to assess CIPN [29,30]. A high correlation was found for the NCI-CTCAE and the EORTC QLQ-CIPN [29,30]. Furthermore, we did expect a high prevalence of sensory symptoms, and not motor symptoms, since OX is mainly associated with chronic sensory CIPN [1,31]. Although motor symptoms were also commonly reported in our study, it should be noted that the severity of motor symptoms was relatively low in the present study (mean score 12.5 versus 20.8 for sensory symptoms).

In the present study, we found that a higher magnesium intake was associated with a lower severity of chronic CIPN, whereas no association for calcium was found. Both magnesium and calcium are involved in electric excitability of neurons and muscle contraction [8]. A potential explanation for the association between magnesium and the severity of CIPN is the role of magnesium in the neuromuscular system and nervous tissue conduction [32]. It has been supposed that CIPN is caused by the stimulating effect of OX on neural excitability due to re-configuration of sodium channels in the cell membrane [33]. Magnesium (and calcium) are hypothesized to decrease OX-induced hyper-excitability [34,35], thereby limiting damage of neurons. In addition, magnesium specifically plays a role in membrane integrity and stability [32].

In the present study, we focused for the first time on dietary intake of magnesium and calcium in relation to CIPN. It should be noted that magnesium levels in blood are tightly regulated [36]. When circulating levels of magnesium are low, other tissues such as bone and muscle provide magnesium to restore circulating magnesium levels. With a low magnesium intake, body stores of magnesium could be depleted, while circulating levels are still in the healthy range [3,37]. Among our study population, 65% of the patients had an intake below the estimated average requirement of 350 mg/day for men and 265 mg/day for women [28] during chemotherapy. Hypothetically, especially patients with a low intake of magnesium could benefit from additional intake of magnesium, as a higher intake could restore depleted body stores of magnesium and thereby increases availability of magnesium in muscles and nerves. Stratified analyses for age showed a stronger association in patients aged 65 years and older. In this group the percentages of patients with a magnesium intake below the estimated average requirement was higher compared to participants younger than 65. In addition, during chemotherapy more participants had a magnesium intake below the estimated average requirement compared to before and after chemotherapy. These results indicate that an optimal magnesium status throughout treatment is important. Further studies are needed to confirm these findings and to determine the clinical relevance of the reported association between magnesium and CIPN.

The present study has some limitations. First, intake from dietary supplements was not considered because of the relative limited number of supplement users. In addition detailed data on dosage, frequency and compliance was lacking and supplement use was not consistent over the study duration. Also, the mineral content of the drinking water was not considered. Magnesium and calcium from drinking water contribute to the total magnesium and calcium intake. In the Netherlands, magnesium and calcium content in the tap water ranges from 1.7–26.2 mg/L (1–8% of the total intake) and 15–157 mg/L (1–17% of the total intake), respectively [38]. Second, although we explored the possible interaction between magnesium or calcium and many nutrients like B vitamins, calcium, vitamin D, vitamin E and alcohol, we could not exclude the possibility that other nutrients or bioactive compounds contributed to the observed effects. Third, the prevalence of pre-existing CIPN was not taken into account. Pre-existing CIPN is a risk factor for developing chronic CIPN [1]. Diabetes mellitus is an important cause of peripheral neuropathy [39]. However, in the present study, adjustment for self-reported diabetes mellitus did not influence the observed associations. In addition, we have not been able to take specific information on treatment-related factors, such as cumulative dose of chemotherapy and use of specific medications that may have influenced magnesium status into account. However, in the specific setting of studies focusing on long-term (chronic) toxicities, dose is a complicated factor. Patients who received a low (cumulative) dose may have experienced severe (acute) toxicities which have resulted in a dose reduction or premature discontinuation of therapy. Because of severe toxicities, among which potentially CIPN, an increased risk of chronic CIPN on the long-term may be expected. On the other hand, patients who completed their scheduled treatment, and hence received a high (cumulative) dose, may also have an increased risk of CIPN because of extensive exposure to the cytotoxic regimens. Furthermore, although information on clinical and socio-demographic characteristics of patients who did not fill out the QLQ-CIPN16 ($n = 67, 23$%) was available, it remains unknown why they did not fill out the questionnaires. It could be that these patients suffered from CIPN symptoms in their hands, resulting in selection which theoretically could decrease the validity of the present study. However, we do not expect that these non-responses had a major impact on the results of our study as the overall response rate was high (77%). The sample size of this study was relatively small ($n = 196$) and restricted to CRC patients and therefore we cannot state yet if generalization of our results to other cancer patients or chemotherapeutic agents is justified. Finally, we did not measure blood levels of magnesium and calcium. It should be noted, however, that the specific objective of this study was to investigate the association between dietary intake of magnesium and CIPN. Next to that, circulating levels are tightly regulated and not representative for magnesium levels in muscles and bone [37].

The present study also has important strengths. First of all, this is the first prospective cohort study which assessed the association between habitual dietary intake of magnesium or calcium and CIPN. Our data extend and complement existing evidence regarding the association between magnesium, calcium and neuropathy. Previous studies focusing on infusions with magnesium and calcium showed inconsistent findings and relied on acute exposure, while we assessed habitual, long-term intake of magnesium and calcium. In addition, previous studies focused on acute CIPN (during and directly after chemotherapy), while we focused on chronic and persistent CIPN. Therefore, this study provides an important contribution to the limited knowledge on chronic CIPN and its association with diet before, during and after chemotherapy. Furthermore, in the present study we used the 16 items of the QLQ-CIPN20 that are considered to be valid and reliable [22]. This approach resulted in a clinically relevant estimation of the prevalence and severity of CIPN compared to the QLQ-CIPN20 [22]. Due the availability of detailed data on diet and other clinical and lifestyle factors, we could adjust for the most plausible confounders, although residual confounding can never be fully excluded.

5. Conclusions

The results of this study showed that a higher dietary magnesium intake was associated with a lower prevalence and less severe CIPN symptoms among CRC patients who received adjuvant chemotherapy. Further studies are needed to confirm our findings and to provide a solid basis for future recommendations directed towards the intake of magnesium before and during chemotherapy.

Acknowledgments: The authors would like to thank the co-workers from the following hospitals for their involvement in recruitment for the COLON study: Hospital Gelderse Vallei, Ede; RadboudUMC, Nijmegen; Slingeland Hospital, Doetinchem,; Canisius Wilhelmina Hospital, Nijmegen; Rijnstate Hospital, Arnhem; Gelre Hospitals, Apeldoorn/Zutphen; Hospital Bernhoven, Uden; Isala, Zwolle; ZGT, Almelo; Martini Hospital, Groningen; Admiraal de Ruyter Hospital, Goes/Vlissingen, all in The Netherlands. Sources of support: This project is sponsored by Wereld Kanker Onderzoek Fonds (WCRF-NL) & World Cancer Research Fund International (WCRF International 2014/1179); Alped'Huzes / Dutch Cancer Society (UM 2012–5653, UW 2013–5927; UW 2015-7946).

Author Contributions: E.W., R.M.W., E.K. and D.E.G.K. contributed to the conception and design of this study. B.M.E.H., H.K.v.H. and H.d.W. contributed to the recruitment of participants. M.v.Z., H.v.B., A.J.M.R.G. and E.W. contributed to recruitment of participants and the data collection. Statistical data analyses were done and interpreted by E.W. The manuscript was drafted by E.W. and D.E.G.K., who also had primary responsibility, and all authors critically read and revised the manuscript. All authors approved the final version of the manuscript. The datasets used and analyzed during the current study are available from the corresponding author on reasonable request.

Conflicts of Interest: The authors declare no conflict of interest. The founding sponsors had no role in the design of the study; in the collection, analyses, or interpretation of data; in the writing of the manuscript, and in the decision to publish the results.

References

1. Argyriou, A.A.; Polychronopoulos, P.; Iconomou, G.; Chroni, E.; Kalofonos, H.P. A review on oxaliplatin-induced peripheral nerve damage. *Cancer Treat. Rev.* **2008**, *34*, 368–377. [CrossRef] [PubMed]

2. Staff, N.P.; Grisold, A.; Grisold, W.; Windebank, A.J. Chemotherapy-Induced Peripheral Neuropathy: A Current Review. *Ann. Neurol.* **2017**, *81*, 772–781. [CrossRef] [PubMed]

3. Vincenzi, B.; Frezza, A.M.; Schiavon, G.; Spoto, C.; Silvestris, N.; Addeo, R.; Catalano, V.; Graziano, F.; Santini, D.; Tonini, G. Identification of clinical predictive factors of oxaliplatin-induced chronic peripheral neuropathy in colorectal cancer patients treated with adjuvant Folfox IV. *Support. Care Cancer* **2013**, *21*, 1313–1319. [CrossRef] [PubMed]

4. Attal, N.; Bouhassira, D.; Gautron, M.; Vaillant, J.N.; Mitry, E.; Lepère, C.; Rougier, P.; Guirimand, F. Thermal hyperalgesia as a marker of oxaliplatin neurotoxicity: A prospective quantified sensory assessment study. *Pain* **2009**, *144*, 245–252. [CrossRef] [PubMed]

5. André, T.; de Gramont, A.; Vernerey, D.; Chibaudel, B.; Bonnetain, F.; Tijeras-Raballand, A.; Scriva, A.; Hickish, T.; Tabernero, J.; Van Laethem, J.L.; et al. Adjuvant Fluorouracil, Leucovorin, and Oxaliplatin in Stage II to III Colon Cancer: Updated 10-Year Survival and Outcomes According to BRAF Mutation and Mismatch Repair Status of the MOSAIC Study. *J. Clin. Oncol.* **2015**, *33*, 4176–4187. [CrossRef] [PubMed]

6. De Gramont, A.; Figer, A.; Seymour, M.; Homerin, M.; Hmissi, A.; Cassidy, J.; Boni, C.; Cortes-Funes, H.; Cervantes, A.; Freyer, G.; et al. Leucovorin and fluorouracil with or without oxaliplatin as first-line treatment in advanced colorectal cancer. *J. Clin. Oncol.* **2000**, *18*, 2938–2947. [CrossRef] [PubMed]

7. Extra, J.M.; Marty, M.; Brienza, S.; Misset, J.L. Pharmacokinetics and safety profile of oxaliplatin. *Semin. Oncol.* **1998**, *25*, 13–22. [PubMed]

8. Laires, M.J.; Monteiro, C.P.; Bicho, M. Role of cellular magnesium in health and human disease. *Front. Biosci.* **2004**, *9*, 262–276. [CrossRef] [PubMed]

9. Gamelin, L.; Boisdron-Celle, M.; Delva, R.; Guérin-Meyer, V.; Ifrah, N.; Morel, A.; Gamelin, E. Prevention of oxaliplatin-related neurotoxicity by calcium and magnesium infusions: A retrospective study of 161 patients receiving oxaliplatin combined with 5-Fluorouracil and leucovorin for advanced colorectal cancer. *Clin. Cancer Res.* **2004**, *10*, 4055–4061. [CrossRef] [PubMed]

10. Knijn, N.; Tol, J.; Koopman, M.; Werter, M.J.B.P.; Imholz, A.L.T.; Valster, F.A.A.; Mol, L.; Vincent, A.D.; Teerenstra, S.; Punt, C.J.A. The effect of prophylactic calcium and magnesium infusions on the incidence of neurotoxicity and clinical outcome of oxaliplatin-based systemic treatment in advanced colorectal cancer patients. *Eur. J. Cancer* **2011**, *47*, 369–374. [CrossRef] [PubMed]

11. Kono, T.; Mamiya, N.; Chisato, N.; Ebisawa, Y.; Yamazaki, H.; Watari, J.; Yamamoto, Y.; Suzuki, S.; Asama, T.; Kamiya, K. Efficacy of Goshajinkigan for Peripheral Neurotoxicity of Oxaliplatin in Patients with Advanced or Recurrent Colorectal Cancer. *Evid.-Based Complement. Altern. Med.* **2011**, *2011*, 418481. [CrossRef] [PubMed]

12. Grothey, A.; Nikcevich, D.A.; Sloan, J.A.; Kugler, J.W.; Silberstein, P.T.; Dentchev, T.; Wender, D.B.; Novotny, P.J.; Chitaley, U.; Alberts, S.R.; et al. Intravenous calcium and magnesium for oxaliplatin-induced sensory neurotoxicity in adjuvant colon cancer: NCCTG N04C7. *J. Clin. Oncol.* **2011**, *29*, 421–427. [CrossRef] [PubMed]

13. Hochster, H.S.; Grothey, A.; Hart, L.; Rowland, K.; Ansari, R.; Alberts, S.; Chowhan, N.; Ramanathan, R.K.; Keaton, M.; Hainsworth, J.D.; et al. Improved time to treatment failure with an intermittent oxaliplatin strategy: Results of CONcePT. *Ann. Oncol.* **2014**, *25*, 1172–1178. [CrossRef] [PubMed]

14. Loprinzi, C.L.; Qin, R.; Dakhil, S.R.; Fehrenbacher, L.; Flynn, K.A.; Atherton, P.; Seisler, D.; Qamar, R.; Lewis, G.C.; Grothey, A. Phase III randomized, placebo-controlled, double-blind study of intravenous calcium and magnesium to prevent oxaliplatin-induced sensory neurotoxicity (N08CB/Alliance). *J. Clin. Oncol.* **2014**, *32*, 997–1005. [CrossRef] [PubMed]

15. Ishibashi, K.; Okada, N.; Miyazaki, T.; Sano, M.; Ishida, H. Effect of calcium and magnesium on neurotoxicity and blood platinum concentrations in patients receiving mFOLFOX6 therapy: A prospective randomized study. *Int. J. Clin. Oncol.* **2010**, *15*, 82–87. [CrossRef] [PubMed]

16. Chay, W.-Y.; Tan, S.-H.; Lo, Y.-L.; Ong, S.Y.-K.; Ng, H.-C.; Gao, F.; Koo, W.-H.; Choo, S.-P. Use of calcium and magnesium infusions in prevention of oxaliplatin induced sensory neuropathy. *Asia Pac. J. Clin. Oncol.* **2010**, *6*, 270–277. [CrossRef] [PubMed]

17. Albers, J.W.; Chaudhry, V.; Cavaletti, G.; Donehower, R.C. Interventions for preventing neuropathy caused by cisplatin and related compounds. In *Cochrane Database of Systematic Reviews*; Albers, J.W., Ed.; John Wiley & Sons, Ltd.: Chichester, UK, 2014; p. CD005228.

18. Winkels, R.M.; Heine-Bröring, R.C.; van Zutphen, M.; van Harten-Gerritsen, S.; Kok, D.E.G.; van Duijnhoven, F.J.B.; Kampman, E. The COLON study: Colorectal cancer: Longitudinal, Observational study on Nutritional and lifestyle factors that may influence colorectal tumour recurrence, survival and quality of life. *BMC Cancer* **2014**, *14*, 374. [CrossRef] [PubMed]

19. Van Leersum, N.J.; Snijders, H.S.; Henneman, D.; Kolfschoten, N.E.; Gooiker, G.A.; ten Berge, M.G.; Eddes, E.H.; Wouters, M.W.J. M.; Tollenaar, R.A.E.M.; Bemelman, W.A.; et al. The Dutch Surgical Colorectal Audit. *Eur. J. Surg. Oncol.* **2013**, *39*, 1063–1070. [CrossRef] [PubMed]

20. Netherlands Nutrition Center: NEVO Nederlandse Voedingsmiddelen Tabel 2011 (In Englisch: Dutch Food Composition Table). Available online: http://nevo-online.rivm.nl/ (accessed on 10 May 2016).

21. Willett, W.C.; Howe, G.R.; Kushi, L.H. Adjustment for total energy intake in epidemiologic studies. *Am. J. Clin. Nutr.* **1997**, *65*, 1220S–1228S. [CrossRef] [PubMed]

22. Lavoie Smith, E.M.; Barton, D.L.; Qin, R.; Steen, P.D.; Aaronson, N.K.; Loprinzi, C.L. Assessing patient-reported peripheral neuropathy: The reliability and validity of the European Organization for Research and Treatment of Cancer QLQ-CIPN20 Questionnaire. *Qual. Life Res.* **2013**, *22*, 2787–2799. [CrossRef] [PubMed]

23. Mols, F.; van de Poll-Franse, L.V.; Vreugdenhil, G.; Beijers, A.J.; Kieffer, J.M.; Aaronson, N.K.; Husson, O. Reference data of the European Organisation for Research and Treatment of Cancer (EORTC) QLQ-CIPN20 Questionnaire in the general Dutch population. *Eur. J. Cancer* **2016**, *69*, 28–38. [CrossRef] [PubMed]

24. Roth, P.L. Missing Data in Multiple Item Scales: A Monte Carlo Analysis of Missing Data Techniques. *Organ. Res. Methods* **1999**, *2*, 211–232. [CrossRef]

25. Tamhane, A.R.; Westfall, A.O.; Burkholder, G.A.; Cutter, G.R. Prevalence odds ratio versus prevalence ratio: Choice comes with consequences. *Stat. Med.* **2016**, *35*, 5730–5735. [CrossRef] [PubMed]

26. Bewick, V.; Cheek, L.; Ball, J. Statistics review 8: Qualitative data—Tests of association. *Crit. Care* **2004**, *8*, 46–53. [CrossRef] [PubMed]

27. Institute of Medicine (US). Standing Committee on the Scientific Evaluation of Dietary Reference Intakes. Chapter 6 Magnesium; In *Dietary Reference Intakes for Calcium, Phosphorus, Magnesium, Vitamin D, and Fluoride*; National Academies Press US: Washington, DC, USA, 1997; pp. 71–145. ISBN 978-0-309-06403-3.

28. Institute of Medicine (US). Standing Committee on the Scientific Evaluation of Dietary Reference Intakes. Chapter 4 Calcium; In *Dietary Reference Intakes for Calcium, Phosphorus, Magnesium, Vitamin D, and Fluoride*; National Academies Press US: Washington, DC, USA, 1997; pp. 190–249. ISBN 978-0-309-06403-3.

29. Alberti, P.; Rossi, E.; Cornblath, D.R.; Merkies, I.S.J.; Postma, T.J.; Frigeni, B.; Bruna, J.; Velasco, R.; Argyriou, A.A.; Kalofonos, H.P.; et al. Physician-assessed and patient-reported outcome measures in chemotherapy-induced sensory peripheral neurotoxicity: Two sides of the same coin. *Ann. Oncol.* **2014**, *25*, 257–264. [CrossRef] [PubMed]

30. Le-Rademacher, J.; Kanwar, R.; Seisler, D.; Pachman, D.R.; Qin, R.; Abyzov, A.; Ruddy, K.J.; Banck, M.S.; Lavoie Smith, E.M.; Dorsey, S.G.; et al. Patient-reported (EORTC QLQ-CIPN20) versus physician-reported (CTCAE) quantification of oxaliplatin- and paclitaxel/carboplatin-induced peripheral neuropathy in NCCTG/Alliance clinical trials. *Support. Care Cancer* **2017**, *25*, 3537–3544. [CrossRef] [PubMed]

31. Cavaletti, G.; Cornblath, D.R.; Merkies, I.S.J.; Postma, T.J.; Rossi, E.; Frigeni, B.; Alberti, P.; Bruna, J.; Velasco, R.; Argyriou, A.A.; et al. The chemotherapy-induced peripheral neuropathy outcome measures standardization study: From consensus to the first validity and reliability findings. *Ann. Oncol.* **2013**, *24*, 454–462. [CrossRef] [PubMed]

32. Hoenderop, J.G.J.; Bindels, R.J.M. Epithelial Ca^{2+} and Mg^{2+} Channels in Health and Disease. *J. Am. Soc. Nephrol.* **2004**, *16*, 15–26. [CrossRef] [PubMed]

33. Gamelin, E.; Gamelin, L.; Bossi, L.; Quasthoff, S. Clinical aspects and molecular basis of oxaliplatin neurotoxicity: Current management and development of preventive measures. *Semin. Oncol.* **2002**, *29*, 21–33. [CrossRef] [PubMed]

34. Bara, M.; Guiet-Bara, A.; Durlach, J. Regulation of sodium and potassium pathways by magnesium in cell membranes. *Magnes. Res.* **1993**, *6*, 167–177. [PubMed]

35. Miltenburg, N.C.; Boogerd, W. Chemotherapy-induced neuropathy: A comprehensive survey. *Cancer Treat. Rev.* **2014**, *40*, 872–882. [CrossRef] [PubMed]

36. De Baaij, J.H.F.; Hoenderop, J.G.J.; Bindels, R.J.M. Regulation of magnesium balance: Lessons learned from human genetic disease. *Clin. Kidney J.* **2012**, *5*, i15–i24. [CrossRef] [PubMed]

37. Elin, R.J. Magnesium: The Fifth but Forgotten Electrolyte. *Am. J. Clin. Pathol.* **1994**, *102*, 616–622. [CrossRef] [PubMed]

38. Leurs, J.L.; Schouten, L.J.; Mons, M.N.; Goldbohm, R.A.; van den Brandt, P. Relationship between Tap Water Hardness, Magnesium, and Calcium Concentration and Mortality Due to Ischemic Heart Disease or Stroke in the Netherlands. *Environ. Health Perspect.* **2010**, *118*, 414–420. [CrossRef] [PubMed]

39. Wolf, S.; Barton, D.; Kottschade, L.; Grothey, A.; Loprinzi, C. Chemotherapy-induced peripheral neuropathy: Prevention and treatment strategies. *Eur. J. Cancer* **2008**, *44*, 1507–1515. [CrossRef] [PubMed]

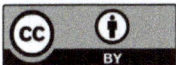

nutrients

MDPI

Article

Changes of Blood Pressure and Hemodynamic Parameters after Oral Magnesium Supplementation in Patients with Essential Hypertension—An Intervention Study

Nikolina Banjanin * and Goran Belojevic

Institute of Hygiene and Medical Ecology, Faculty of Medicine, University of Belgrade, 11000 Belgrade, Serbia; goran.belojevic@med.bg.ac.rs
* Correspondence: nikolina.banjanin@med.bg.ac.rs; Tel.: +381-11-3612-762

Received: 13 April 2018; Accepted: 6 May 2018; Published: 8 May 2018

Abstract: The objective of this study was to examine the changes of blood pressure and hemodynamic parameters after oral magnesium supplementation in patients with essential hypertension. The single-arm non-blinded intervention study comprised 48 patients (19 men; 29 women) whose antihypertensive therapy was not changed for at least one month. The participants were asked to consume (daily at home) 300 mg of oral magnesium-oxide supplementation product for one month and to have their blood pressure and hemodynamic parameters (thoracic fluid content, stroke volume, stroke index, cardiac output, cardiac index, acceleration index, left cardiac work index and systemic vascular resistance index, heart rate) measured in the hospital before and after the intervention. Measurements were performed with impedance cardiography. After magnesium supplementation, systolic and diastolic pressures were significantly decreased (mean ± standard deviation (SD)/mmHg/from 139.7 ± 15.0 to 130.8 ± 13.4 and from 88.0 ± 10.4 to 82.2 ± 9.0, respectively; both $p < 0.001$). The two significant hemodynamic changes were the decrease of systemic vascular resistance index (dyn s m^2/cm^5) and left cardiac work index (kg m/m^2)/mean ± SD from 2319.3 ± 753.3 to 2083.0 ± 526.9 and from 4.8 ± 1.4 to 4.4 ± 0.9, respectively; both $p < 0.05$). The observed hemodynamic changes may explain lowering blood pressure after magnesium supplementation.

Keywords: magnesium; dietary supplements; hypertension; systemic vascular resistance; cardiac output

---

1. Introduction

Magnesium is an important cation for the activity of many enzymes related to energy metabolism, e.g., serine racemase [1], ATP diphosphohydrolase [2] or myosin ATPase [3]. In addition, elevated levels of serum magnesium may lead to smooth muscle relaxation and vasodilatation due to antagonistic action on calcium receptors and channels [4]. On the other hand, the reduction of extracellular magnesium causes vasospasm, particularly important pathogenic factor for sudden death in ischemic heart disease [5] and for glaucoma and diabetic retinopathy [6]. Elevated extracellular magnesium leads to decrease of blood pressure through stimulated production of prostacyclin in endothelial cells and vascular smooth muscle cells [7] and the inhibition of norepinephrine release from nerve endings [8].

An intervention study of a 6-month supplementation with magnesium aspartate hydrochloride among patients on a diuretic therapy for hypertension showed a significant reduction of both systolic and diastolic blood pressure [9]. On the other hand, a double-blind randomized study reported no effect of a three-month magnesium supplementation on blood pressure when compared with placebo treatment [10]. A recent meta-analysis of randomized double-blind placebo controlled trials showed that a daily supplementation with a dose of 300 mg magnesium of at least one month duration significantly reduced blood pressure [11]. The discrepancies in the presented studies may be explained by the differences regarding the study designs, study protocols, ways, form or duration of supplement application, age and race of participants, patients' compliance, the instruments of measurement and the inclusion and exclusion criteria.

Due to conflicting results there is a lack of definitive conclusion and consensus on the effectiveness of magnesium in the treatment of hypertension. Besides blood pressure there is a need for further investigation of the effects of magnesium on other hemodynamic parameters that may explain the Mg-hypertension relationship. The aim of this intervention study was to examine the changes of blood pressure and hemodynamic parameters after oral magnesium supplementation in patients with essential hypertension. We hypothesized that magnesium supplementation would lead to lowering blood pressure and other compatible hemodynamic changes.

2. Materials and Methods

This study was performed in the collaboration between the Institute of Hygiene with Medical Ecology, Faculty of Medicine, and the Multidisciplinary Center for Polyclinic Diagnostics, Assessment and Treatment of Blood Pressure Disorders, Clinic for Cardiology, Clinical Center of Serbia. The study has been registered by The Iranian Registry of Clinical Trials (www.irct.ir; Registration number: IRCT2017081535716N1). All subjects signed their informed consent for inclusion before they participated in the study. The study was conducted in accordance with the declaration of Helsinki, and the protocol was approved by the Ethics Committee of the Clinical Center of Serbia, Belgrade (code 1322/1) and by the Ethics Committee of the Faculty of Medicine, University of Belgrade, Serbia (code 29/VII-16).

The investigation was designed as a single-arm non-blinded intervention study due to an expected limited pool of patients that would fulfill all inclusion and exclusion criteria [12]. The recruitment of patients was performed from September to November 2014 and comprised all patients aged 24–65 years with essential hypertension who came for a regular blood pressure check-up. Among them, only patients whose antihypertensive therapy was not changed for at least one month were eligible for the intervention study. The patients were not allowed to change their blood pressure medication during the trial. The exclusion criteria for participation in the study were: renal diseases, gastrointestinal diseases, diabetes mellitus, diseases of adrenal, thyroid and parathyroid glands, angina pectoris, myocardial infarction, coronary revascularization, congestive heart failure, aortic coarctation, food and drug allergy, pregnancy and lactation, transitory ischemic attack and oral intake of magnesium supplements in the previous month.

The minimum sample size of 43 patients was calculated based on previously reported clinically significant reduction of mean values of systolic and diastolic pressure of 3 mmHg and 2 mmHg, respectively, and effect size of 0.44 after magnesium supplementation [13]. The calculation was performed online using the input values of a power of 80% and a two sided level of significance of 5% [14].

The eligible participants ($n = 68$, 27 men and 41 women) were asked to consume 300 mg of oral magnesium-oxide supplementation product for one month and to have their blood pressure and hemodynamic parameters measured in hospital settings at baseline and at the end of the intervention. The participants were given a dietary supplement ("Magnezijum 300 Direkt", Hermes Arzneimittel GmbH, Wolfratshausen, Germany) which is approved by the Ministry of Health of the Republic of Serbia (Number: 1708/2011). All participants were informed how to use this product, were warned not to exceed the daily recommended dose, and were advised not to change their dietary habits. The participants did not report adverse effects that might be related to magnesium supplementation. They were not informed about the expected changes of blood pressure and hemodynamic parameters after magnesium supplementation.

At baseline, the participants underwent a detailed medical examination and completed a questionnaire that included personal data (age, gender), duration of hypertension (years), hypertension in the family (coded as: 1-any family member diagnosed with hypertension; 0-none), physical activity of at least 30 min most days per week (coded as: 1-Yes; 0-No) and smoking habits (coded as: 0-non-smoker;1-current smoker; 2-ex-smoker). Data on antihypertensive treatment were obtained from patient's medical records. Antihypertensive treatment included: ACE inhibitors (23 patients; 48%); calcium channel blockers (24;50); thiazide diuretics (24;50); beta blockers (35;73) and angiotensin II receptor blockers (10;21). At follow-up after one month, all participants were invited for medical examination. Despite being called several times, 20 participants did not return for check-up (8 men and 12 women), but they did not report adverse effects of magnesium supplementation as the reason. The statistical analysis revealed that the non-responders were significantly younger than the responders (mean age of the non-responders 37.75 ± 12.45 years) with non-significantly shorter duration of hypertension (mean duration of hypertension among the non-responders 5.39 ± 5.19 years). The final sample comprised 48 persons, 19 men and 29 women, aged 47.40 ± 11.30 years, range 24 to 65 years. This sample size was considered sufficient according to afore mentioned calculation.

Average daily magnesium intake from food and drinks was obtained using a 24-h recall questionnaire. The participants were very carefully asked about food and drinks they consumed during 24 h prior to the interview. The questions referred to food types and amounts, time and place of consumption, how the food was prepared (fried, fresh, baked or cooked) and what was used to prepare the food (salt, oil, sugar etc.). A trained physician conducted the interview with the participants. Magnesium intake from food and drinks was calculated from all foodstuffs consumed the previous day using Serbian food tables [15]. Serum magnesium concentration was measured both at baseline and follow up using the photometric method [16]. Blood samples were taken at the central laboratory of the Clinical Center of Serbia between 8 and 9 a.m., after a morning fast. The laboratory is an accredited institution with a strict quality control standards for all laboratory analyses.

Participants had their weight and height measured by a trained physician. Body height was measured to the nearest 0.5 cm. Body weight was measured on a digital scale (TANITA Inner Scan Body Composition Monitor BC-543) to the nearest 0.1 kg. Participants were in light clothes and barefoot. Body mass index (BMI) was calculated as body weight (in kilograms) divided by squared body height (in meters).

Both at baseline and at follow-up participants had their systolic, diastolic and mean arterial blood pressure measured with impedance cardiography (ICG) by CardioScreen® 2000 (Medis. Medizinische Messtechnik GmbH, Ilmenau, Germany). A cuff was placed on patient's left upper arm.

We also used ICG for measurements of hemodynamic parameters at baseline and follow-up. ICG electrodes measure the change in thorax impedance during the flow of the alternating current through the thorax. The following parameters were measured: thoracic fluid content (the electrical conductivity of the chest, L/kOhm), acceleration index (the acceleration of blood in the ascending aorta and the aortic arch, $L/100/s^2$) and heart rate (beats per minute). The following parameters were calculated: stroke volume (the amount of blood pumped by the left ventricle each beat, mL) and cardiac output (stroke volume multiplied by heart rate, L/min). With reference to body surface area the following parameters were calculated: stroke index (stroke volume related to the body surface, mL/m^2), cardiac index (cardiac output related to the body surface, $L/(min\ m^2)$, systemic vascular resistance index (the resistance to the blood flow through the arterial system the heart works against, $dyn\ s\ m^2/cm^5$) and left cardiac work index (an expression for the work of the left ventricle, $kg\ m/m^2$). DuBois formula was used to calculate the body surface area [17].

Descriptive statistic was presented as mean values and standard deviation for numeric variables, or as percent's (relative numbers) for categorical variables. All investigated parameters were tested by Kolmogorov-Smirnov test and almost all observed distributions corresponded to the normal distribution. The differences between men and women were tested with Student's t-test for parametric variables and with Mann-Whitney *U*-test and Chi-square test for non-parametric data. The differences between baseline and follow-up were tested with paired-samples *t*-test. Probability level of less than 0.05 was accepted as significant. Statistical analyses were performed using SPSS 15.0 for Windows software (SPSS Inc., Chicago, IL, USA, 1989–2006).

3. Results

Men and women were of similar age, and had similar body mass index, blood pressure levels, and shared smoking habits, engagement in physical activity and magnesium intake from food and water and serum magnesium concentrations. Men and women had similar duration of hypertension, and had similar family history of hypertension. These results support further analysis regardless of gender (Table 1).

Table 1. Baseline characteristics of the investigated population by gender.

Parameters	Men	Women	Total	*p* Value
Gender (%)	19 (39.6)	29 (60.4)	48 (100.0)	NS (*p* > 0.05) *
Age (years)	43.79 ± 11.11	49.76 ± 10.98	47.40 ± 11.30	NS **
Body mass index (kg/m^2)	27.03 ± 2.48	25.94 ± 5.36	26.38 ± 4.42	NS **
Duration of hypertension (years)	9.50 ± 9.75	7.75 ± 6.99	8.44 ± 8.14	NS ***
Hypertension in the family (%)	15 (83.3)	25 (92.6)	40 (88.9)	NS *
Current smoker (%)	7 (36.8)	9 (31.0)	16 (33.3)	NS *
Regular physical activity (%)	10 (52.6)	18 (64.3)	28 (59.6)	NS *
Systolic pressure (mmHg)	140.74 ± 11.14	139.09 ± 17.26	139.74 ± 15.03	NS **
Diastolic pressure (mmHg)	87.37 ± 11.43	88.50 ± 9.83	88.05 ± 10.39	NS **
Mg intake from food (mg/day)	196.30 ± 114.74	158.73 ± 50.19	173.60 ± 82.99	NS ***
Mg intake from water (mg/day)	12.69 ± 6.44	15.55 ± 8.13	14.42 ± 7.56	NS ***
Total Mg intake (mg/day)	208.89 ± 115.66	174.28 ± 51.72	187.98 ± 83.72	NS ***
Serum magnesium concentration (mmol/L)	0.86 ± 0.05	0.85 ± 0.06	0.85 ± 0.05	NS **

* Chi-square test; ** Student's *t*-test; *** Mann–Whitney *U*-test. NS (not significant)

There was no significant difference between serum magnesium concentrations at baseline and at follow-up (mean ± SD = 0.858 ± 0.054 and 0.847 ± 0.070 mmol/L, respectively; *p* = 0.432). The range of serum magnesium concentrations at baseline and at follow-up was 0.74–0.94 and 0.69–0.96 mmol/L, respectively.

Magnesium supplementation lead to significant decrease in systolic, diastolic and mean arterial blood pressure. Mean systolic pressure was decreased by 8.97 ± 2.01 mmHg; mean diastolic pressure was decreased by 5.87 ± 1.49 mmHg; mean arterial pressure was decreased by 8.06 ± 1.67mmHg (Table 2).

Table 2. Changes of blood pressure after magnesium supplementation in patients with essential hypertension (*N* = 48).

Parameters	At Baseline	At Follow-Up	95% Confidence Interval of the Difference	*p* Value *
Systolic pressure (mmHg)	139.74 ± 15.03	130.77 ± 13.42	4.92–13.02	<0.001
Diastolic pressure (mmHg)	88.05 ± 10.39	82.19 ± 9.00	2.88–8.86	<0.001
Mean pressure (mmHg)	102.13 ± 12.07	94.07 ± 10.11	4.70–11.42	<0.001

* Paired-samples *t*-test.

After one month of supplementation, thoracic fluid content, stroke index, cardiac index acceleration index and heart rate remained stable. On the other hand, systemic vascular resistance index and left cardiac work index were significantly decreased following a month of magnesium supplementation (Table 3). Mean change of left cardiac work index equaled 0.439 ± 0.19 kg m/m^2, whereas mean change of systemic vascular resistance index was 236.29 ± 93.49 dyn s m^2/cm^5.

Table 3. Changes of hemodynamic parameters after magnesium supplementation in patients with essential hypertension (*N* = 48).

Parameters	At Baseline	At Follow-Up	95% Confidence Interval of the Difference	*p* Value *
Thoracic fluid content (L/kOhm)	38.75 ± 8.95	36.57 ± 6.09	−0.67–5.04	0.131
Stroke volume (mL)	101.74 ± 27.90	99.26 ± 24.13	−10.18–15.13	0.686
Stroke index (mL/m^2)	48.77 ± 11.31	48.44 ± 11.09	−5.62–6.28	0.905
Cardiac output (L/min)	6.93 ± 1.42	6.76 ± 1.29	−0.58–0.93	0.636
Cardiac index (L/(min m^2))	3.61 ± 0.95	3.56 ± 0.64	−0.21–0.30	0.727
Acceleration index (L/100/s^2)	105.96 ± 39.64	104.88 ± 40.27	−8.98–11.13	0.831
Left cardiac work index (kg m/m^2)	4.83 ± 1.42	4.39 ± 0.91	0.05–0.82	0.026
Systemic vascular resistance index (dyn s m^2/cm^5)	2319.30 ± 753.31	2083.01 ± 526.95	47.87–424.71	0.015
Heart rate (beat/min)	71.56 ± 11.82	69.55 ± 9.06	−0.83–4.85	0.162

* Paired-samples *t*-test.

4. Discussion

We show a reduction of blood pressure after a one-month magnesium supplementation in hypertensive patients. This effect is compatible with a reduction in two hemodynamic parameters: systemic vascular resistance and left cardiac work.

Our results are in accordance with a meta-analysis of 22 trials which showed that the intake of magnesium supplements exceeding 370 mg daily has a bigger effectiveness in the reduction of systolic and diastolic blood pressures in hypertensive patients than the dose lower than 370 mg daily. The study found that the average reduction of systolic blood pressure was 3–4 mmHg and diastolic 2–3 mmHg after the consumption of magnesium supplements lasting from 3 to 24 weeks (average duration 11.3 weeks) [13]. Another review reported that oral magnesium supplements at a dosage from 10 to 15 mmol per day may reduce blood pressure in hypertensive patients on antihypertensive therapy [18].Additionally, our study points out the changes in hemodynamic parameters after magnesium supplementation that are compatible with lowering blood pressure. But, the results of the studies on the association between magnesium intake and blood pressure are not fully congruent. For example, a double-blind randomized study was conducted in patients with essential hypertension. When treatment with 40 mmol (972 mg) magnesium aspartate supplementation daily was compared with placebo treatment for three months no effect of magnesium supplementation on blood pressure was found [10]. However, this study had a small sample size of 13 patients. Another experimental study conducted in the US showed that magnesium supplementation for 16 weeks in dose of 14 mmol (336 mg) of magnesium had no blood pressure-lowering effect in normotensive women who reported low habitual intake of this mineral in comparison with placebo group [19].

An important magnesium function, the vasodilatation of peripheral arteries [20], may explain the lowering of systemic vascular resistance in our study. Magnesium may achieve its vasodilatatory effect through its impact on: intracellular calcium concentration [21], production of prostacyclin [7], and sensitivity to angiotensin II [22].

Serum magnesium concentration was not significantly changed after magnesium supplementation in our study. This finding is congruent with other intervention studies of a similar duration [23,24]. A significant raise of serum magnesium concentration after a seven-week magnesium supplementation may be expected only in participants with hypomagnesemia (concentrations lower than 0.70 mmol/L) [23] but in our sample the lowest serum magnesium concentration at baseline was 0.74 mmol/L. But, in longer intervention studies of a median duration of 12 weeks a significant elevation of serum magnesium concentrations after magnesium supplementation may be expected even in patients with baseline median serum magnesium concentrations of 0.785 mmol/L [25].

There are several limitations of this study. First, a single-arm non-blinded design was chosen because of a limited pool of patients. We consider that a placebo effect was alleviated by the fact that although the patients knew they were given magnesium supplementation they were not informed about the expected changes in blood pressure and hemodynamic parameters. Second, we did not control the possible effect of thiazide diuretics on magnesium excretion in some patients. Third, we did not check for magnesium concentration in a 24 h urine sample at baseline and at follow-up. Fourth, the intervention period of our study was limited to thirty days. In further investigations it would be useful to examine the effects of different duration (shorter and longer than in our study) of magnesium supplementation on blood pressure and hemodynamic parameters. Fifth, the study was conducted in persons with essential hypertension; the hemodynamic changes in persons with diabetes or kidney diseases would be of great importance for understanding the mechanisms of action of magnesium supplementation. The strength of this study is the use of ICG, which objectively measures both blood pressure and hemodynamic parameters that may explain blood pressure changes after magnesium supplementation.

5. Conclusions

In conclusion, oral magnesium supplementation probably had a positive effect on blood pressure reduction in patients with essential hypertension. The decrease in systemic vascular resistance and left cardiac work may explain the reduction of blood pressure after magnesium supplementation.

Author Contributions: N.B. designed the study, collected data, and wrote the first draft; N.B. and G.B. performed statistical analysis, wrote the manuscript, revised and approved the final version of manuscript and prepared the paper for submission.

Conflicts of Interest: The authors declare no conflict of interest.

References

1. Bruno, S.; Margiotta, M.; Marchesani, F.; Paredi, G.; Orlandi, V.; Faggiano, S.; Ronda, L.; Campanini, B.; Mozzarelli, A. Magnesium and calcium ions differentially affect human serine racemase activity and modulate its quaternary equilibrium toward a tetrameric form. *Biochim. Biophys. Acta* **2017**, *1865*, 381–387. [CrossRef] [PubMed]
2. Sinha, P.; Paswan, R.K.; Kumari, A.; Kumar, S.; Bimal, S.; Das, P.; Lal, C.S. Magnesium-Dependent Ecto-ATP Diphosphohydrolase Activity in *Leishmania donovani. Curr. Microbiol.* **2016**, *73*, 811–819. [CrossRef] [PubMed]
3. Ge, J.; Huang, F.; Nesmelov, Y.E. Metal cation controls phosphate release in the myosin ATPase. *Protein Sci.* **2017**, *26*, 2181–2186. [CrossRef] [PubMed]
4. Odom, M.J.; Zuckerman, S.L.; Mocco, J. The role of magnesium in the management of cerebral vasospasm. *Neurol. Res. Int.* **2013**, *2013*, 943914. [CrossRef] [PubMed]
5. Turlapaty, P.D.; Altura, B.M. Magnesium deficiency produces spasms of coronary arteries: Relationship to etiology of sudden death ischemic heart disease. *Science* **1980**, *208*, 198–200. [CrossRef] [PubMed]
6. Agarwal, R.; Iezhitsa, L.; Agarwal, P. Pathogenetic role of magnesium deficiency inophthalmic diseases. *Biometals* **2014**, *27*, 5–18. [CrossRef] [PubMed]
7. Satake, K.; Lee, J.D.; Shimizu, H.; Uzui, H.; Mitsuke, Y.; Yue, H.; Ueda, T. Effects of magnesium on prostacyclin synthesis and intracellular free calcium concentration in vascular cells. *Magnes. Res.* **2004**, *17*, 20–27. [PubMed]
8. Shimosawa, T.; Takano, K.; Ando, K.; Fujita, T. Magnesium inhibits norepinephrine release by blocking N-type calcium channels at peripheral sympathetic nerve endings. *Hypertension* **2004**, *44*, 897–902. [CrossRef] [PubMed]
9. Dyckner, T.; Wester, P.O.; Widman, L. Effects of peroral magnesium on plasma and skeletal muscle electrolytes in patients on long-term diuretic therapy. *Int. J. Cardiol.* **1988**, *19*, 81–87. [CrossRef]
10. Zemel, P.C.; Zemel, M.B.; Urberg, M.; Douglas, F.L.; Geiser, R.; Sowers, J.R. Metabolic and hemodynamic effects of magnesium supplementation in patients with essential hypertension. *Am. J. Clin. Nutr.* **1990**, *51*, 665–669. [CrossRef] [PubMed]
11. Zhang, X.; Li, Y.; Del Gobbo, L.C.; Rosanoff, A.; Wang, J.; Zhang, W.; Song, Y. Effects of Magnesium Supplementation on Blood Pressure: A Meta-Analysis of Randomized Double-Blind Placebo-Controlled Trials. *Hypertension* **2016**, *68*, 324–333. [CrossRef] [PubMed]
12. Evans, S.R. Clinical trial structures. *J. Exp. Stroke Transl. Med.* **2010**, *3*, 8–18. [CrossRef] [PubMed]

13. Kass, L.; Weekes, J.; Carpenter, L. Effect of magnesium supplementation on blood pressure: a meta-analysis. *Eur. J. Clin. Nutr.* **2012**, *66*, 411–418. [CrossRef] [PubMed]

14. Dhand, N.K.; Khatkar, M.S. Statulator: An Online Statistical Calculator. Sample Size Calculator for Comparing Two Paired Means 2014. Available online: http://statulator.com/SampleSize/ss2PM.html (accessed on 10 April 2018).

15. Jokić, N. *Calories in Daily Life 5000 Groceries-Dishes and Natural Mineral Waters*, 1st ed.; Institute for Textbooks: Belgrade, Serbia, 2007; ISBN 978-86-17-14449-2. (In Serbian)

16. Wong, H.K.C. Fully automated procedure for serum magnesium. *Clin. Chem.* **1975**, *21*, 169. [PubMed]

17. DuBois, D.; DuBois, E.F. A formula to estimate the approximate surface area if height and weight be known. *Arch. Intern. Med.* **1916**, *17*, 863–871. [CrossRef]

18. Rosanoff, A. Importance of magnesium dose in the treatment of hypertension. In *Advances in Magnesium Research: New Data*; Porr, P.J., Nechifor, M., Durlach, J., Eds.; Èditions John Libbey Eurotext: Montrouge, France, 2006; pp. 97–103. ISBN 2-7420-0606-0.

19. Sacks, F.M.; Willett, W.C.; Smith, A.; Brown, L.E.; Rosner, B.; Moore, T.J. Effect on blood pressure of potassium, calcium, and magnesium in women with low habitual intake. *Hypertension* **1998**, *31*, 131–138. [CrossRef] [PubMed]

20. Gröber, U.; Schmidt, J.; Kisters, K. Magnesium in Prevention and Therapy. *Nutrients* **2015**, *7*, 8199–8226. [CrossRef] [PubMed]

21. D'Angelo, E.K.; Singer, H.A.; Rembold, C.M. Magnesium relaxes arterial smooth muscle by decreasing intracellular Ca^{2+} without changing intracellular Mg^{2+}. *J. Clin. Investig.* **1992**, *89*, 1988–1994. [CrossRef] [PubMed]

22. Altura, B.M.; Turlapaty, P.D. Withdrawal of magnesium enhances coronary arterial spasms produced by vasoactive agents. *Br. J. Pharmacol.* **1982**, *77*, 649–659. [CrossRef] [PubMed]

23. Nielsen, F.H.; Johnson, L.K.; Zeng, H. Magnesium supplementation improves indicators of low magnesium status and inflammatory stress in adults older than 51 years with poor quality sleep. *Magnes. Res.* **2010**, *23*, 158–168. [CrossRef] [PubMed]

24. Asemi, Z.; Karamali, M.; Jamilian, M.; Foroozanfard, F.; Bahmani, F.; Heidarzadeh, Z.; Benisi-Kohansal, S.; Surkan, P.J.; Esmaillzadeh, A. Magnesium supplementation affects metabolic status and pregnancy outcomes in gestational diabetes: A randomized, double-blind, placebo-controlled trial. *Am. J. Clin. Nutr.* **2015**, *102*, 222–229. [CrossRef] [PubMed]

25. Costello, R.B.; Elin, R.J.; Rosanoff, A.; Wallace, T.C.; Guerrero-Romero, F.; Hruby, A.; Lutsey, P.L.; Nielsen, F.H.; Rodriguez-Moran, M.; Song, Y.; et al. Perspective: The Case for an Evidence-Based Reference Interval for Serum Magnesium: The Time Has Come. *Adv. Nutr.* **2016**, *7*, 977–993. [CrossRef] [PubMed]

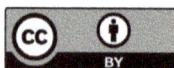

nutrients

MDPI

Article

Longitudinal Study of the Role of Epidermal Growth Factor on the Fractional Excretion of Magnesium in Children: Effect of Calcineurin Inhibitors

Kristien J. Ledeganck [1,*], Charlotte Anné [1], Amandine De Monie [1], Sarang Meybosch [1], Gert A. Verpooten [1], Marleen Vinckx [1], Koen Van Hoeck [1,2], Annelies Van Eyck [1], Benedicte Y. De Winter [1] and Dominique Trouet [1,2]

[1] Laboratory of Experimental Medicine and Pediatrics, University of Antwerp, Universiteitsplein 1, T3.34, 2610 Antwerp, Belgium; charlotte.anne@student.uantwerpen.be (C.A.); amandine.demonie@student.uantwerpen.be (A.D.M.); sarang.meybosch@student.uantwerpen.be (S.M.); gert.verpooten@uantwerpen.be (G.A.V.); marleen.vinckx@uantwerpen.be (M.V.); Koen.vanhoeck@uza.be (K.V.H.); annelies.vaneyck@uantwerpen.be (A.V.E.); benedicte.dewinter@uantwerpen.be (B.Y.D.W); Dominique.trouet@uza.be (D.T.)
[2] Department of Pediatric Nephrology, Antwerp University Hospital, Wilrijkstraat 10, 2650 Edegem, Belgium
*   Correspondence: kristien.ledeganck@uantwerp.be; Tel.:+32(0)32652573

Received: 30 April 2018; Accepted: 21 May 2018; Published: 27 May 2018

Abstract: Background: It was shown in animal models and adults that the epidermal growth factor (EGF) is involved in the pathophysiology of calcineurin inhibitor (CNI) induced renal magnesium loss. In children, however, the exact mechanism remains unclear, which was set as the purpose of the present study. Methods: Children with nephrotic syndrome and renal transplant children treated with CNI (n = 50) and non-CNI treated children (n = 46) were included in this study. Urine and serum samples were collected at three time points to determine magnesium, creatinine, and EGF. The magnesium intake was calculated from a food frequency questionnaire. Results: Serum Mg^{2+} and urinary EGF/creatinine were significantly lower in the CNI treated children, with significantly more CNI-treated children developing hypomagnesaemia. In the latter patients, the fractional excretion of magnesium (FE Mg^{2+}) was significantly higher. Urinary EGF, age, renal function, and serum magnesium were independent predictors of the FE Mg^{2+}. Only 29% of the children reached the recommended daily intake of magnesium. The magnesium intake did not differ between hypomagnesemic and normomagnesemic patients and was not a predictor of the FE Mg^{2+}. Conclusions: In CNI-treated children who developed hypomagnesemia, the FE Mg^{2+} was increased. The urinary EGF concentration, age, and renal function are independent predictors of the FE Mg^{2+}.

Keywords: epidermal growth factor; magnesium; children; magnesium intake; fractional excretion; calcineurin inhibitor; kidney transplantation; nephrotic syndrome

---

1. Introduction

Magnesium (Mg^{2+}) is an intracellular cation with roles in multiple physiologic processes, such as parathyroid metabolism, cardiovascular tone, nerve conduction, and the proper function of adenosine triphosphate complexes [1]. Furthermore, it also plays an important role in bone metabolism [2]. In the growing child, it is, therefore, essential to maintain a positive Mg^{2+} balance so that the amount of Mg^{2+} needed for growth and metabolic needs is ensured [2]. This balance requires interaction between the gut, the kidney, and the bone. Mg^{2+} is absorbed from the food in the gut and stored in the bone, while Mg^{2+} excess is excreted by the kidneys in the feces [3].

The recommended Mg^{2+} intake in children depends on their age, with increasing needs during adolescence to meet pubertal growth needs. The recommended intake approximates 130–150 mg/day for ages 4–8 year [2], 240 mg/day for ages 9–13 year, and 340 mg/day for boys and 300 mg/day for girls aged 14–18 year [4]. Magnesium deficiency is rare in healthy subjects as Mg^{2+} is widely present in food sources, such as dairy, nuts, whole cereal grains, green vegetables, dark chocolate, and legumes [5–7]. However, in a Cypriot population, none of the children aged 6–19 year met the recommended Mg^{2+} intake, with the highest prevalence of insufficiency in the adolescents [8]. Additionally, in chronic kidney disease (CKD) patients, magnesium intake has been shown to be below the recommended level [9]. The main nutrition-related goals for CKD patients involve slowing of the kidney failure progression rate, maintaining good nutritional status, and minimizing CKD complications, such as metabolic disorders and proteinuria. The nutrition requirements differ among patients with various stages of kidney function and proper nutrition is, therefore, difficult to fulfil in CKD patients [10]. Hypomagnesemia is defined as a serum Mg^{2+} concentration below 0.7 mmoL/L [11]. Most cases of hypomagnesemia in clinical practice, however, are asymptomatic. The clinical manifestation may depend more on the total body Mg^{2+} deficit rather than on the actual serum Mg^{2+} levels. Personality changes, muscle weakness, tremor, and dysphagia may occur at concentrations of <1.45 mg/dL, while confusion and a decreased consciousness develop at concentrations of $\leq$1.00 mg/dL [12]. Hypomagnesemia has been reported in children with malignancy and in those being treated for malnutrition [1]. In hospitalized children at the pediatric intensive care unit, a 20% to 60% incidence of hypomagnesemia has been reported [1].

Calcineurin inhibitors (CNIs), especially cyclosporine-A (CsA) and tacrolimus (TAC), are widely used immunosuppressive agents. Since the 1970s, CNIs are commonly administered to kidney transplant recipients or after other solid organ transplantation to reduce the rejection rate and improve early graft survival, although long-term nephrotoxicity is a serious side effect [13]. CNIs are also used for the treatment of steroid-resistant or steroid-dependent idiopathic nephrotic syndrome [13].

Besides nephrotoxicity, CNIs also induce functional alterations and ion homeostasis disturbances, such as hypomagnesemia and renal magnesium wasting, hyponatremia, hyperkalemia, hyperchloremic metabolic acidosis, and hyperuricemia [14,15]. Two ion channels play an important role in the Mg^{2+} homeostasis, TRPM6 and TRPM7. TRPM6 has an expression pattern predominantly present in absorbing epithelia. In the kidney, TRPM6 is expressed in the distal convoluted tubule, known as the main site of active transcellular Mg^{2+} reabsorption along the nephron. TRPM7 is ubiquitously expressed and implicated in cellular Mg^{2+} homeostasis, cell death, and cell cycle regulation [16,17]. A decade ago, it was demonstrated that epidermal growth factor (EGF) plays a crucial role in the stimulation of the renal Mg^{2+} channel TRPM6 [18,19]. Our research group demonstrated in a rat model that a combined decrease in the expression of renal EGF and the Mg^{2+} channel TRPM6 is responsible for CsA-induced renal Mg^{2+} loss [20]. In a translational clinical setting in adults, an increased FE Mg^{2+} was observed in CsA-treated patients who developed hypomagnesemia associated with decreased urinary renal EGF levels [21].

Besides its role in magnesium homeostasis, EGF is involved in many biological responses, including cell proliferation, differentiation, and migration, as well as pathophysiological events, such as tissue repair including ulcer and wound healing, or tissue repair, after ischemia/reperfusion injury [22,23]. EGF is also involved in inflammation, showing protective effects in animal models of pancreatitis [24]. Moreover, the correlation between EGF and other growth factors, such as transforming growth factor β (TGF-β) and platelet derived growth factor, needs to be considered [25,26].

In the present study, we aimed to investigate if children who were treated with CNIs developed hypomagnesemia and/or renal Mg^{2+} loss, and if the urinary EGF expression level is related to the fractional excretion of Mg^{2+} (FE Mg^{2+}). Furthermore, we investigated whether Mg^{2+} intake was related to the serum Mg^{2+} level and the FE Mg^{2+} in patients treated with CNIs.

2. Materials and Methods

2.1. Study Design

We performed a longitudinal observational clinical trial. Patients were included between March 2016 and February 2018 at the Antwerp University Hospital. Ninety-six patients were recruited in this study and divided into 2 subgroups. Group 1: Patients treated with CNI ($n = 50$); subdivided into renal transplant patients treated with CNI ($n = 23$; group 1A) and patients with nephrotic syndrome treated with CNI ($n = 27$; group 1B). Group 2: Non-CNI treated patients ($n = 46$); subdivided into patients with CKD as a control group for group 1A ($n = 24$; group 2A) and patients with nephrotic syndrome not treated with CNI as a control group for group 1B ($n = 22$; group 2B). Exclusion criteria were an estimated glomerular filtration rate (eGFR) < 20 mL/min/1.73 m^2, use of cisplatin, diuretics or aminoglycosides, diabetes mellitus, and an active urinary tract infection.

At 3 time points, with an interval of at least 1 month, blood and urine samples were collected from each patient to determine creatinine, magnesium, and EGF (urine). In the nephrotic syndrome patients, samples were collected during a period of remission. At one time point during the study, a Food Frequency Questionnaire was performed to obtain the frequency and portion size information.

A healthy control group ($n = 103$ healthy children) was included to determine serum and urine EGF reference values in children. From these patients, age, gender, weight, and length were obtained. From 42 patients, at 1 time point, both urine and serum were sampled, from 31 patients, only urine was sampled, and from 30 patients, only serum was sampled.

The study was conducted in accordance with the *Declaration of Helsinki* and the principles of Good Clinical Practice. The study protocol was approved by the Ethics Committee of the Antwerp University Hospital (file number 9/44/231). All patients and their parents and/or legal guardians gave a written informed consent.

2.2. Magnesium Intake Questionnaire and Nubel®

A Food Frequency Questionnaire was performed to obtain standardized information on food intake, with special attention to the frequency and portion size information. This information was then entered into the dietary software program Nubel® food planner (Nubel v.z.w. Eurostation, Brussels, Belgium) to analyse the daily Mg^{2+} intake. Nubel® is a Belgian non-profit organization responsible for the management of the nutritional and scientific information of food products in Belgium [27]. In patients treated with magnesium supplements, the amount of magnesium substitution was added to the daily magnesium intake from the food to calculate the total magnesium intake. The magnesium intake was then calculated as a percentage of the reference daily intake (RDI; Nubel) and thus corrected for age.

2.3. Determination of Creatinine, Magnesium, and CsA Levels

Serum and urine creatinine and magnesium, and whole blood CsA levels were analyzed with the Dimension Vista system (Siemens Healthcare Diagnostics, Deerfield, MA, USA) using an ECREA, Mg, or CsA flex® reagent cartridge, respectively. FE Mg^{2+} was calculated using the following equation: $FE_{Mg} = 100 \times (U_{Mg} \times S_{Cr})/[(0.8 \times S_{Mg}) \times U_{Cr}]$, with U_{Mg} urinary excretion of Mg^{2+} (mg/dL), S_{Cr} serum creatinine (mg/dL), S_{Mg} serum Mg^{2+} (mg/dL), and U_{Cr} urinary excretion of creatinine (mg/dL). The serum Mg^{2+} concentration was multiplied by 0.8, since, in children, only 80% of the serum Mg^{2+} is freely filtered by the glomerulus, with the remaining part being protein-bound [28].

Creatinine clearance was calculated using the Bedside Swartz equation, which is the recommended equation to estimate the GFR in children [29].

Since it is known that estradiol might influence renal magnesium reabsorption [30], serum estradiol levels were measured in female children using the Elecsys Estradiol III Assay (Cobas®, Roche Diagnostics GmbH, Mannheim, Germany). TAC levels were measured with the Elecsys Tacrolimus Assay.

2.4. Determination of Urinary EGF

Urinary EGF was measured using an EGF human Elisa kit® (Invitrogen, Waltham, MA, USA), according to the manufacturer's guidelines. The detection limit of this assay was 3.9 pg/mL. A preliminary experiment ($n = 10$) was performed to test the intra- and inter-variability of the EGF human Elisa kit®, showing a mean intra-assay coefficient of variance of 9.82% and an inter-assay coefficient of variation of 9.81%.

2.5. Statistical Analysis

All data were analysed using SPSS (version 24.0). Statistical significance was predetermined as p-value < 0.05. Normality of cross-sectional data (such as magnesium intake) was tested by applying the Kolmogorov-Smirnov test. Parametric data are expressed as mean $\pm$ standard deviation (SD) and non-parametric data are expressed as median (minimum-maximum). The correlation of magnesium intake with other variables was tested with a Pearson or Spearman correlation test for parametric or skewed data, respectively. Generalized Estimating Equations (GEE) were used to analyse the data collected per visit since the groups had unequal sample sizes. Moreover, the number of visits per patient varied from 1 to 3. GEEs were used to calculate the estimated means of variables and to compare them between groups. Models were constructed to study the time-dependency of the variables and to determine the relationship between outcome variables, such as FE Mg^{2+} and urinary EGF excretion, and a number of other predictors.

3. Results

3.1. Population Demographics

Group Descriptions

From 89% of the patients, three consecutive samples were collected, while from 9% of the patients only two samples were collected, and from 2% of the patients only one sample was collected. In the entire study population, the median age was 12.0 year (2.3–20.3 year). Seventy-one percent of the patients were male, the mean weight was 43.0 $\pm$ 18.0 kg, the median length was 147.5 cm (88–190 cm), and the median BMI z-score was 0.16 (−2.24–2.82).

The demographic data per group are displayed in Table 1.

Table 1. Demographic data of the study groups.

Group	Renal Tx + CNI (n = 23)	CKD − CNI (n = 24)	NS + CNI (n = 27)	NS − CNI (n = 22)
Age (year)	13.4 (2.2–20.3)	11.1 (3.2–18.9)	12.5 (3.1–19.5)	12.3 (3.7–18.7)
Gender (M/F; %)	87/13	62/38	71/29	64/36
Length (cm)	151 (88–183)	145 (95–176)	149 (92–190)	149 (101–183)
Weight (kg)	43 $\pm$ 17	42 $\pm$ 16	46 $\pm$ 23	42 $\pm$ 15
BMI z-score	0.40 (−2.10–1.13)	0.24 (−2.24–2.05)	0.17 (−1.57–2.12)	−0.09 (−1.86–2.82)
Mg^{2+} intake (% of RDI)	89 (37–684)	86 (63–436)	87 (45–299)	86 (41–383)
Patients who exceeded the RDI for Mg^{2+} intake (%)	27.3	30.4	30.8	42.1
Mg^{2+} supplements (%)	13.0	8.0	13.8	25.0

Normally distributed variables are presented as mean $\pm$ SD; skewed data are presented as median (minimum-maximum). None of the presented variables significantly differed between the groups. Tx: Transplantation; CNI: Calcineurin inhibitor, CKD: Chronic kidney disease, NS: Nephrotic syndrome, RDI: Reference daily intake (corrected for age).

3.2. Kidney Function, Magnesium, EGF, and CNI Levels

In the entire study population, the median serum creatinine was 0.77 mg/dL (0.27–2.97 mg/dL), the creatinine clearance was 80 mL/min/1.73 m^2 (19–180 mL/min/1.73 m^2), serum Mg^{2+} was 0.80 mg/dL (0.42–1.22 mg/dL), and the FE Mg^{2+} was 4.70% (0.16–21.47%). From all the patients, 29.3% developed hypomagnesemia at least at 1 time point during the study. The mean urinary EGF was 10.51 ng/mL (1.14–182.70 ng/mL) and the mean serum EGF was 811.73 pg/mL (33.07–2014.33 pg/mL). A detailed overview per group is shown in Table 2.

In the female patients (n = 28), the median estrogen level was 34.86 pg/mL (2.5–268.3 pg/mL) and did not differ between groups. From these patients, 29.6% had serum estrogen levels below the detection limit.

Table 2. Urine and serum analyses; data are presented in 4 groups.

Group	Renal Tx + CNI (n = 23)	CKD – CNI (n = 24)	NS + CNI (n = 28)	NS – CNI (n = 22)
Serum Creatinine (mg/dL)	1.11 (0.08) §#	1.27 (0.14) #§	0.72 (0.07) #$*	0.54 (0.03) $*§
Creatinine clearance (mL/min/1.73 m^2)	59 (3) §#	62 (6) #§	98 (5) #$*	117 (4) $*§
Urinary protein/creatinine (mg/g)	347.4 (71.8) $	613.2 (115.0) *	848.0 (333.9)	544.9 (215.8)
Serum Mg^{2+} (mg/dL)	0.76 (0.02) #$	0.82 (0.02) *§	0.78 (0.02) #$	0.84 (0.01) *§
HypoMg (%)	39.1 $#	16.0 *§	44.8 $#	10.0 *§
FE Mg^{2+} (%)	7.82 (0.84) §#	7.76 (0.84)	3.95 (0.32) *$	3.57 (0.28) *$
CsA levels (ng/mL)	666 (45)	-	579 (38)	-
Tacrolimus levels (ng/mL)	8.62 (0.91)	-	7.71 (0.79)	-
Serum EGF (pg/mL)	776.6 (39.9)	742.1 (47.8) §	865.5 (40.7) $	817.2 (55.0)
Urine EGF (ng/mL)	7.0 (1.1) #§	11.5 (2.4) #§	35.4 (6.0) $*§	47.7 (6.6) *$
Urine EGF/creatinine (ng/mg)	0.11 (0.01) $#§	0.19 (0.03) #*§	0.33 (0.05) #$*	0.51 (0.07) $*§

The renal Tx patients treated with CNI, the CKD patients, the nephrotic syndrome patients treated with CNI, and the nephrotic syndrome patients not treated with CNI. Data were analysed with GEE and, therefore, presented as mean (SE). Tx: Transplantation, CNI: Calcineurin inhibitor, CKD: Chronic kidney disease, NS: Nephrotic syndrome, CsA: Cyclosporine, EGF: Epidermal growth factor, FE: Fractional excretion. # p < 0.05 vs NS-CNI; $ p < 0.05 vs CKD-CNI; * p < 0.05 vs Renal Tx + CNI; § p < 0.05 vs NS+CNI.

Patients with Hypomagnesemia versus Patients with Normomagnesemia (presented in Table 3)

Twenty-nine percent of the patients developed hypomagnesemia. Patients who developed hypomagnesemia showed a higher FE Mg^{2+} when treated with CNI. The FE Mg^{2+} was 10.4% (1.8%) in the renal Tx group and 5.9% (1.7%) in the CKD group (p = 0.073), and 4.9% (0.6%) in the nephrotic syndrome group treated with CNI compared to 3.5% (<0.1%) in the nephrotic syndrome group not treated with CNI (p = 0.023). There was no difference in magnesium intake between hypomagnesemic patients treated with CNI and both control groups (p = 0.243).

Table 3. Comparison of clinical and laboratory data between patients who developed hypomagnesemia and nomomagnesemic patients.

Group	Normomagnesemic Patients (n = 69)	Hypomagnesemic Patients (n = 28)	p-Value
Age (year)	11.79 (3.20–18.66)	13.91 (3.14–19.53)	0.492
Length (cm)	147 (94.5–190)	155.4 (92–77.5)	0.582
Weight (kg)	42.95 ± 18.39	43.61 ± 19.31	0.683
BMI z-score	0.14 (−2.24–2.82)	0.13 (−1.66–2.12)	0.418
Mg^{2+} intake (% of RDI)	87 (41–436)	88 (37–684)	0.692
Patients who exceeded the RDI for Mg^{2+} intake (%)	31.3	34.6	0.419
Serum Creatinine (mg/dL)	0.88 (0.06)	1.01 (0.11)	0.287
Creatinine clearance (mL/min/1.73 m^2)	86 (4)	75 (6)	0.122
Urinary protein/creatinine (mg/g)	625.2 (155.8)	561.7 (120.5)	0.747
Serum estradiol (pg/mL)	60.28 (15.83)	67.24 (37.75)	0.865
Serum Mg^{2+} (mg/dL)	0.83 (0.01)	0.70 (0.01)	<0.001
FE Mg^{2+} (%)	5.41 (0.43)	6.55 (0.72)	0.178
CsA levels (ng/mL)	566.13 (30.70)	685.75 (53.56)	0.053
Tacrolimus levels (ng/mL)	6.90 (0.64)	8.55 (0.99)	0.163
Serum EGF (pg/mL)	802.77 (27.93)	795.60 (40.08)	0.883
Urine EGF (ng/mL)	27.46 (3.50)	18.58 (4.52)	0.120
Urine EGF/creatinine (ng/mg)	0.31 (0.03)	0.22 (0.05)	0.120

Cross-sectional data were analysed with Mann-Whitney-U test and presented as the median (minimum-maximum) or Student's t-test (mean ± SD). Longitudinal data were analysed with GEE and, therefore, presented as the mean (SE). RDI: Reference daily intake, EGF: Epidermal growth factor, FE: Fractional excretion, CsA: cyclosporine.

3.3. Magnesium Intake

The median amount of magnesium intake was 87% (37–684%) of the reference daily intake (RDI, corrected for age). Only 29% of all patients exceeded the RDI. Although the median magnesium intake remained stable from 8 year on, the number of children that reached the RDI for magnesium intake was decreasing with age: 63.2% of the children < 8 year exceeded the RDI for magnesium intake (median amount was 119% (62–684%)), while this was only 17.9% of children between 8–12 year (77% (41–151%)), 33.3% between 12–16 year (80% (56–436%), and 21.1% of the >16 year old children and adolescents (86% (37–323%)).

Magnesium intake was significantly correlated with age (Figure 1A; p < 0.001; r = −0.375), weight (p = 0.009; r = −0.272), and length (p = 0.002; r = −0.318). The use of Mg^{2+} supplements was negatively correlated with magnesium intake (p = 0.095; r = −0.177). Magnesium intake did not correlate with other variables, such as the BMI z-score, sex, serum Mg levels (Figure 1B), renal function, serum or urinary EGF concentration, or the presence of hypomagnesemia.

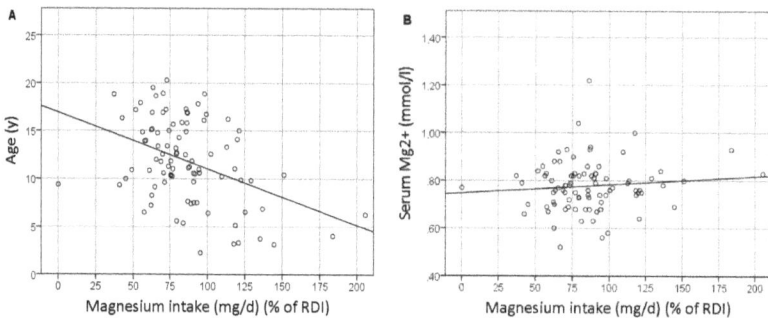

Figure 1. Correlation between the magnesium intake and age (**A**) and the serum magnesium level (**B**). RDI: Recommended daily intake.

3.4. The Healthy Control Group

The median age in the healthy control group was 13.2 year (3.3–17.9 year). Fifty-four percent of the healthy control children were male and length, weight, and BMI z-score was comparable to the study groups.

The serum creatinine was 0.54 mg/dL (0.32–1.09 mg/dL), the creatinine clearance was 108 mL/min/1.73 m^2 (66–143 mL/min/1.73 m^2), serum Mg^{2+} was 0.92 mg/dL (0.80–1.07 mg/dL), and the FE Mg^{2+} was 3.45% (0.81–5.82%). None of the patients developed hypomagnesemia.

The median urinary EGF was 67.4 ng/mL (17.9–218.8 ng/mL) and the median serum EGF was 807.7 pg/mL (141.6–2087.0 pg/mL). The urinary and serum EGF strongly correlated with age ($p < 0.001$; $r = -0.406$ for urinary EGF and $r = -0.447$ for serum EGF). Urinary EGF also correlated with creatinine clearance ($p = 0.011$; $r = 0.408$), but not with sex ($p = 0.514$; $r = -0.079$), FE Mg^{2+} ($p = 0.819$; $r = 0.038$), serum Mg^{2+} ($p = 0.478$; $r = 0.119$), or serum EGF ($p = 0.405$; $r = 0.135$). Serum EGF also correlated with the BMI z-score ($p = 0.001$; $r = 0.369$) but not with sex ($p = 0.054$; $r = 0.231$), creatinine clearance ($p = 0.520$; $r = 0.108$), serum Mg^{2+} ($p = 0.478$; $r = 0.119$), or FE Mg^{2+} ($p = 0.231$; $r = -0.199$).

3.5. Predictors of FE Mg^{2+}

In a univariate GEE analysis, the FE Mg^{2+} was predicted by the urinary EGF concentration, with $r = -0.57$ and $p < 0.001$ (depicted in Figure 2).

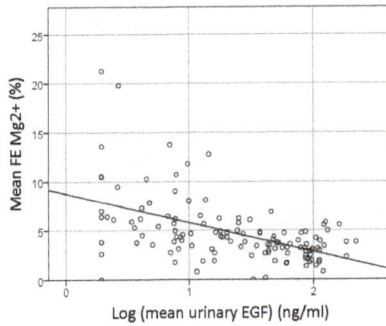

Figure 2. Correlation between the EGF and fractional excretion (FE) of magnesium. Logarithmic normalized data of the EGF are presented.

Urinary EGF, age, sex, renal function, serum magnesium concentration, the urinary protein/creatinine ratio, and Mg^{2+} intake were tested in a multivariate GEE model as predictors of FE Mg^{2+}. Except for sex ($p = 0.747$), urinary protein/creatinine ratio ($p = 0.192$), and Mg^{2+} intake ($p = 0.593$), the other factors appeared to be independent predictors of FE Mg^{2+} (data presented in Table 4).

Table 4. Log EGF as a predictor of FE Mg^{2+}.

	β	*p*-Value	95% CI	
			Lower	Upper
Log Urinary EGF (ng/mL)	−2.084	<0.001	−3.153	−1.015
eGFR (mL/min/1.73 m^2)	−0.049	<0.001	−0.067	−0.032
Serum Mg^{2+} (mg/dL)	−6.239	0.034	−12.014	−0.463
Age (year)	−0.239	0.001	−0.384	−0.094
Constant	20.078	<0.001		

In this population, the FE Mg^{2+} can be calculated using the following formula: FE Mg^{2+} = 20.078 − 2.084 × log Urinary EGF − 0.049 × eGFR − 0.239 × Age − 6.239 × serum Mg^{2+}. eGFR: estimated glomerular filtration rate, EGF: epidermal growth factor.

4. Discussion

This clinical study revealed several new insights into magnesium homeostasis in children: (1) Children treated with calcineurin inhibitors had lower serum magnesium levels and, more frequently, developed hypomagnesemia; (2) In children who developed hypomagnesemia, the FE Mg^{2+} was increased in patients treated with calcineurin inhibitors; (3) The urinary EGF concentration and the FE Mg^{2+} were inversely correlated in all research groups; (4) We defined a predictive model for the FE Mg^{2+} in children, including the urinary EGF concentration, age, renal function, and the serum magnesium concentration; (5) We found that only 29% of the children exceeded the RDI for magnesium intake, which further decreased with age; and (6) Magnesium intake was negatively correlated with the use of magnesium supplements.

In this study, we found that children treated with CNI showed significantly lower serum magnesium levels and that they were significantly more likely to develop hypomagnesemia. This is in line with previous findings in children [31–34] and adults [21]. In adults and animal models, it was shown that hypomagnesemia is caused by renal magnesium wasting [20,21,35]. CNI treatment lead to a decreased renal EGF production, resulting in a decreased magnesium channel TRPM6 expression in the distal convoluted tubule and, thus, a decreased renal magnesium reabsorption [20,35]. However, in children the pathogenesis of CNI induced hypomagnesemia is less clear as few studies have found a normal FE Mg^{2+} after CNI treatment, despite the development of hypomagnesemia [31,36]. In the present study, we demonstrated for the first time that the FE Mg^{2+} increased in children who developed hypomagnesemia when treated with CNI. This effect was independent from the magnesium intake as children who developed hypomagnesemia had an equal magnesium intake compared to normomagnesemic children. In addition to this finding, the urinary EGF concentration and the FE Mg^{2+} were inversely correlated, thus supporting the role of EGF in the renal magnesium reabsorption in children. In a multivariate model, EGF remained a significant predictor of the FE Mg^{2+}. Our results pinpoint to a similar mechanism of renal magnesium reabsorption in children as was demonstrated in adults and rats: Renal EGF stimulates the magnesium reabsorption via the TRPM6 channel in the distal convoluted tubule. To strengthen this hypothesis, a study should be conducted investigating EGF and TRPM6 in renal biopsies. However, as this would indicate an invasive procedure in children, ethical approval can never be obtained in a study context alone.

Additionally, from the multivariate model, age also appeared to be an independent predictor of the FE Mg^{2+} in children, with a positive correlation coefficient. In healthy children, it was shown that the FE Mg^{2+} did not correlate with age [37]. In the present study, only children with an underlying kidney disease were included. Several kidney diseases are accompanied by renal magnesium wasting in children, such as genetic disorders [38] or tubular dysfunction after acute tubular necrosis, or post-obstructive diuresis [39,40]. From our data, the FE Mg^{2+} increases with age in this population, which might indicate that the duration of the kidney disease is of importance in the development of renal magnesium wasting. As we did not go into detail on this finding, this would be an interesting topic for further research.

In children, the renal function also predicts the FE Mg^{2+}. A few other studies have already established a relation between the FE Mg^{2+} and the renal function. In children who recovered from ischemic acute tubular necrosis, it was shown that the FE Mg^{2+} declined, while the renal function improved [41]. This accords with the physiological principles as the FE Mg^{2+} is calculated from the serum creatinine (which is higher in patients with renal failure) and the urinary creatinine (which is lower in patients with renal failure). Therefore, an improvement of creatinine clearance would mathematically result in a decrease in the FE Mg^{2+}. To overcome this mathematical issue, biomarkers of kidney function other than creatinine should be determined, such as urine neutrophil gelatinase-associated lipocalin (NGAL), chromium-51 EDTA, or cystatin-C, which have been shown to be reliable markers of acute kidney injury as well as chronic kidney disease [42–44]. In the present study, the renal function of the children with CKD (the CKD group) was also determined with chromium-51 EDTA analysis (data not shown), which showed a significant relation with the FE Mg^{2+}. Also in

Nutrients **2018**, *10*, 677

pediatric patients after kidney transplantation, FE Mg^{2+} was negatively correlated with the renal function [45,46]. In adult patients, the renal function did not predict FE Mg^{2+} [21]. In that study, both the renal transplant group and the CKD control group were matched for renal function, which might explain why the relation was not found. In the present study, children with a decreased renal function (renal transplant group and CKD group), as well as children with a normal creatinine clearance (both nephrotic syndrome groups), were included.

The protein/creatinine ratio was increased in all groups in this study population, however, below the nephrotic range proteinuria. Normal protein/creatinine ratios up to 340 mg/g were reported in healthy children [47], while nephrotic range proteinuria is defined as protein/creatinine ratio >2 g/g creatinine [48]. The protein/creatinine ratio did not differ between patients with and without hypomagnesemia and was not independently related to the FE Mg^{2+}, suggesting that renal magnesium loss is not due to proteinuria.

Only 29% of the children reached the recommended amount of magnesium intake, which negatively correlated with age, with a higher magnesium intake more likely at a younger age. A few other European studies also found that older children had a higher prevalence of inadequate magnesium intake compared to younger children [8,49,50]. The average magnesium intake was the highest in the youngest children (<8 year), while the lowest intake was in the 8 to 12 year old children. From then on, the average magnesium intake increased with age which was also found in one other report [50]. In our study cohort, this was explained by the use of magnesium supplements, a treatment that is prescribed to patients with hypomagnesemia or patients susceptible to the development of hypomagnesemia. Our findings contrasted with a study of white and African-American girls, in which the magnesium intake decreased with age [51].

Our study has several strengths that led to new insights into the pathogenesis of CNI-induced magnesium loss in children. Despite the low incidence of nephrotic syndrome and renal transplantation in children, we were able to include sufficient numbers of patients. The longitudinal study design, with a low drop-out rate and age, gender, and renal function, matched the control groups and enabled us to draw sound conclusions. The most important limitation of the present study is that the CNI treated patients were included when they were already on treatment with CNI, sometimes for several years already. It would be of interest to include the patients at the moment CNIs are initiated and perform a long-term follow-up study over several years to study the time course influence of CNI on the renal EGF expression and renal magnesium loss. However, as CNI treatment is rare in children, with the low incidence of CNI-dependent nephrotic syndrome and kidney transplantation, the inclusion of sufficient children would take years.

5. Conclusions

In CNI-treated children who developed hypomagnesemia, the FE Mg^{2+} was increased. The urinary EGF concentration was an independent predictor of the FE Mg^2, as were age and renal function.

Author Contributions: Conceptualization, K.J.L., B.Y.D.W. and D.T.; Data curation, C.A., A.D.M., S.M. and M.V.; Formal analysis, K.J.L., C.A., S.M. and G.A.V.; Funding acquisition, D.T.; Investigation, K.J.L.; Methodology, K.J.L., A.V.E., B.Y.D.W. and D.T.; Project administration, K.J.L., A.D.M., M.V. and A.V.E.; Resources, K.V.H. and D.T.; Software, K.J.L.; Supervision, D.T.; Writing-original draft, K.J.L. and C.A.; Writing-review & editing, G.A.V., K.V.H., A.V.E., B.Y.D.W. and D.T.

Acknowledgments: We thank the nursing staff and all patients for making this observational study possible. We also like to thank Petra Aerts, Ilse Goolaerts, Angelika Jürgens and Lieve Vits for the technical assistance.

Conflicts of Interest: The authors declare no conflict of interest.

References

1. Narayanan, S.; Scalici, P. Serum magnesium levels in pediatric inpatients: A study in laboratory overuse. *Hosp. Pediatr.* **2015**, *5*, 9–17. [CrossRef] [PubMed]
2. Abrams, S.A.; Chen, Z.; Hawthorne, K.M. Magnesium metabolism in 4-year-old to 8-year-old children. *J. Bone Miner. Res.* **2014**, *29*, 118–122. [CrossRef] [PubMed]
3. Jahnen-Dechent, W.; Ketteler, M. Magnesium basics. *Clin. Kidney J.* **2012**, *5*, i3–i14. [CrossRef] [PubMed]
4. Weaver, C.M. Calcium and magnesium requirements of children and adolescents and peak bone mass. *Nutrition* **2000**, *16*, 514–516. [CrossRef]
5. Kris-Etherton, P.M.; Hu, F.B.; Ros, E.; Sabate, J. The role of tree nuts and peanuts in the prevention of coronary heart disease: Multiple potential mechanisms. *J. Nutr.* **2008**, *138*, 1746S–1751S. [CrossRef] [PubMed]
6. Heaney, R.P. Dairy and bone health. *J. Am. Coll. Nutr.* **2009**, *28* (Suppl. 1), 82S–90S. [CrossRef] [PubMed]
7. Hurrell, R.F. Influence of vegetable protein sources on trace element and mineral bioavailability. *J. Nutr.* **2003**, *133*, 2973S–2977S. [CrossRef] [PubMed]
8. Tornaritis, M.J.; Philippou, E.; Hadjigeorgiou, C.; Kourides, Y.A.; Panayi, A.; Savva, S.C. A study of the dietary intake of cypriot children and adolescents aged 6–18 years and the association of mother's educational status and children's weight status on adherence to nutritional recommendations. *BMC Public Health* **2014**, *14*, 13. [CrossRef] [PubMed]
9. Sanchez, C.; Aranda, P.; Perez de la Cruz, A.; Llopis, J. Magnesium and zinc status in patients with chronic renal failure: Influence of a nutritional intervention. *Magnes. Res.* **2009**, *22*, 72–80. [PubMed]
10. Gluba-Brzozka, A.; Franczyk, B.; Rysz, J. Vegetarian diet in chronic kidney disease-a friend or foe. *Nutrients* **2017**, *9*, 374. [CrossRef] [PubMed]
11. Lameris, A.L.; Monnens, L.A.; Bindels, R.J.; Hoenderop, J.G.J. Drug-induced alterations in mg2+ homoeostasis. *Clin. Sci.* **2012**, *123*, 1–14. [CrossRef] [PubMed]
12. Milbouw, S.; Verhaegen, J.; Verrijken, A.; Schepens, T.; De Winter, B.Y.; Van Gaal, L.F.; Ledeganck, K.J.; De Block, C.E.M. Predictors of insulin resistance in obesity and type 2 diabetes mellitus—The role of magnesium. *J. Metab. Syndr.* **2017**, *6*, 235. [CrossRef]
13. Liu, F.; Mao, J.H. Calcineurin inhibitors and nephrotoxicity in children. *World J. Pediatr.* **2018**, *14*, 121–126. [CrossRef] [PubMed]
14. Burdmann, E.A.; Andoh, T.F.; Lindsley, J.; Houghton, D.C.; Bennett, W.M. Effects of oral magnesium supplementation on acute experimental cyclosporin nephrotoxicity. *Nephrol. Dial. Transplant.* **1994**, *9*, 16–21. [PubMed]
15. Higgins, R.; Ramaiyan, K.; Dasgupta, T.; Kanji, H.; Fletcher, S.; Lam, F.; Kashi, H. Hyponatraemia and hyperkalaemia are more frequent in renal transplant recipients treated with tacrolimus than with cyclosporin. Further evidence for differences between cyclosporin and tacrolimus nephrotoxicities. *Nephrol. Dial. Transplant.* **2004**, *19*, 444–450. [CrossRef] [PubMed]
16. Hoenderop, J.G.J.; Bindels, R.J.M. Epithelial ca2+ and mg2+ channels in health and disease. *J. Am. Soc. Nephrol.* **2005**, *16*, 15–26. [CrossRef] [PubMed]
17. Schlingmann, K.P.; Waldegger, S.; Konrad, M.; Chubanov, V.; Gudermann, T. Trpm6 and trpm7—Gatekeepers of human magnesium metabolism. *Biochim. Biophys. Acta* **2007**, *1772*, 813–821. [CrossRef] [PubMed]
18. Thebault, S.P.; Alexander, R.T.; Tiel Groenestege, W.M.; Hoenderop, J.G.; Bindels, R.J. Egf increases trpm6 activity and surface expression. *J. Am. Soc. Nephrol.* **2009**, *20*, 78–85. [CrossRef] [PubMed]
19. Groenestege, W.M.; Thebault, S.; van der Wijst, J.; van den Berg, D.; Janssen, R.; Tejpar, S.; van den Heuvel, L.P.; van Cutsem, E.; Hoenderop, J.G.; Knoers, N.V.; et al. Impaired basolateral sorting of pro-egf causes isolated recessive renal hypomagnesemia. *J. Clin. Invest.* **2007**, *117*, 2260–2267. [CrossRef] [PubMed]
20. Ledeganck, K.J.; Boulet, G.A.; Horvath, C.A.; Vinckx, M.; Bogers, J.J.; Van den Bossche, R.; Verpooten, G.A.; De Winter, B.Y. Expression of renal distal tubule transporters trpm6 and ncc in a rat model of cyclosporine nephrotoxicity and effect of egf treatment. *Am. J. Physiol. Renal Physiol.* **2011**, *301*, F486–F493. [CrossRef] [PubMed]
21. Ledeganck, K.J.; De Winter, B.Y.; Van den Driessche, A.; Jurgens, A.; Bosmans, J.L.; Couttenye, M.M.; Verpooten, G.A. Magnesium loss in cyclosporine-treated patients is related to renal epidermal growth factor downregulation. *Nephrol. Dial. Transplant.* **2013**, *29*, 1097–1102. [CrossRef] [PubMed]

22. Zeng, F.; Harris, R.C. Epidermal growth factor, from gene organization to bedside. *Semin. Cell Dev. Biol.* **2014**, *28*, 2–11. [CrossRef] [PubMed]

23. Tomaszewska, R.; Dembinski, A.; Warzecha, Z.; Ceranowicz, P.; Konturek, S.J.; Stachura, J. The influence of epidermal growth factor on the course of ischemia-reperfusion induced pancreatitis in rats. *J. Physiol. Pharmacol.* **2002**, *53*, 183–198. [PubMed]

24. Warzecha, Z.; Dembinski, A.; Konturek, P.C.; Ceranowicz, P.; Konturek, S.J. Epidermal growth factor protects against pancreatic damage in cerulein-induced pancreatitis. *Digestion* **1999**, *60*, 314–323. [CrossRef] [PubMed]

25. Konturek, P.C.; Dembinski, A.; Warzecha, Z.; Ceranowicz, P.; Konturek, S.J.; Stachura, J.; Hahn, E.G. Expression of transforming growth factor-beta 1 and epidermal growth factor in caerulein-induced pancreatitis in rat. *J. Physiol. Pharmacol.* **1997**, *48*, 59–72. [PubMed]

26. Bennett, S.P.; Griffiths, G.D.; Schor, A.M.; Leese, G.P.; Schor, S.L. Growth factors in the treatment of diabetic foot ulcers. *Br. J. Surg.* **2003**, *90*, 133–146. [CrossRef] [PubMed]

27. Huysentruyt, K.; Laire, D.; Van Avondt, T.; De Schepper, J.; Vandenplas, Y. Energy and macronutrient intakes and adherence to dietary guidelines of infants and toddlers in belgium. *Eur. J. Nutr.* **2016**, *55*, 1595–1604. [CrossRef] [PubMed]

28. Cochat, P. *Espn Handbook*; European Society for Paediatric Nephrology; Medcom: Lyon, France, 2002.

29. Schwartz, G.J.; Munoz, A.; Schneider, M.F.; Mak, R.H.; Kaskel, F.; Warady, B.A.; Furth, S.L. New equations to estimate gfr in children with ckd. *J. Am. Soc. Nephrol.* **2009**, *20*, 629–637. [CrossRef] [PubMed]

30. Cao, G.; van der Wijst, J.; van der Kemp, A.; van Zeeland, F.; Bindels, R.J.; Hoenderop, J.G. Regulation of the epithelial mg2+ channel trpm6 by estrogen and the associated repressor protein of estrogen receptor activity (rea). *J. Biol. Chem.* **2009**, *284*, 14788–14795. [CrossRef] [PubMed]

31. Nozue, T.; Kobayashi, A.; Kodama, T.; Uemasu, F.; Endoh, H.; Sako, A.; Takagi, Y. Pathogenesis of cyclosporine-induced hypomagnesemia. *J. Pediatr.* **1992**, *120*, 638–640. [CrossRef]

32. Riva, N.; Schaiquevich, P.; Caceres Guido, P.; Halac, E.; Dip, M.; Imventarza, O. Pharmacoepidemiology of tacrolimus in pediatric liver transplantation. *Pediatr. Transplant.* **2017**, *21*. [CrossRef] [PubMed]

33. Hayes, W.; Boyle, S.; Carroll, A.; Bockenhauer, D.; Marks, S.D. Hypomagnesemia and increased risk of new-onset diabetes mellitus after transplantation in pediatric renal transplant recipients. *Pediatr. Nephrol.* **2017**, *32*, 879–884. [CrossRef] [PubMed]

34. Yanik, G.; Levine, J.E.; Ratanatharathorn, V.; Dunn, R.; Ferrara, J.; Hutchinson, R.J. Tacrolimus (fk506) and methotrexate as prophylaxis for acute graft-versus-host disease in pediatric allogeneic stem cell transplantation. *Bone Marrow Transplant.* **2000**, *26*, 161–167. [CrossRef] [PubMed]

35. Nijenhuis, T.; Hoenderop, J.G.; Bindels, R.J. Downregulation of ca(2+) and mg(2+) transport proteins in the kidney explains tacrolimus (fk506)-induced hypercalciuria and hypomagnesemia. *J. Am. Soc. Nephrol.* **2004**, *15*, 549–557. [CrossRef] [PubMed]

36. Freundlich, M. Bone mineral content and mineral metabolism during cyclosporine treatment of nephrotic syndrome. *J. Pediatr.* **2006**, *149*, 383–389. [CrossRef] [PubMed]

37. Ariceta, G.; Rodriguez-Soriano, J.; Vallo, A. Renal magnesium handling in infants and children. *Acta Paediatr.* **1996**, *85*, 1019–1023. [CrossRef] [PubMed]

38. Viering, D.; de Baaij, J.H.F.; Walsh, S.B.; Kleta, R.; Bockenhauer, D. Genetic causes of hypomagnesemia, a clinical overview. *Pediatr. Nephrol.* **2017**, *32*, 1123–1135. [CrossRef] [PubMed]

39. Whang, R. Magnesium deficiency: Pathogenesis, prevalence, and clinical implications. *Am. J. Med.* **1987**, *82*, 24–29. [CrossRef]

40. Agus, Z.S. Mechanisms and causes of hypomagnesemia. *Curr. Opin. Nephrol. Hypertens.* **2016**, *25*, 301–307. [CrossRef] [PubMed]

41. Gheissari, A.; Andalib, A.; Labibzadeh, N.; Modarresi, M.; Azhir, A.; Merrikhi, A. Fractional excretion of magnesium (femg), a marker for tubular dysfunction in children with clinically recovered ischemic acute tubular necrosis. *Saudi J. Kidney Dis. Transpl.* **2011**, *22*, 476–481. [PubMed]

42. Zylka, A.; Gala-Bladzinska, A.; Dumnicka, P.; Ceranowicz, P.; Kuzniewski, M.; Gil, K.; Olszanecki, R.; Kusnierz-Cabala, B. Is urinary ngal determination useful for monitoring kidney function and assessment of cardiovascular disease? A 12-month observation of patients with type 2 diabetes. *Dis. Markers* **2016**, *2016*, 8489543. [CrossRef] [PubMed]

43. Shlipak, M.G.; Mattes, M.D.; Peralta, C.A. Update on cystatin c: Incorporation into clinical practice. *Am. J. Kidney Dis.* **2013**, *62*, 595–603. [CrossRef] [PubMed]

44. Geist, B.K.; Diemling, M.; Staudenherz, A. Glomerular filtration rate and error calculation based on the slope-intercept method with chromium-51 ethylenediaminetetraacetic acid via a new clinical software: Gfrcalc. *Med. Princ. Pract.* **2016**, *25*, 368–373. [CrossRef] [PubMed]

45. Uslu Gokceoglu, A.; Comak, E.; Dogan, C.S.; Koyun, M.; Akbas, H.; Akman, S. Magnesium excretion and hypomagnesemia in pediatric renal transplant recipients. *Ren. Fail.* **2014**, *36*, 1056–1059. [CrossRef] [PubMed]

46. Osorio, J.M.; Bravo, J.; Perez, A.; Ferreyra, C.; Osuna, A. Magnesemia in renal transplant recipients: Relation with immunosuppression and posttransplant diabetes. *Transplant. Proc.* **2010**, *42*, 2910–2913. [CrossRef] [PubMed]

47. Slev, P.R.; Bunker, A.M.; Owen, W.E.; Roberts, W.L. Pediatric reference intervals for random urine calcium, phosphorus and total protein. *Pediatr. Nephrol.* **2010**, *25*, 1707–1710. [CrossRef] [PubMed]

48. Ariceta, G. Clinical practice: Proteinuria. *Eur. J. Pediatr.* **2011**, *170*, 15–20. [CrossRef] [PubMed]

49. Lopez-Sobaler, A.M.; Aparicio, A.; Gonzalez-Rodriguez, L.G.; Cuadrado-Soto, E.; Rubio, J.; Marcos, V.; Sanchidrian, R.; Santos, S.; Perez-Farinos, N.; Dal Re, M.A.; et al. Adequacy of usual vitamin and mineral intake in spanish children and adolescents: Enalia study. *Nutrients* **2017**, *9*, 131. [CrossRef] [PubMed]

50. Manios, Y.; Moschonis, G.; Mavrogianni, C.; Bos, R.; Singh-Povel, C. Micronutrient intakes among children and adults in greece: The role of age, sex and socio-economic status. *Nutrients* **2014**, *6*, 4073–4092. [CrossRef] [PubMed]

51. Affenito, S.G.; Thompson, D.R.; Franko, D.L.; Striegel-Moore, R.H.; Daniels, S.R.; Barton, B.A.; Schreiber, G.B.; Schmidt, M.; Crawford, P.B. Longitudinal assessment of micronutrient intake among african-american and white girls: The national heart, lung, and blood institute growth and health study. *J. Am. Diet. Assoc.* **2007**, *107*, 1113–1123. [CrossRef] [PubMed]

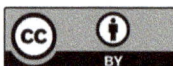

nutrients

MDPI

Review

Serum Magnesium after Kidney Transplantation: A Systematic Review

Anne-Sophie Garnier [1,2], Agnès Duveau [1,2], Martin Planchais [1,2], Jean-François Subra [1,2,3], Johnny Sayegh [1,2] and Jean-François Augusto [1,2,3,*]

[1] LUNAM Université, 49180 Angers, France; AnneSophie.Garnier@chu-angers.fr (A.-S.G.); agnes.duveau@chu-angers.fr (A.D.); martin.planchais@chu-angers.fr (M.P.); jfsubra@chu-angers.fr (J.-F.S.); josayegh@chu-angers.fr (J.S.)
[2] Université Angers, CHU Angers, Service de Néphrologie-Dialyse-Transplantation, CHU d'Angers, 49933 Angers CEDEX 9, France
[3] CRCINA, INSERM, Université de Nantes, Université d'Angers, LabEx IGO Immunotherapy, Graft, Oncology, 44007 Angers, France
* Correspondence: jfaugusto@chu-angers.fr; Tel.: +33-241-353-934; Fax: +33-241-354-892

Received: 25 April 2018; Accepted: 31 May 2018; Published: 6 June 2018

Abstract: Magnesium (Mg) status has recently drawn close attention in chronic kidney disease and in kidney transplant recipients. This review aims to evaluate the body of evidence linking hypomagnesemia to clinical consequences in these specific populations. After a brief summary of the main mechanisms involved in Mg regulation and of Mg status in end-stage renal disease, the review focuses on the relationship between hypomagnesemia and cardiovascular risk in kidney transplant recipients. A body of evidence in recent studies points to a negative impact of hypomagnesemia on post-transplant diabetes mellitus (PTDM) and cardiovascular risk, which currently represent the main threat for morbidity and mortality in kidney transplantation. Deleterious biological mechanisms induced by hypomagnesemia are also discussed. While data analysis enables us to conclude that hypomagnesemia is linked to the development of PTDM, studies prospectively evaluating the impact of hypomagnesemia correction after kidney transplantation are still lacking and needed.

Keywords: Magnesium-Kidney; transplantation-New-onset; diabetes after transplantation-cardiovascular risk

1. Magnesium: Physiology

Magnesium (Mg) is the fourth cation of the body and the second most prevalent intracellular cation [1]. Approximately half of total body Mg is located in bone [2], the remainder being contained in skeletal muscles and soft tissues [1]. Extracellular Mg represents only 1% of total body Mg [3] and is mostly found in serum with concentrations ranging between 0.65 to 1.05 mmol/L [4] and in red blood cells [3]. It is present in three different states: ionized Mg (55–70%), protein-bound Mg (20–30%), and Mg complexed with anions such as bicarbonate or phosphate (5–15%) [1].

Mg homeostasis is mainly dependent on intestinal absorption and renal excretion. In the intestine, absorption is modulated by luminal Mg concentration, at high concentrations, Mg is regulated by an active transcellular transport and passive paracellular diffusion; whereas in low concentrations, Mg is absorbed by an active transcellular pathway involving a Transient Receptor Potential Melastatin 6 (TRPM6) channel expressed on the small intestine cells [5].

In patients with normal kidney function, around 70 to 80% of plasma Mg is ultra-filtrable. About 40% of the filtered Mg is reabsorbed in the proximal tubule by paracellular uptake, while 50% is absorbed in the ascending limb of the loop of Henle and 5% is absorbed in the distal tubule by an active transport. Thus, only 5% of filtered Mg is excreted in final urine, but this excretion can vary widely from 0.5 to 70% to keep plasma Mg concentration within the normal range [6]. Figure 1 summarizes Mg exchange in nephron.

Hypomagnesemia is frequently associated with hypokalemia [7]. This is mainly due to common disorders leading to ion wasting, such as through diuretic intake or diarrhea.

However, reduction of intracellular Mg concentration induces a decline in ATP activity that in turn affects potassium ATP-dependent channels located in the ascending limb and cortical collecting tubule, leading to urinary potassium loss [8,9]. This mechanism may explain the common resistance to hypokalemia correction until hypomagnesemia is normalized.

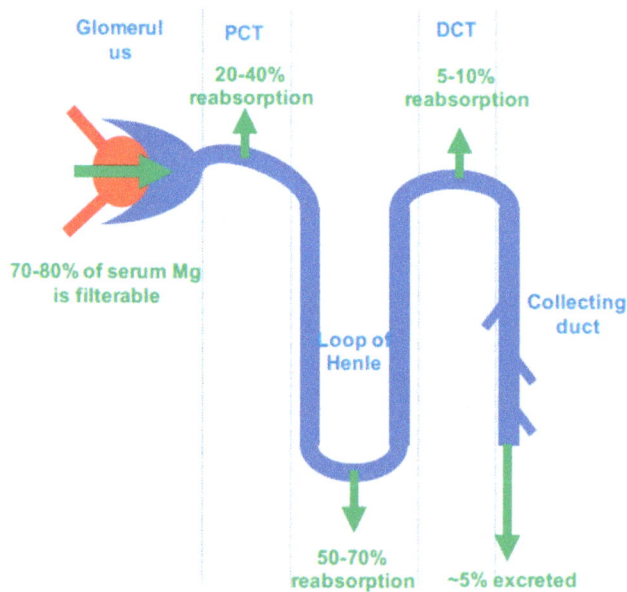

Figure 1. Magnesium exchanges in nephron. PCT, proximal convoluted tubule; DCT, distal convoluted tubule.

2. Clinical Signs and Etiologies of Hypomagnesemia

Clinical manifestations of hypomagnesemia are quite unspecific. Early signs include nausea, vomiting, anorexia and weakness [1]. Neuromuscular signs can also be present, including numbness, tingling, cramps, fasciculation seizures and neuropsychological disorders [1]. Severe hypomagnesemia has been associated with cardiac arrhythmia and coronary spasm [10]. Mg depletion can induce changes in electrocardiogram readings from pointed T waves in mild hypomagnesemia to widening of the QRS complex, prolongation of the PR interval and ventricular arrhythmias in patients with severe Mg depletion. Arrhythmias are more frequently observed in the setting of an acute ischemic event [11], congestive heart failure—partly due to the administration of diuretics—or after a cardiopulmonary bypass [12]. Some authors showed that administration of magnesium after a cardiopulmonary bypass may prevent postoperative arrhythmias [13].

Hypomagnesemia results mainly from gastrointestinal and renal losses. Gastrointestinal losses can arise from diarrhea, malabsorption, steatorrhea, small bowel bypass surgery, acute pancreatitis and dietary deprivation [14]. Rarely, hypomagnesemia may occur due to a selective defect in the intestinal Mg absorption, also known as primary intestinal hypomagnesemia. Urinary Mg losses can be induced by loop or thiazide-type diuretics, volume expansion, alcohol, hypercalcemia, nephrotoxins such as aminoglycoside antibiotics, cisplatin or cyclosporine. Urinary Mg wasting can also be due to loop of Henle or distal tubule dysfunction, after acute tubular necrosis, post-obstructive diuresis or kidney transplantation [1,14]. Lastly, primary renal Mg wasting was observed in Bartter and Gitelman syndromes, in which hypomagnesemia is associated with hypercalciuria and hypocalciuria respectively [14].

3. Magnesium Status in CKD Patients

Chronic kidney disease (CKD) is frequently associated with hypermagnesaemia, which is usually mild or asymptomatic until end-stage renal disease (ESRD). In moderate CKD patients, increased fractional excretion of Mg compensates for a decline in renal function, providing a stable serum Mg within the normal range. However, in CKD stages IV-V, this compensatory mechanism becomes insufficient which results in hypermagnesaemia [6]. Thus, in this setting, dietary Mg intake and administration of Mg-containing drugs, such as laxatives or antacids, can more easily induce hypermagnesaemia [6]. Alternatively, Mg balance may be negative in some ESRD patients on high doses of diuretics, with reduced gastrointestinal uptake induced by severe metabolic acidosis or reduced albumin levels [5].

Dialysate Mg concentration has a significant impact on Mg balance in hemodialysis (HD) or peritoneal dialysis (PD) patients. Indeed, Mg has a significant diffusion across dialysis membranes and its elimination depends on ultrafiltration and the diffusible gradient between the serum and dialysate concentration. A significant reduction in serum Mg concentration has been observed in HD patients, probably due to the Gibbs–Donnan effect [15]. Conversely, mild hypermagnesemia is frequently observed in PD patients, because Mg concentration of PD "standard dialysate" is about 0.75 mmol/L [16]. Interestingly, bone appears as the greatest Mg reservoir in CKD patients. To support this, a 70% increase in both cortical and trabecular bone Mg content has been reported in uremic patients, compared to non-uremic patients, suggesting that dialysis induces positive net Mg balance in ESRD patients.

4. Magnesium and Cardiovascular Risk in CKD Patients

Several studies have shown an association between Mg status and survival in ESRD patients. Indeed, Ishimura et al. investigated the prognostic value of serum Mg concentration in 515 patients on maintenance hemodialysis (60 ± 12 years, 306 males and 209 females; 24% diabetics). Mortality was significantly higher in the lower Mg group (<2.77 mg/dL, i.e., <1.14 mmol/L, $n = 261$), compared to the higher Mg group (≥2.77 mg/dL, $n = 254$) ($p < 0.001$). Thus, serum Mg was predictive of mortality (HR (per 1 mg/dL increase), 0.485 (95% CI, 0.241–0.975), $p = 0.0424$), particularly of non-cardiovascular mortality (HR 0.318 (95% CI, 0.132 to 0.769), $p = 0.0110$), after adjustment on confounding factors, including age, gender, hemodialysis duration and presence of diabetes [17]. Likewise, in a nationwide registry-based cohort of 142,555 hemodialysis patients, Sakaguchi et al. moreover observed a U-shaped relation with higher all-cause and cardiovascular mortality of patients in both the lowest Mg sextile (<0.95 mmol/L) and the highest (>1.27 mmol/L) [18].

Several studies maintain that the increased cardiovascular mortality in hypomagnaesemic ESRD patients may be related to accelerated atherosclerosis. In an observational study, PD patients who developed arterial calcifications had significantly lower serum Mg levels ($p < 0.001$) [19]. Similar results were found in a retrospective cohort of 390 non-diabetic and hemodialysis patients. Serum Mg was significantly lower in patients with vascular calcification than in those without (2.69 ± 0.28 vs. 2.78 ± 0.33 mg/dL, $p < 0.05$). Serum Mg concentration appeared as an independent risk factor of vascular calcification (OR 0.28, 95% CI 0.09–0.92/1 mg/dL increase in serum magnesium, $p = 0.036$) after adjustments for age, gender, duration of hemodialysis, calcium, phosphate and intact parathyroid hormone concentrations [20]. Given these observations, some authors investigated the effect of Mg supplementation in ESRD patients. In one study, 47 hemodialysis patients were randomized to one group receiving oral Mg citrate (610 mg per day) and oral calcium acetate, and the other oral calcium acetate and a placebo. After 2 months, patients receiving Mg had a significant decrease in intima-media thickness (0.70 vs. 0.97 mm, $p = 0.001$ and 0.78 vs. 0.95 mm, $p = 0.002$ for left and right carotid arteries respectively) [21]. In another work, hemodialysis patients were randomized to receive low (0.5 mmol/L) or high (0.75 mmol/L) dialysate Mg and were followed-up for 3 years. No difference was observed for all-cause mortality between groups, but an increase in cardiovascular mortality was observed after 3 years in the low dialysate Mg group (14.5% vs. 0%, $p = 0.042$) in HDM group [22].

5. Magnesium Status after Kidney Transplantation and Relation with Graft Function

Hypomagnesemia is frequently observed after kidney transplantation, in part to immunosuppressive regimens including calcineurin inhibitors (CNI) that induce Mg urinary waste. Hypomagnesemia was observed in 6.6% of patients treated with tacrolimus and in 1.5% of patients on cyclosporine [23]. The mechanisms leading to hypomagnesemia are not fully understood, but it has been shown that CNI induce a down-regulation of renal expression of the epidermal growth factor [24] and TRMP6 in the distal collecting tubule [25], leading to decreased Mg reabsorption. Sirolimus might induce hypomagnesemia through inhibition of Na-K-Cl co-transporter 2 expression in the thick ascending loop of Henle [26]. Renal Mg wasting has been shown to be similar between rats treated with sirolimus and those treated with cyclosporine or tacrolimus [27]. Many other factors influence Mg levels after kidney transplantation, such as post-transplantation volume expansion, metabolic acidosis, insulin resistance, decreased gastro-intestinal absorption due to diarrhea, low Mg intake and medication such as diuretics or proton pump inhibitors [28].

Hypomagnesemia was reported to develop frequently within the first few weeks following transplantation [29], with a serum Mg level nadir in the second month post-transplantation [30]. Hypomagnesemia may persist for several years after kidney transplantation. In a cohort of 49 kidney transplant recipients, 22.4% of patients had hypomagnesemia 6 years after transplantation [31]. As observed in the general population, serum Mg levels were inversely correlated with glomerular filtration rate [32].

The relationship between serum Mg and graft function has been poorly evaluated in literature. In a cohort study published in 2005, 320 kidney recipients were divided into two groups, based on median Mg level in the entire cohort: the low serum Mg group ($n = 29$, 0.74 (0.68–0.78) mmol/L) compared to the normal Mg group ($n = 31$, 0.9 (0.82–0.98) mmol/L, $p < 0.05$). The authors showed that hypomagnesemia was associated with a greater decline in allograft function and an increased risk of graft loss for patients with ciclosporine-induced nephropathy [33]. In animals studies, hypomagnesemia is associated with glomerular dysfunction and the development of chronic fibrotic lesions [34]. In mice treated with cyclosporine, Mg supplementation improved renal function and decreased kidney fibrotic lesions [35]. Likewise, Mg supplementation in cyclosporine-treated rats was associated with a reduction in tubular atrophy and interstitial fibrosis and prevented kidney function decline [34].

In murine studies, Mg supplementation has been shown to exert an effect using several mechanisms, including innate immune pathways. Indeed, Mg supplementation inhibits monocyte and macrophage recruitment, partly by abolishing expression of chemoattractant proteins (osteopontin and monocyte chemoattractant protein-1), fibrogenic molecules and extracellular matrix proteins [36]. Moreover, Mg induces down-regulation of endothelin-1 expression [36] and decreased nuclear factor kappa-light-chain-enhancer of activated B cells (NFkB) activation [37].

These data in human and mice converge to suggest that hypomagnesemia is not only associated with accelerated decline of graft function but is also an active contributor to renal lesions. Thus, prospective studies are needed to analyze the potential benefits of Mg supplements on graft function after kidney transplantation.

6. Serum Magnesium and New-Onset Diabetes Mellitus after Transplantation

6.1. Serum Magnesium and Diabetes Mellitus in the General Population

Hypomagnesemia has been reported to occur in 13.5 to 47.7% of non-hospitalized patients with type-2 diabetes [38]. Poor dietary Mg intake, glomerular hyperfiltration, osmotic diuresis, recurrent metabolic acidosis, hypophosphataemia and hypokalemia are all potential contributing factors for hypomagnesemia in diabetic patients [38,39]. A higher incidence of hypomagnesemia was reported in females as compared to males on a 2-to-1 ratio [40]. Several authors showed an inverse correlation between Mg intake and the risk of developing diabetes mellitus [41–44]. Moreover, in a study including 39,345 US women followed-up for 6 years, the protective role of high Mg intake was higher in the subgroup of overweight women [42]. In the Atherosclerosis Risk in Communities Study, low serum Mg level was an independent risk factor for incident diabetes mellitus [44].

The diabetogenic effects of hypomagnesemia are not yet well understood and have been attributed to several mechanisms. Data supporting the fact that hypomagnesemia may induce altered cellular glucose transport, reduced pancreatic insulin secretion, defective post-receptor insulin signaling and/or altered insulin–insulin receptor interactions have been reported. Dietary-induced Mg deficiency increased urinary thromboxane concentration and enhanced angiotensin-induced aldosterone synthesis, resulting in resistance to the effect of insulin [45]. This may be due to changes of tyrosine kinase expression on insulin receptor level and/or induction of inflammation and oxidative stress [46]. Conversely, it is interesting to note that oral Mg supplementation during a 16-week period showed an improvement in insulin sensitivity and a better metabolic control in type-2 diabetic patients [47].

6.2. Serum Magnesium and New-Onset Diabetes Mellitus after Transplantation

After transplantation, diabetes mellitus is frequently observed, with incidences ranging from 10 to 30%, depending on the criteria used for diagnosis and the length of follow-up [48,49]. Post-transplant diabetes mellitus (PTDM) affects both patient and graft survival [50], highlighting the importance of identifying potentially modifiable risk factors. Several risk factors for PTDM have already been identified, such as older age, male gender, ethnicity, acute rejection, hepatitis C, higher body mass index, higher pre-transplant glucose levels and higher trough tacrolimus levels [51–53], some of them being common risk factors for type-2 diabetes in the general population. Hypomagnesemia has recently been identified as an independent risk factor for PTDM, however with some conflicting data in literature. Van Laecke et al., in a retrospective study, were the first to identify a relationship between PTDM and post-transplant Mg level in a cohort of 254 kidney transplant recipients. Serum Mg values were recorded at months 1 and 2 after transplantation. 29.5% of recipients developed PTDM after a mean time of 90 ± 80 days post-transplantation. Patients with PTDM had significantly lower Mg levels compared to those without ($p < 0.001$). Post-transplant Mg appeared as an independent predictor of PTDM after adjustment on classical risk factors and on CNI use. Moreover, the association between the use of CNI and PTDM disappeared after adjustments to Mg levels in the multivariate analysis, suggesting that the diabetogenic effect of CNI may be more related to hypomagnesemia itself than to CNI [53]. In another study recently published, the association between serum Mg level and PTDM was examined in a retrospective cohort study of 948 non-diabetic kidney transplant recipients. The authors used multivariable Cox proportional hazards models to evaluate the risk of PTDM as a function of baseline (at 1 month post-transplantation), time-varying (every 3 months) and rolling-average (mean for 3 months moving at 3-month intervals). Hypomagnesemia, defined as a serum Mg concentration below 0.74 mmol/L, was significantly associated with an increased risk of PTDM in baseline (HR, 1.58; 95% CI, 1.07 to 2.34; $p = 0.02$), time-varying (HR, 1.78; 95% CI, 1.29 to 2.45; $p = 0.001$) and rolling-average models (HR, 1.83; 95% CI, 1.30 to 2.57; $p = 0.001$) [54].

The association between hypomagnesemia and PTDM was also studied in pediatric kidney recipients. In a retrospective cohort of 173 young recipients with a median age of 7 years at transplantation, 20 patients developed PTDM at 9 days post transplantation on average. Hypomagnesemia and high tacrolimus levels were significant and independent risk factors for PTDM ($p = 0.01$ and $p < 0.001$, respectively). No association between hypomagnesemia and tacrolimus levels was observed, suggesting that both risk factors were independent from each other [55]. Conversely, in a cohort study of 451 pediatric solid organ transplant recipients, Chanchlani et al. failed to identify an association between hypomagnesemia and PTDM. However, lack of close Mg monitoring and frequent Mg supplementation in their cohort (75% of children) make the study difficult to interpret [56]. Two other studies failed to demonstrate a significant difference in Mg levels between PTDM and non-PTDM adult recipients [57,58]. Osorio et al. analyzed 589 kidney recipients and did not identify a relationship between Mg levels and occurrence of PTDM in patients receiving CNI treatment [57]. Santos et al. observed similar results in a cohort of 205 kidney recipients [58]. However, again, in these studies, no information was given about immunosuppressive regimens, which also limits their interpretation.

In order to minimize the possible effect of post-transplant confounders, our group evaluated the relationship between pre-transplant hypomagnesemia and the risk of PTDM in a cohort of 154 kidney transplant recipients. 28 patients (18.2%) developed a PTDM within the first year of transplantation, and in most patients within the first 2 months. Patients who developed PTDM were older, had a higher body mass index and a higher pre-transplant glucose level, compared to patients without PTDM. The pre-transplant Mg level was significantly lower in patients that developed PTDM ($p = 0.014$). Moreover, a pre-transplant Mg level <2 mg/dL compared to >2.3 mg/dL was associated with a higher risk of PTDM within the first year of transplantation (HR, 2.99; 95% CI, 1.07–8.37, $p = 0.037$) [49]. In the field of liver transplantation, a retrospective cohort of 169 patients showed that both pre-transplant and month 1 post-transplant Mg levels were independent risk factors for PTDM [59]. In these studies, patients were free of diabetes mellitus at inclusion, thus hypomagnesemia was not the result of Mg wasting induced by diabetes.

Based on these observations, Van Laecke et al. investigated the effect of Mg supplementation on post-transplant glucose metabolism [60,61]. In a single-center parallel group study, 54 patients with serum Mg level ≤1.7 mg/dL were randomized to receive 450 mg oral Mg oxide (MgO) one to three times daily, aiming for an Mg concentration of >1.9 mg/dL ($n = 27$) or no treatment ($n = 27$). The primary outcome was a fasting serum glucose concentration at 3 months post-transplantation. Secondary outcomes were the 2 h area under the curve (AUC) for glycaemia and insulin resistance, assessed by a homeostasis model assessment-estimated insulin-resistance index (HOMA_IR) at month 3 post-transplantation. Six patients in the control group received MgO (450 mg daily) as serum Mg concentration dropped below to 1.2 mg/dL. Fasting serum glucose concentration was lower in the Mg group compared to the control group (95% CI; 1.7–21.3; $p = 0.02$), even after adjustment on tacrolimus concentrations. No differences were observed between groups for 2 h-AUC glucose and HOMA-IR. The authors suggest that a disparity in the timing of supplementation and consequent drug exposure along with the use of tacrolimus versus cyclosporine can explain the smaller effect of their intervention compared with other trials [60]. Similar results were observed in another study including 52 renal transplant recipients on tacrolimus with chronic hypomagnesemia. Recipients were randomized to the Mg group ($n = 26$), with a similar Mg supplementation as previously described, or the control group ($n = 26$). No differences between the groups were observed in first-phase insulin release, in second-phase insulin release, HbA1c and HOMA-IR index at month 6 post-transplantation [61]. The main limitation of this study was that oral Mg supplementation failed to increase both serum and intracellular Mg significantly over the concentrations observed in the control group. Thus, it was impossible to draw conclusions on the effects of Mg supplementation on insulin resistance and glucose metabolism.

While most studies converge to confirm that hypomagnesemia is an independent risk factor for PTDM, the impact of hypomagnesemia correction after kidney transplantation has not yet been fully explored. Literature analysis also highlights the need for studies in order to determine the best routes for Mg supplementation, formulations and doses to achieve normal serum Mg concentration in these patients.

An important issue is the impact of immunosuppressive regimen according to diabetes risk and their impact on post-transplant Mg status. As underline above, CNI induce renal Mg wasting which contributes to hypomagnesemia. In the study from Van Laecke et al., the association between CNI and PTDM disappeared after adjustment on Mg levels, suggesting that the diabetogenic effect of CNI was at least partially related to CNI-induced hypomagnesemia [53]. The switch from CNI to mTOR inhibitors has been shown to result in serum Mg increase [62]. Thus, the early use of mTOR inhibitors soon after transplantation could be an interesting approach to decrease PTDM risk. However, several reports have shown a diabetogenic effect of mTOR inhibitors, and in the study from Van Laecke et al., sirolimus appeared as an independent risk factor of PTDM [53,63]. Moreover, the use of mTOR inhibitors soon after kidney transplantation has been shown to be associated with a higher risk of allograft rejection [64]. For these reasons, mTOR inhibitor in replacement of CNI may not be an interesting approach to reduce PTDM risk.

7. Magnesium Status and Cardiovascular Risk before and after Kidney Transplantation

PTDM-associated mortality is mainly related to cardiovascular events, which are today the main causes of death in kidney transplant patients [65]. Hypomagnesemia has been shown to play a role in the pathogenesis of arterial hypertension, endothelial dysfunction, dyslipidemia and inflammation, with all these factors contributing to coronary heart disease (CHD).

In vitro, exposure of endothelial cells to low Mg concentrations reversibly inhibits endothelial proliferation and was associated with an up-regulation of interleukin-1, Vascular Cell Adhesion Molecule-1 and Plasminogen Activator Inhibitor-1 [66]. In vivo, hypomagnesemia is associated with increased CRP levels, leukocyte and macrophage activation, NFKB/cytokines activation and platelet aggregation. Furthermore, inbred mice with low intracellular Mg levels have significantly impaired endothelial function together with decreased endothelial NO synthase expression [67].

The relationship between CHD and serum Mg concentrations was studied in a cohort of 13,922 middle-age adults. In this study, after adjustment, the relative risk of CHD across quartiles of serum Mg was 1.00, 0.92, 0.48, and 0.44 (*p* for trend = 0.009) among women and 1.00, 1.32, 0.95, and 0.73 (*p* for trend = 0.07) among men. Moreover, patients who developed CHD had a lower serum Mg concentration than the controls, suggesting that low serum Mg was an independent risk factor for CHD [68].

In a Japanese cohort of 728 subjects, lower serum Mg was significantly and independently associated with mean intima-media thickness (*p* = 0.004) and risk of $\geq$2 carotid plaques (*p* = 0.03) [69]. Hypomagnesemia was also reported to directly or indirectly affect vascular stiffness in the general population [70]. In another study, Mg supplementation improved endothelial dysfunction in patients with CHD [71]. In parallel, hypomagnesemia may play a role in the promotion and progression of vascular calcification as underlined earlier. Indeed, Mg is known to prevent tissue calcification by increasing natural inhibitors of calcification such as fetuin A, carboxylated matrix Gla protein (MGP), osteopontin and the inorganic inhibitory compound pyrophosphate [72].

Few studies investigated the association between Mg levels and cardiovascular risk after kidney transplantation. In a small crossover trial published in 1998, 15 renal transplant patients were randomized in a 6-week treatment period with either placebo or Mg oxide (MgO) 2 g per os with a 2-week washout interval, then 6-weeks of the alternative agent (placebo or MgO). There was no reduction in systolic or diastolic blood pressure in either cholesterol or triglyceride level with magnesium supplementation [73].

Finally, the association between serum Mg level and cardiovascular risk after kidney transplantation has been poorly studied. A small crossover trial, including 15 kidney transplant patients randomized in a 6-week treatment period with either the placebo or Mg oxide (MgO) 2 g per os with a 2-week washout interval, then 6-weeks of the alternative agent (placebo or MgO), was published 1998. No change in metabolic profile, including systolic or diastolic blood pressure control, or cholesterol or triglyceride levels was observed with Mg supplementation [73]. The relationship between hypomagnesemia and vascular stiffness was investigated in a study published in 2011. An evaluation was conducted in 512 renal transplant recipients, by determination of carotid-femoral pulse wave velocity. Serum Mg was an independent risk factor for arterial stiffness, but this association was attenuated after adjustment on the use of sirolimus ($p = 0.054$). After stratification according to the median age of 55 years and adjustment with covariates, Mg remained an independent predictor of pulse wave velocity ($p = 0.024$) [74].

8. Conclusions

Despite relying on retrospective studies, a body of evidence links hypomagnesemia to PTDM and cardiovascular risk in kidney transplant patients (Figure 2). Given the frequency of PTDM and its relationship with cardiovascular risk, correcting hypomagnesemia soon after transplantation could translate into a significant decrease in vascular disease, which today is the primary cause of death in kidney transplant recipients. Thus, prospective studies to evaluate the impact of hypomagnesemia correction after kidney transplantation, as well as the best ways of achieving correction are needed.

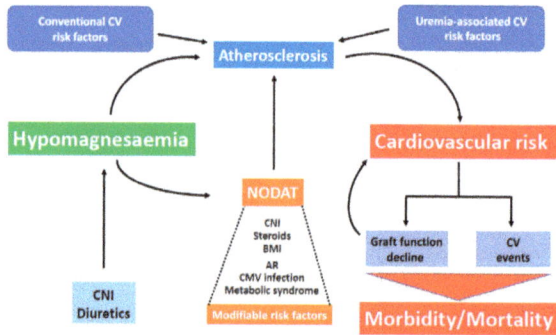

Figure 2. Deleterious effects of hypomagnesaemia after kidney transplantation. Several studies support that posttransplant hypomagnesaemia increases cardiovascular (CV) risk by increasing the risk of post-transplant diabetes mellitus (PTDM) development and by favoring accelerated atherosclerosis, along with other more conventional risk factors. We suggest that hypomagnesaemia correction soon after kidney transplantation may allow to decrease CV risk and result in less CV-related morbidity and mortality in kidney transplant recipients.

Author Contributions: A.-S.G., wrote and revised the manuscript. A.D., revised the manuscript. M.P., revised the manuscript. J.-F.S., revised the manuscript. J.S., revised the manuscript. J.-F.A., corresponding author wrote and revised the manuscript.

Conflicts of Interest: The authors declare no conflicts of interest.

Abbreviations

AUC	Area under the curve
CKD	Chronic kidney disease
CNI	Calcineurin inhibitors
ESRD	End-stage renal disease
HD	Hemodialysis
HOMA_IR	Homeostasis model assessment-estimated insulin-resistance index
Mg	Magnesium
PD	Peritoneal dialysis
PTDM	Post-transplant diabetes mellitus
TRPM6	Transient Receptor Potential Melastatin 6

References

1. Jahnen-Dechent, W.; Ketteler, M. Magnesium basics. *Clin. Kidney J.* **2012**, *5*, i3–i14. [CrossRef] [PubMed]
2. Weisinger, J.R.; Bellorín-Font, E. Magnesium and phosphorus. *Lancet* **1998**, *352*, 391–396. [CrossRef]
3. Fawcett, W.J.; Haxby, E.J.; Male, D.A. Magnesium: Physiology and pharmacology. *Br. J. Anaesth.* **1999**, *83*, 302–320. [CrossRef] [PubMed]
4. Tietz, N.W.; Rinker, A.D.; Morrison, S.R. When is a serum iron really a serum iron? The status of serum iron measurements. *Clin. Chem.* **1994**, *40*, 546–551. [PubMed]
5. Kanbay, M.; Goldsmith, D.; Uyar, M.E.; Turgut, F.; Covic, A. Magnesium in chronic kidney disease: Challenges and opportunities. *Blood Purif.* **2010**, *29*, 280–292. [CrossRef] [PubMed]
6. Cunningham, J.; Rodríguez, M.; Messa, P. Magnesium in chronic kidney disease Stages 3 and 4 and in dialysis patients. *Clin. Kidney J.* **2012**, *5*, i39–i51. [CrossRef] [PubMed]
7. Whang, R.; Ryder, K.W. Frequency of hypomagnesemia and hypermagnesemia. Requested vs. routine. *JAMA* **1990**, *263*, 3063–3064. [CrossRef] [PubMed]
8. Nichols, C.G.; Ho, K.; Hebert, S. Mg(2+)-dependent inward rectification of ROMK1 potassium channels expressed in Xenopus oocytes. *J. Physiol. (Lond.)* **1994**, *476*, 399–409. [CrossRef]
9. Agus, Z.S.; Kelepouris, E.; Dukes, I.; Morad, M. Cytosolic magnesium modulates calcium channel activity in mammalian ventricular cells. *Am. J. Physiol.* **1989**, *256*, C452–C455. [CrossRef] [PubMed]
10. Hashizume, N.; Mori, M. An analysis of hypermagnesemia and hypomagnesemia. *Jpn. J. Med.* **1990**, *29*, 368–372. [CrossRef] [PubMed]
11. Kafka, H.; Langevin, L.; Armstrong, P.W. Serum magnesium and potassium in acute myocardial infarction. Influence on ventricular arrhythmias. *Arch. Intern. Med.* **1987**, *147*, 465–469. [CrossRef] [PubMed]
12. Aglio, L.S.; Stanford, G.G.; Maddi, R.; Boyd, J.L.; Nussbaum, S.; Chernow, B. Hypomagnesemia is common following cardiac surgery. *J. Cardiothorac. Vasc. Anesth.* **1991**, *5*, 201–208. [CrossRef]
13. England, M.R.; Gordon, G.; Salem, M.; Chernow, B. Magnesium administration and dysrhythmias after cardiac surgery. A placebo-controlled, double-blind, randomized trial. *JAMA* **1992**, *268*, 2395–2402. [CrossRef] [PubMed]
14. Agus, Z.S. Hypomagnesemia. *J. Am. Soc. Nephrol.* **1999**, *10*, 1616–1622. [PubMed]
15. Truttmann, A.C.; Faraone, R.; Von Vigier, R.O.; Nuoffer, J.M.; Pfister, R.; Bianchetti, M.G. Maintenance hemodialysis and circulating ionized magnesium. *Nephron* **2002**, *92*, 616–621. [CrossRef] [PubMed]
16. Blumenkrantz, M.J.; Kopple, J.D.; Moran, J.K.; Coburn, J.W. Metabolic balance studies and dietary protein requirements in patients undergoing continuous ambulatory peritoneal dialysis. *Kidney Int.* **1982**, *21*, 849–861. [CrossRef] [PubMed]
17. Ishimura, E.; Okuno, S.; Yamakawa, T.; Inaba, M.; Nishizawa, Y. Serum magnesium concentration is a significant predictor of mortality in maintenance hemodialysis patients. *Magnes. Res.* **2007**, *20*, 237–244. [PubMed]
18. Sakaguchi, Y.; Fujii, N.; Shoji, T.; Hayashi, T.; Rakugi, H.; Isaka, Y. Hypomagnesemia is a significant predictor of cardiovascular and non-cardiovascular mortality in patients undergoing hemodialysis. *Kidney Int.* **2014**, *85*, 174–181. [CrossRef] [PubMed]
19. Meema, H.E.; Oreopoulos, D.G.; Rapoport, A. Serum magnesium level and arterial calcification in end-stage renal disease. *Kidney Int.* **1987**, *32*, 388–394. [CrossRef] [PubMed]
20. Ishimura, E.; Okuno, S.; Kitatani, K.; Tsuchida, T.; Yamakawa, T.; Shioi, A.; Inaba, M.; Nishizawa, Y. Significant association between the presence of peripheral vascular calcification and lower serum magnesium in hemodialysis patients. *Clin. Nephrol.* **2007**, *68*, 222–227. [CrossRef] [PubMed]
21. Turgut, F.; Kanbay, M.; Metin, M.R.; Uz, E.; Akcay, A.; Covic, A. Magnesium supplementation helps to improve carotid intima media thickness in patients on hemodialysis. *Int. Urol. Nephrol.* **2008**, *40*, 1075–1082. [CrossRef] [PubMed]
22. Schmaderer, C.; Braunisch, M.C.; Suttmann, Y.; Lorenz, G.; Pham, D.; Haller, B.; Angermann, S.; Matschkal, J.; Renders, L.; Baumann, M.; et al. Reduced Mortality in Maintenance Haemodialysis Patients on High versus Low Dialysate Magnesium: A Pilot Study. *Nutrients* **2017**, *9*, 926. [CrossRef] [PubMed]
23. Margreiter, R. European Tacrolimus vs. Ciclosporin Microemulsion Renal Transplantation Study Group Efficacy and safety of tacrolimus compared with ciclosporin microemulsion in renal transplantation: A randomised multicentre study. *Lancet* **2002**, *359*, 741–746. [CrossRef]

24. Ledeganck, K.J.; De Winter, B.Y.; Van den Driessche, A.; Jürgens, A.; Bosmans, J.-L.; Couttenye, M.M.; Verpooten, G.A. Magnesium loss in cyclosporine-treated patients is related to renal epidermal growth factor downregulation. *Nephrol. Dial. Transplant.* **2014**, *29*, 1097–1102. [CrossRef] [PubMed]

25. Nijenhuis, T.; Hoenderop, J.G.J.; Bindels, R.J.M. Downregulation of Ca(2+) and Mg(2+) transport proteins in the kidney explains tacrolimus (FK506)-induced hypercalciuria and hypomagnesemia. *J. Am. Soc. Nephrol.* **2004**, *15*, 549–557. [CrossRef] [PubMed]

26. Da Silva, C.A.; de Bragança, A.C.; Shimizu, M.H.M.; Sanches, T.R.; Fortes, M.A.Z.; Giorgi, R.R.; Andrade, L.; Seguro, A.C. Rosiglitazone prevents sirolimus-induced hypomagnesemia, hypokalemia, and downregulation of NKCC2 protein expression. *Am. J. Physiol. Renal Physiol.* **2009**, *297*, F916–F922. [PubMed]

27. Andoh, T.F.; Burdmann, E.A.; Fransechini, N.; Houghton, D.C.; Bennett, W.M. Comparison of acute rapamycin nephrotoxicity with cyclosporine and FK506. *Kidney Int.* **1996**, *50*, 1110–1117. [CrossRef] [PubMed]

28. Van Laecke, S.; Van Biesen, W. Hypomagnesaemia in kidney transplantation. *Transplant. Rev.* **2015**, *29*, 154–160. [CrossRef] [PubMed]

29. Barton, C.H.; Vaziri, N.D.; Martin, D.C.; Choi, S.; Alikhani, S. Hypomagnesemia and renal magnesium wasting in renal transplant recipients receiving cyclosporine. *Am. J. Med.* **1987**, *83*, 693–699. [CrossRef]

30. Stevens, R.B.; Lane, J.T.; Boerner, B.P.; Miles, C.D.; Rigley, T.H.; Sandoz, J.P.; Nielsen, K.J.; Skorupa, J.Y.; Skorupa, A.J.; Kaplan, B.; Wrenshall, L.E. Single-dose rATG induction at renal transplantation: Superior renal function and glucoregulation with less hypomagnesemia: RATGS minimizes glucose dysregulation. *Clin. Transplant.* **2012**, *26*, 123–132. [CrossRef] [PubMed]

31. Van de Cauter, J.; Sennesael, J.; Haentjens, P. Long-term evolution of the mineral metabolism after renal transplantation: A prospective, single-center cohort study. *Transplant. Proc.* **2011**, *43*, 3470–3475. [CrossRef] [PubMed]

32. Rodrigues, N.; Santana, A.; Guerra, J.; Neves, M.; Nascimento, C.; Gonçalves, J.; da Costa, A.G. Serum Magnesium and Related Factors in Long-Term Renal Transplant Recipients: An Observational Study. *Transplant. Proc.* **2017**, *49*, 799–802. [CrossRef] [PubMed]

33. Holzmacher, R.; Kendziorski, C.; Michael Hofman, R.; Jaffery, J.; Becker, B.; Djamali, A. Low serum magnesium is associated with decreased graft survival in patients with chronic cyclosporin nephrotoxicity. *Nephrol. Dial. Transplant.* **2005**, *20*, 1456–1462. [CrossRef] [PubMed]

34. Miura, K.; Nakatani, T.; Asai, T.; Yamanaka, S.; Tamada, S.; Tashiro, K.; Kim, S.; Okamura, M.; Iwao, H. Role of hypomagnesemia in chronic cyclosporine nephropathy. *Transplantation* **2002**, *73*, 340–347. [CrossRef] [PubMed]

35. Yuan, J.; Zhou, J.; Chen, B.C.; Zhang, X.; Zhou, H.M.; Du, D.F.; Chang, S.; Chen, Z.K. Magnesium supplementation prevents chronic cyclosporine nephrotoxicity via adjusting nitric oxide synthase activity. *Transplant. Proc.* **2005**, *37*, 1892–1895. [CrossRef] [PubMed]

36. Asai, T.; Nakatani, T.; Yamanaka, S.; Tamada, S.; Kishimoto, T.; Tashiro, K.; Nakao, T.; Okamura, M.; Kim, S.; Iwao, H.; et al. Magnesium supplementation prevents experimental chronic cyclosporine a nephrotoxicity via renin-angiotensin system independent mechanism. *Transplantation* **2002**, *74*, 784–791. [CrossRef] [PubMed]

37. Asai, T.; Nakatani, T.; Tamada, S.; Kuwabara, N.; Yamanaka, S.; Tashiro, K.; Nakao, T.; Komiya, T.; Okamura, M.; Kim, S.; et al. Activation of transcription factors AP-1 and NF-kappaB in chronic cyclosporine A nephrotoxicity: Role in beneficial effects of magnesium supplementation. *Transplantation* **2003**, *75*, 1040–1044. [CrossRef] [PubMed]

38. Pham, P.-C.T.; Pham, P.-M.T.; Pham, S.V.; Miller, J.M.; Pham, P.-T.T. Hypomagnesemia in Patients with Type 2 Diabetes. *Clin. J. Am. Soc. Nephrol.* **2007**, *2*, 366–373. [CrossRef] [PubMed]

39. Geiger, H.; Wanner, C. Magnesium in disease. *Clin. Kidney J.* **2012**, *5*, i25–i38. [CrossRef] [PubMed]

40. Pham, P.C.T.; Pham, P.M.T.; Pham, P.a.T.; Pham, S.V.; Pham, H.V.; Miller, J.M.; Yanagawa, N.; Pham, P.T.T. Lower serum magnesium levels are associated with more rapid decline of renal function in patients with diabetes mellitus type 2. *Clin. Nephrol.* **2005**, *63*, 429–436. [CrossRef] [PubMed]

41. Lopez-Ridaura, R.; Willett, W.C.; Rimm, E.B.; Liu, S.; Stampfer, M.J.; Manson, J.E.; Hu, F.B. Magnesium intake and risk of type 2 diabetes in men and women. *Diabetes Care* **2004**, *27*, 134–140. [CrossRef] [PubMed]

42. Song, Y.; Manson, J.E.; Buring, J.E.; Liu, S. Dietary magnesium intake in relation to plasma insulin levels and risk of type 2 diabetes in women. *Diabetes Care* **2004**, *27*, 59–65. [CrossRef] [PubMed]

43. Fang, X.; Wang, K.; Han, D.; He, X.; Wei, J.; Zhao, L.; Imam, M.U.; Ping, Z.; Li, Y.; Xu, Y.; et al. Dietary magnesium intake and the risk of cardiovascular disease, type 2 diabetes, and all-cause mortality: A dose-response meta-analysis of prospective cohort studies. *BMC Med.* **2016**, *14*, 210. [CrossRef] [PubMed]
44. Kao, W.H.; Folsom, A.R.; Nieto, F.J.; Mo, J.P.; Watson, R.L.; Brancati, F.L. Serum and dietary magnesium and the risk for type 2 diabetes mellitus: The Atherosclerosis Risk in Communities Study. *Arch. Intern. Med.* **1999**, *159*, 2151–2159. [CrossRef] [PubMed]
45. Nadler, J.L.; Buchanan, T.; Natarajan, R.; Antonipillai, I.; Bergman, R.; Rude, R. Magnesium deficiency produces insulin resistance and increased thromboxane synthesis. *Hypertension* **1993**, *21*, 1024–1029. [CrossRef] [PubMed]
46. Van Laecke, S.; Van Biesen, W.; Vanholder, R. Hypomagnesaemia, the kidney and the vessels. *Nephrol. Dial. Transplant.* **2012**, *27*, 4003–4010. [CrossRef] [PubMed]
47. Rodriguez-Moran, M.; Guerrero-Romero, F. Oral Magnesium Supplementation Improves Insulin Sensitivity and Metabolic Control in Type 2 Diabetic Subjects: A randomized double-blind controlled trial. *Diabetes Care* **2003**, *26*, 1147–1152. [CrossRef] [PubMed]
48. Kasiske, B.L.; Snyder, J.J.; Gilbertson, D.; Matas, A.J. Diabetes mellitus after kidney transplantation in the United States. *Am. J. Transplant.* **2003**, *3*, 178–185. [CrossRef] [PubMed]
49. Augusto, J.-F.; Subra, J.-F.; Duveau, A.; Rakotonjanahary, J.; Dussaussoy, C.; Picquet, J.; Croue, A.; Villemain, F.; Onno, C.; Sayegh, J. Relation between Pretransplant Magnesemia and the Risk of New Onset Diabetes After Transplantation within the First Year of Kidney Transplantation. *Transplantation* **2014**, *97*, 1155–1160. [CrossRef] [PubMed]
50. Yates, C.J.; Fourlanos, S.; Hjelmesaeth, J.; Colman, P.G.; Cohney, S.J. New-onset diabetes after kidney transplantation-changes and challenges. *Am. J. Transplant.* **2012**, *12*, 820–828. [CrossRef] [PubMed]
51. Mazali, F.C.; Lalli, C.A.; Alves-Filho, G.; Mazzali, M. Posttransplant diabetes mellitus: Incidence and risk factors. *Transplant. Proc.* **2008**, *40*, 764–766. [CrossRef] [PubMed]
52. Maes, B.D.; Kuypers, D.; Messiaen, T.; Evenepoel, P.; Mathieu, C.; Coosemans, W.; Pirenne, J.; Vanrenterghem, Y.F.C. Posttransplantation Diabetes Mellitus in Fk-506-Treated Renal Transplant Recipients: Analysis of Incidence and Risk Factors. *Transplantation* **2001**, *72*, 1655–1661. [CrossRef] [PubMed]
53. Van Laecke, S.; Van Biesen, W.; Verbeke, F.; De Bacquer, D.; Peeters, P.; Vanholder, R. Posttransplantation hypomagnesemia and its relation with immunosuppression as predictors of new-onset diabetes after transplantation. *Am. J. Transplant.* **2009**, *9*, 2140–2149. [CrossRef] [PubMed]
54. Huang, J.W.; Famure, O.; Li, Y.; Kim, S.J. Hypomagnesemia and the Risk of New-Onset Diabetes Mellitus after Kidney Transplantation. *J. Am. Soc. Nephrol.* **2016**, *27*, 1793–1800. [CrossRef] [PubMed]
55. Hayes, W.; Boyle, S.; Carroll, A.; Bockenhauer, D.; Marks, S.D. Hypomagnesemia and increased risk of new-onset diabetes mellitus after transplantation in pediatric renal transplant recipients. *Pediatr. Nephrol.* **2017**, *32*, 879–884. [CrossRef] [PubMed]
56. Chanchlani, R.; Joseph Kim, S.; Kim, E.D.; Banh, T.; Borges, K.; Vasilevska-Ristovska, J.; Li, Y.; Ng, V.; Dipchand, A.I.; Solomon, M.; et al. Incidence of hyperglycemia and diabetes and association with electrolyte abnormalities in pediatric solid organ transplant recipients. *Nephrol. Dial. Transplant.* **2017**, *32*, 1579–1586. [CrossRef] [PubMed]
57. Osorio, J.M.; Bravo, J.; Pérez, A.; Ferreyra, C.; Osuna, A. Magnesemia in Renal Transplant Recipients: Relation With Immunosuppression and Posttransplant Diabetes. *Transplant. Proc.* **2010**, *42*, 2910–2913. [CrossRef] [PubMed]
58. Santos, L.; Rodrigo, E.; Piñera, C.; Robledo, C.; Palomar, R.; Gómez-Alamillo, C.; González-Cotorruelo, J.; Arias, M. Elevated serum gamma-glutamyltransferase and hypomagnesemia are not related with new-onset diabetes after transplantation. *Transplant. Proc.* **2010**, *42*, 2914–2916. [CrossRef] [PubMed]
59. Van Laecke, S.; Desideri, F.; Geerts, A.; Van Vlierberghe, H.; Berrevoet, F.; Rogiers, X.; Troisi, R.; de Hemptinne, B.; Vanholder, R.; Colle, I. Hypomagnesemia and the risk of new-onset diabetes after liver transplantation. *Liver Transplant.* **2010**, *16*, 1278–1287. [CrossRef] [PubMed]
60. Van Laecke, S.; Nagler, E.V.; Taes, Y.; Van Biesen, W.; Peeters, P.; Vanholder, R. The effect of magnesium supplements on early post-transplantation glucose metabolism: A randomized controlled trial. *Transpl. Int.* **2014**, *27*, 895–902. [CrossRef] [PubMed]

61. Van Laecke, S.; Caluwe, R.; Huybrechts, I.; Nagler, E.V.; Vanholder, R.; Peeters, P.; Van Vlem, B.; Van Biesen, W. Effect of Magnesium Supplements on Insulin Secretion After Kidney Transplantation: A Randomized Controlled Trial. *Ann. Transplant.* **2017**, *22*, 524–531. [CrossRef] [PubMed]
62. Sánchez-Fructuoso, A.I.; Santín Cantero, J.M.; Pérez Flores, I.; Valero San Cecilio, R.; Calvo Romero, N.; Vilalta Casas, R. Changes in magnesium and potassium homeostasis after conversion from a calcineurin inhibitor regimen to an mTOR inhibitor-based regimen. *Transplant. Proc.* **2010**, *42*, 3047–3049. [CrossRef] [PubMed]
63. Murakami, N.; Riella, L.V.; Funakoshi, T. Risk of metabolic complications in kidney transplantation after conversion to mTOR inhibitor: A systematic review and meta-analysis. *Am. J. Transplant.* **2014**, *14*, 2317–2327. [CrossRef] [PubMed]
64. Grimbert, P.; Thaunat, O. mTOR inhibitors and risk of chronic antibody-mediated rejection after kidney transplantation: Where are we now? *Transpl. Int.* **2017**, *30*, 647–657. [CrossRef] [PubMed]
65. Zhang, R.; Kumar, P.; Reisin, E.; Ramcharan, T. Kidney Transplantation: The Evolving Challenges. *Am. J. Med. Sci.* **2004**, *328*, 156–161. [CrossRef] [PubMed]
66. Maier, J.A.M.; Malpuech-Brugère, C.; Zimowska, W.; Rayssiguier, Y.; Mazur, A. Low magnesium promotes endothelial cell dysfunction: Implications for atherosclerosis, inflammation and thrombosis. *Biochim. Biophys. Acta* **2004**, *1689*, 13–21. [CrossRef] [PubMed]
67. Paravicini, T.M.; Yogi, A.; Mazur, A.; Touyz, R.M. Dysregulation of Vascular TRPM7 and Annexin-1 is Associated with Endothelial Dysfunction in Inherited Hypomagnesemia. *Hypertension* **2009**, *53*, 423–429. [CrossRef] [PubMed]
68. Liao, F.; Folsom, A.R.; Brancati, F.L. Is low magnesium concentration a risk factor for coronary heart disease? The Atherosclerosis Risk in Communities (ARIC) Study. *Am. Heart J.* **1998**, *136*, 480–490. [CrossRef]
69. Hashimoto, T.; Hara, A.; Ohkubo, T.; Kikuya, M.; Shintani, Y.; Metoki, H.; Inoue, R.; Asayama, K.; Kanno, A.; Nakashita, M.; et al. Serum Magnesium, Ambulatory Blood Pressure, and Carotid Artery Alteration: The Ohasama Study. *Am. J. Hypertens.* **2010**, *23*, 1292–1298. [CrossRef] [PubMed]
70. Kisters, K.; Gremmler, B.; Hausberg, M. Magnesium and arterial stiffness. *Hypertension* **2006**, *47*, e3. [CrossRef] [PubMed]
71. Shechter, M.; Sharir, M.; Labrador, M.J.; Forrester, J.; Silver, B.; Bairey Merz, C.N. Oral magnesium therapy improves endothelial function in patients with coronary artery disease. *Circulation* **2000**, *102*, 2353–2358. [CrossRef] [PubMed]
72. Massy, Z.A.; Drüeke, T.B. Magnesium and outcomes in patients with chronic kidney disease: Focus on vascular calcification, atherosclerosis and survival. *Clin. Kidney J.* **2012**, *5*, i52–i61. [CrossRef] [PubMed]
73. Nguyen, T.; Steiner, R.W. A trial of oral magnesium supplementation in renal transplant recipients receiving cyclosporine. *Transplant. Proc.* **1998**, *30*, 4317–4319. [CrossRef]
74. Van Laecke, S.; Maréchal, C.; Verbeke, F.; Peeters, P.; Van Biesen, W.; Devuyst, O.; Jadoul, M.; Vanholder, R. The relation between hypomagnesaemia and vascular stiffness in renal transplant recipients. *Nephrol. Dial. Transplant.* **2011**, *26*, 2362–2369. [CrossRef] [PubMed]

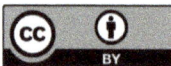

nutrients

MDPI

Review

The Role of Magnesium in Neurological Disorders

Anna E. Kirkland [1], Gabrielle L. Sarlo [1] and Kathleen F. Holton [2,3,*]

1   Department of Psychology, Behavior, Cognition and Neuroscience Program, American University, Washington, DC 20016, USA; ak0698a@american.edu (A.E.K.); gs0703a@american.edu (G.L.S.)
2   Department of Health Studies, American University, Washington, DC 20016, USA
3   Center for Behavioral Neuroscience, American University, Washington, DC 20016, USA
*   Correspondence: holton@american.edu; Tel.: +1-202-885-3797

Received: 2 May 2018; Accepted: 4 June 2018; Published: 6 June 2018

Abstract: Magnesium is well known for its diverse actions within the human body. From a neurological standpoint, magnesium plays an essential role in nerve transmission and neuromuscular conduction. It also functions in a protective role against excessive excitation that can lead to neuronal cell death (excitotoxicity), and has been implicated in multiple neurological disorders. Due to these important functions within the nervous system, magnesium is a mineral of intense interest for the potential prevention and treatment of neurological disorders. Current literature is reviewed for migraine, chronic pain, epilepsy, Alzheimer's, Parkinson's, and stroke, as well as the commonly comorbid conditions of anxiety and depression. Previous reviews and meta-analyses are used to set the scene for magnesium research across neurological conditions, while current research is reviewed in greater detail to update the literature and demonstrate the progress (or lack thereof) in the field. There is strong data to suggest a role for magnesium in migraine and depression, and emerging data to suggest a protective effect of magnesium for chronic pain, anxiety, and stroke. More research is needed on magnesium as an adjunct treatment in epilepsy, and to further clarify its role in Alzheimer's and Parkinson's. Overall, the mechanistic attributes of magnesium in neurological diseases connote the macromineral as a potential target for neurological disease prevention and treatment.

Keywords: magnesium; excitotoxicity; glutamate; migraine; chronic pain; epilepsy; Alzheimer's; Parkinson's; stroke

1. Introduction

Magnesium is a very important macromineral in the diet with a multitude of roles in the human body, including serving as a cofactor in more than 300 enzymatic reactions. Magnesium is essential for regulation of muscle contraction (including that of the heart), blood pressure, insulin metabolism, and is required for the synthesis of DNA, RNA, and proteins [1]. In the nervous system, magnesium is important for optimal nerve transmission and neuromuscular coordination, as well as serving to protect against excitotoxicity (excessive excitation leading to cell death) [1,2].

One of the main neurological functions of magnesium is due to magnesium's interaction with the N-methyl-D-aspartate (NMDA) receptor. Magnesium serves as a blockade to the calcium channel in the NMDA receptor (Figure 1), and must be removed for glutamatergic excitatory signaling to occur [3]. Low magnesium levels may theoretically potentiate glutamatergic neurotransmission, leading to a supportive environment for excitotoxicity, which can lead to oxidative stress and neuronal cell death [4]. Abnormal glutamatergic neurotransmission has been implicated in many neurological and psychiatric disorders [5] including: migraine, chronic pain, epilepsy, Alzheimer's, Parkinson's, and stroke, in addition to depression and anxiety, which are commonly comorbid with these neurological disorders. Molecular studies [6] and animal studies [7] have shown neuronal protection from pre-treatment with magnesium, making this mineral of intense interest for its potential neuroprotective role in humans.

Thus, magnesium could be an important dietary factor in the prevention and/or treatment of the above conditions.

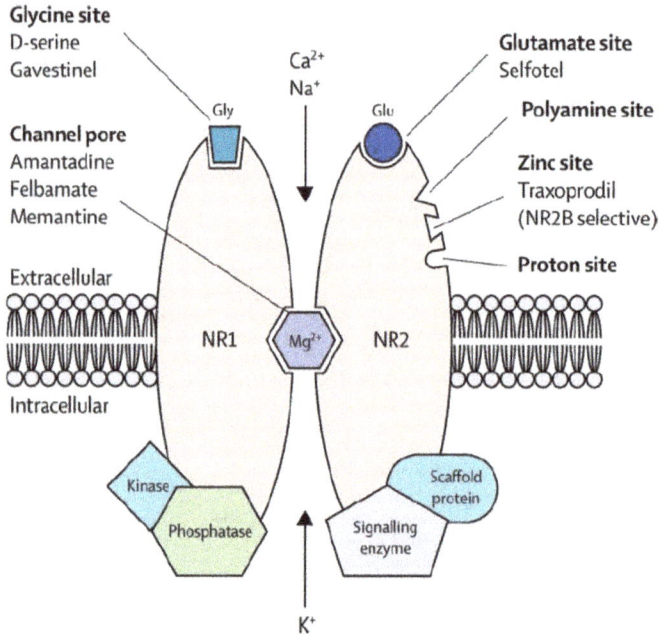

Figure 1. Glutamatergic N-methyl-D-aspartate receptor with magnesium block of calcium channel. Reprinted from [8] with permission from Elsevier.

It has been estimated that approximately half of the US population is consuming inadequate amounts of magnesium [9]. Due to the wide-ranging functions of magnesium, inadequate intake could predispose individuals to multiple health issues, including those related to neurological conditions. This review aims to summarize the recent human literature on what is known about magnesium and the following neurological disorders: migraine, chronic pain, epilepsy, Alzheimer's, Parkinson's, and stroke, as well as anxiety and depression. Recommendations will also be made for future research directions.

2. Materials and Methods

A search was completed using PubMed, MEDLINE, PsychINFO, and Wiley-Blackwell Cochrane Library. Abstracts were pulled for all available literature and were then reviewed by all three authors and a consensus decision was made about which papers met inclusion criteria. Studies of adult human populations from any year were included if they were written in English. Papers were reviewed for every article that met the review criteria, including magnesium levels (e.g., blood serum, cerebrospinal fluid, etc.) or magnesium treatment in human populations with migraine, chronic pain, anxiety, depression, epilepsy, Alzheimer's disease, Parkinson's disease, and stroke. Search strings included the neurological or commonly comorbid disorder AND "magnesium", "intravenous magnesium", "oral magnesium", or "magnesium treatment". Reviews and meta-analyses were used to gain an understanding of where the current literature stands in magnesium research across neurological disorders. The most recent reviews and meta-analyses are discussed in order to reduce duplication and provide a wide scope of the literature previously reviewed. New studies are described in detail to provide an update on the literature. If there was not a review or meta-analysis, like in the case of

Parkinson's disease, available research was compiled and reviewed. Figure 2 summarizes the search strategy and demonstrates the disparity in the number of magnesium research studies ranging from the most studied (i.e., migraine) to the least studied (i.e., Parkinson's disease).

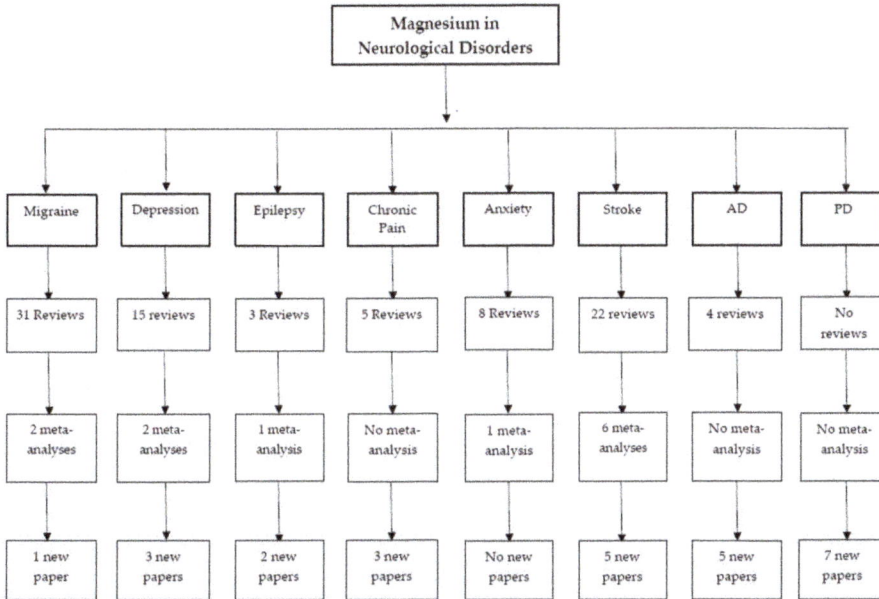

Figure 2. Flow chart of magnesium in neurological disorders literature. New papers refer to published research not included in previously-published reviews and meta-analyses. AD = Alzheimer's Disease; PD = Parkinson's Disease.

3. Results

3.1. Migraine

Migraine is the most common neurological disorder in the United Sates with a prevalence rate of 16.2% [10]. It is classified by recurrent moderate to severe headaches with or without aura, often lasting between 4 and 27 h with many associated symptoms, including nausea, vomiting, and sensitivity to various environmental stimuli [11,12]. Although the exact mechanisms are not yet fully understood, alterations in the excitability of the central nervous system, spontaneous neuronal depolarization, and abnormal mitochondria functioning have been connected to migraines. Since glutamate is the most abundant excitatory neurotransmitter, it is often linked to etiological, prevention, and treatment discussions concerning migraines [13]. Magnesium has been a proposed treatment option for migraines due to its blockade of the glutamatergic N-methyl-D-aspartate (NMDA) receptor, a receptor known to be an active contributor to pain transmission and cortical spreading depression [14]. Magnesium is also known to be a key metabolic factor in mitochondrial functioning and lowers membrane permeability reducing the possibility of spontaneous neuronal depression due to hyperexcitability [15]. Past research has shown that significantly lower levels of magnesium have been reported in serum, saliva, and cerebrospinal fluid of individuals with migraines during, and between, migraine attacks [12,16–18], along with evidence suggesting lower brain concentrations of magnesium based on MR spectroscopy [18].

Oral and intravenous magnesium administration has been proposed as a treatment option for migraines since the late 1980s and the results have been analyzed by several meta-analyses and reviews over the past three decades. In 2014, Choi and Parmer completed a meta-analysis using odds ratio (OR) on 5 randomized controlled trials published between 2000 and 2005 [19–23] and did not find strong evidence for magnesium as an effective treatment. It was concluded that i.v. magnesium resulted in a 7% lower relief rate 30 min post administration than the control groups (OR = −0.07), 37% greater side effect response rate (OR = 0.37), and no significant difference between the use of i.v. magnesium, placebo, or other migraine medications tested. However, 1 study included in the meta-analysis showed differences between migraines with and without aura; i.v. magnesium was significantly more effective at migraine relief in individuals with aura than placebo at 60 min post administration ($p < 0.05$) [24]. A more recent meta-analysis by Chiu et al. in 2016, reviewed a larger sample of randomized clinical trials with 11 studies investigating the effects of intravenous magnesium on acute migraines [19–21,25–30] and 10 studies investigating the effects of oral magnesium on migraine prophylaxis [16,31–39]. Using odds ratios, it was concluded that i.v. magnesium treatment for acute migraines resulted in significant relief across 15–45 min (OR = 0.23), 120 min (OR = 0.20), and 24 h (OR = 0.27) post magnesium administration. Similarly, oral magnesium treatment resulted in significantly reduced frequency of migraine attacks (OR = 0.20) and intensity of the attacks (OR = 0.27). Overall, this meta-analysis presents evidence for the usefulness of magnesium in both i.v. or oral forms on the treatment of migraines [40]. It also expands on the previous meta-analysis since it included randomized clinical trials published in English and Chinese investigating i.v. magnesium or oral magnesium treatment. This broadened the scope, sample size, and external validity of their work.

One quasi-experimental study has been published since the most current review comparing 2 g of i.v. magnesium sulfate compared to 60 mg of caffeine citrate on individuals presenting with a migraine at two hospitals. While both groups displayed improved pain scores over 1 hour, the magnesium group had significantly greater improvement when compared to the group receiving caffeine ($p < 0.001$) [41].

The beneficial use of magnesium in the prevention of migraine and the quality of life improvement has a Grade C evidence classification, meaning it is possibly an effective treatment based on current data. This classification is based on finding a reduction in migraine days between 22–43% across five clinical trials reviewed from 1990–2016. It is suggested that 600 mg of magnesium daily may be a safe and cost effective component of migraine care [42]. While Grade C evidence is not ideal, evidence of the effectiveness for the prevention and treatment of migraines using oral or i.v. magnesium may very well become stronger over time with the publication of more intervention and prospective cohort studies. Overall, while recent evidence does point towards i.v. and oral magnesium as potentially effective treatment options, randomized controlled clinical trials with larger sample sizes and standardized experimental designs need to be conducted in order to have more confidence in the efficacy of magnesium treatment for migraines, and to better understand how magnesium compares to current pharmaceuticals used in the prevention and treatment of migraines.

3.2. Chronic Pain

Pain is a universal sensation that can be presented in several different forms, ranging from acute to chronic. Chronic pain is broadly defined as persistent pain lasting at least three months often spurred on by central pain amplification, although the exact mechanism of pain can vary (e.g., nociceptive, neuropathic, central, etc.) or is sometimes unidentified [43]. It is estimated that chronic regional pain may be present in 20–25% of the population and chronic widespread pain may be present in 10% of the population [44]. As discussed earlier, magnesium blocks the NMDA receptor channels limiting the influx of calcium. Therefore, moderate doses of magnesium may be able to reduce the risk of excitotoxicity [45]. It is proposed that the pain relieving effects of magnesium may be dependent on the blockade of NMDA receptors in the spinal cord [46]. Magnesium is thought to produce antinociceptive and analgesic effects in patients with chronic pain and has been studied as a treatment target for chronic pain in several forms [45].

Research exploring the analgesic use of magnesium in chronic pain disorders is limited by the type and severity of chronic pain evaluated. A review on the use of magnesium as an alternative treatment for chronic pain was recently published [47]. Chronic pain was defined as pain lasting more than three months in any body part, including chronic complex regional pain syndrome, chronic low back pain, fibromyalgia, neuropathy, or pain of vascular origin. Two double-blind randomized clinical trials on complex regional pain syndrome (CRPS) [48,49] and 1 double-blind randomized clinical trial on chronic low back pain [50] were reviewed. The studies used intravenous, intradermal, and oral magnesium administration compared to placebo. The 2 CRPS randomized clinical trials had conflicting results; Fischer et al. reported no differences in CRPS pain between patients who received i.v. magnesium and those who received a placebo using several outcome measures [48]. However, van de Plas reported significant differences between intramuscular magnesium administration and a placebo on the numeric rating scale (NRS) pain assessment scores, but not on the McGill Pain Questionnaire [49]. Both studies reported more adverse effects in the groups receiving magnesium than placebo. Yousef and Al-deeb investigated the use of i.v. magnesium followed by oral magnesium compared to a placebo on chronic lower back pain over six months using NRS pain assessment scores. Beginning at two weeks, and continuing throughout the six months of follow up, the group receiving magnesium treatment had significantly improved scores from baseline measurements. Furthermore, the magnesium group had significantly lower pain scores than the placebo group at six months [50]. Based on the review of these studies, magnesium may be a viable treatment option for some types of chronic pain. A protocol was published in 2015 describing a clinical trial that is currently investigating the effects of oral magnesium administration in patients with peripheral arterial occlusive disease [51]. This trial will add much needed evidence on the potential validity of using oral magnesium as a treatment for chronic pain.

Fibromyalgia was initially considered a rheumatic disorder, but is now known to be a neurological condition, with intense widespread pain and tenderness coupled with other unpleasant symptoms, such as severe fatigue, cognitive dysfunction, memory loss, headache, and sleep problems [52,53]. As with other chronic widespread pain conditions, it is thought that pain neurotransmission occurs through glutamate's action on the NMDA receptor [54]; thus, magnesium is likely to play a protective role. It has also been proposed that fibromyalgia may be a result of insufficient levels of substances necessary for ATP synthesis, such as oxygen, magnesium, ADP, and inorganic phosphate. Magnesium is a key component within this process as it is needed for both aerobic and anaerobic glycolysis. It also aids in maintaining low cytosolic calcium in order to limit the inhibition of ATP synthesis within the mitochondria, ultimately reducing the chances of cell death caused by mitochondrial calcification [55]. Due to the overlap in symptomatology and the mechanistic actions of magnesium, researchers have studied magnesium levels in individuals with fibromyalgia, resulting in conflicting findings between modes of magnesium detection. Erythrocyte [56–59] and intracellular muscle magnesium levels [60] are decreased in fibromyalgia patients while there has been evidence that plasma and serum levels remain in normal ranges [57–59,61]. However, other studies have shown significantly decreased magnesium serum levels in fibromyalgia patients, as compared to controls [53,62,63]. Based on these findings, a recent study examined the effects of 300 mg magnesium citrate and 10 mg of amitriptyline, alone and in combination, in 60 women with fibromyalgia and 20 age- and sex-matched controls over eight weeks. Both erythrocyte and serum magnesium levels were significantly lower in the fibromyalgia group. Furthermore, the group receiving the combination of magnesium and amitriptyline reported significantly decreased pain across various pain and tenderness index scores, while magnesium alone resulted in an improvement in the number of tender points and the intensity of fibromyalgia pain [53]. Another study reported improved scores on the Fibromyalgia Impact Questionnaire-Revised (FIQR) after 8 weeks of transdermal magnesium chloride solution use [64].

It is too early to conclude whether or not magnesium is a viable treatment option for general or specific forms of chronic pain. However, the preliminary data concerning varying levels of systemic magnesium and supplementation of magnesium orally, transdermally, and intravenously for fibromyalgia and other forms of chronic pain, suggest the potential for magnesium to be an important player in the treatment and prevention of chronic pain.

3.3. Anxiety and Depression

Anxiety and depression are both common comorbid conditions with neurological illness [65] especially with chronic pain conditions [66], including migraine [67]. Anxiety and depression are also similarly mediated by altered glutamatergic neurotransmission, which may account for this comorbidity [68,69]. Since magnesium has the ability to modulate glutamatergic neurotransmission through its action at the N-methyl-D-asparate (NMDA) receptor [70], it may be possible for hypomagnesaemia to contribute to both the neurological symptoms, as well as the psychiatric symptoms.

With a lifetime prevalence rate of 15% in the general population, anxiety is considered the most pervasive psychiatric affective disorder [71]. Magnesium is involved in several physiological processes in the psychoneuroendrocrine system and modulates the hypothalamic pituitary adrenal (HPA) axis, along with blocking the calcium influx of NMDA glutamatergic receptors, all of which help prevent feelings of stress and anxiety [72]. While the data on serum and cerebrospinal fluid levels of magnesium are limited, these concentrations have been shown to be modified by exposing individuals to various types of stress, resulting in a reduction in serum magnesium due to excretion by the kidneys [73], and increasing serum levels when magnesium is administered resulting in anxiolytic-like effects [74]. Dietary intake of magnesium was also found to have a slight inverse relationship with subjective anxiety scores in a large community-based sample [75]. However, one study found no difference between the serum magnesium concentrations in patients with Generalized Anxiety Disorders when compared to controls [76].

In 2017, Boyle and Dye published a review on the available studies investigating the effects of magnesium, alone or in combination, on the experience of subjective anxiety or stress (i.e., mild anxiety, premenstrual syndrome, postpartum status, and hypertension) in adult populations [72]. Eight studies were reviewed which focused on the treatment of mild anxiety with magnesium alone [77], magnesium in combination with vitamin B$_6$ [78–81], magnesium with fermented cow's drink with protein hydrolysate [82], or magnesium in combination with Hawthorn extract and California poppy [83]. Modest evidence of the beneficial use of various forms of magnesium for treatment of mild to moderate anxiety was found. However, limitations were present including the occurrence of significant placebo effects and the inability to know the exact effects of magnesium when studying multiple combined compounds. Of the 7 studies which were reviewed for anxiety associated with PMS, 5 investigated the effects of oral or i.v. magnesium administration alone [84–87] and 2 investigated the effects of magnesium in combination with vitamin B$_6$ [88,89]. Despite methodological and sample selection issues presented by Boyle and Dye, the authors concluded that there is a potential positive effect of magnesium alone, and even more so in combination with vitamin B$_6$ on PMS. One study was reviewed for the effects of 64.4 mg of oral magnesium on anxiety related to postpartum depression with no significant effects reported [90]. Overall, the summarized findings allow for marginal support of magnesium as a treatment for mild anxiety and anxiety with PMS, with several of the studies reviewed reporting positive outcomes when administering magnesium as the sole or adjunct treatment.

An earlier review by Lakhan and Vieira in 2010 had a similar conclusion: magnesium administration may have a positive impact on the treatment of multiple anxiety disorders. The authors also note that many studies and clinical trials conducted do not look at the effects of magnesium alone, a comment that holds true today [91]. To our knowledge, no new magnesium studies examining the effects of magnesium on anxiety disorders have been published since the 2017 review. There is currently a strong need for methodologically sound clinical trials exploring this treatment option, as it could improve the lives of those with anxiety disorders while eliminating the negative side effects from current medications to treat anxiety.

Depression is a psychiatric disorder that affects hundreds of millions of people around the world, with major depressive disorder (MDD) accounting for 40% of the neuropsychiatric disorders in the United States [92]. Depression is linked to poor quality of life with severe impairments and, as mentioned earlier, often presents with other comorbid disorders. While there are some beneficial biomedical and clinical therapies for depression, dietary magnesium intake could be an important adjunct treatment [93,94].

Restoring the balance of magnesium within patients with depression has been proposed to have anti-depressive effects by protecting brain structures associated with depression by reducing the cascade of cell death caused by excitotoxicity [95–97]. Magnesium may also impact depressive symptoms by interacting with the HPA system, as discussed with anxiety disorders [97,98]. As seen in several other neurological disorders, lower magnesium levels have been associated with depression. One recent study reported a negative correlation between dietary intake of magnesium and depression [93]. Studies have also observed lower cerebrospinal fluid (CSF) and serum magnesium levels in individuals diagnosed with depression as compared to controls [94] along with moderately lower levels of erythrocyte magnesium levels in patients with major depression [99]. Moreover, plasma levels of magnesium were observed to be significantly lower among those with depression, as compared to healthy controls, while also being correlated with treatment response success [100] and the severity of depressive symptoms [101,102]. However, another study reported no differences in CSF, blood, and serum magnesium levels between groups [103]. This latter finding could have been due to inaccurate assessment technique, since 99% of magnesium within the human body is located intracellularly [103].

There is neurobiological evidence to support magnesium supplementation as a treatment for depression, however, the results from the limited number of randomized controlled trials (RCTs) is not clear cut. In 2016, Rechenberg reviewed RCTs examining the use of magnesium in depressed populations. However, only three studies, with limited insight into the potential use of magnesium as a treatment, are discussed due to the lack of literature on the subject [94]. Bhudi and colleagues compared the use of magnesium to a placebo over three months as a neuroprotective agent for patients undergoing cardiac surgery. Depressive symptoms were reported at baseline and three months postsurgery as one of the outcomes measured. While depressive symptoms decreased, no significant differences were noted between the magnesium and placebo groups [104]. An RCT was conducted in 2007 to study the utility of oral magnesium as a treatment for newly-depressed elderly individuals with type 2 diabetes. After establishing the presence of hypomagnesemia, individuals were randomized to either the magnesium or imipramine treatment group for twelve weeks of treatment administration. At follow-up, there was no significant difference between the magnesium treatment group or the imipramine treatment group, with similar improvements in both arms of the clinical trial. Thus, magnesium performed as well as imipramine, an anti-depressant drug [101]. Lastly, Walker et al. showed no significant differences in reported depressive symptoms when administering 200 mg of magnesium or placebo daily, for two menstrual cycles, in a double-blind placebo-controlled crossover study, among individuals who typically report monthly depressive symptoms with PMS [85].

A meta-analysis of 11 studies was recently published examining the relationship between dietary magnesium intake and the risk of depression. Using pooled measurements of relative risk (RR) and a dose-response analysis, the authors concluded that over half of the reviewed studies supported significant effects of dietary magnesium intake in relation to a decreased risk of depression (pooled RR = 0.81) with a distinct nonlinear relationship ($p = 0.0038$) between the two factors. Furthermore, the largest risk reduction was observed with 320 mg/day of magnesium [93]. This meta-analysis adds more evidence to the theory that magnesium supplementation, either through dietary intake or other routes of administration, should be continued to be researched as a potential target for the treatment of depression.

Three newly-published studies were found since the review by Rechenberg [94] and the meta-analysis by Li et al. [93]. One clinical trial studied the use of intravenous magnesium combined with dextrose in adults with treatment-resistant depression as compared to dextrose alone in a crossover study. The authors observed significant differences in serum magnesium levels measured at two time points: baseline compared to day 8 (the last day of administration) and day 2 compared to day 8. However, depression rating scale results were not as substantial as the only difference seen was a reduction on the Patient Health Questionnaire-9 from baseline to day 7 [105]. This study was limited by its short duration of treatment. Tarleton and colleagues performed an open-label randomized trial with 126 adults comparing 248 mg of magnesium to a placebo over six weeks, resulting in the significant improvement of depression scores within the magnesium group. In fact, improvement was noted within the first two weeks of treatment [106]. Lastly, a study of 60 patients with depression and lab-confirmed hypomagnesaemia were randomized to receive either 250 mg of magnesium or a placebo for eight weeks. Using the Beck Depression Inventory-II as an outcome measure, magnesium levels and Beck scores significantly improved in the magnesium group, as compared to the placebo group [107]. It is important to note that the amount of magnesium supplemented in these latter studies was less than the recommended dietary allowance (RDA) for adults of 310–420 mg/day.

Unfortunately, the current research implementing magnesium as a treatment option for depression has not shown consistently significant results, although this does not mean it is not an effective treatment option [103,108]. There is a need for more well-designed randomized clinical trials and prospective studies of longer duration with adequately powered sample sizes to fully understand the effects of magnesium on depression.

3.4. Epilepsy

Epilepsy is a disease classified by seizure occurrence that is believed to affect 50 million people worldwide [109–111]. The widespread and debilitating effects of this disorder have resulted in the investigation of treatments that fall outside the classic treatment with anti-epileptic drugs (AEDs), especially when research suggests that new AEDs are no better at significantly reducing seizures or improving prognosis than older AEDs [112–114]. The search for alternative treatment possibilities has directed some attention towards magnesium. Magnesium is an essential element involved in many bodily processes and, as mentioned earlier, has been found to be deficient in the modern Western diet [114–116]. Moreover, seizure activity has been strongly linked to excessive glutamatergic neurotransmission, thus, magnesium could potentially modulate the excitotoxicity connected to epilepsy [117]. Extracellular magnesium has been reported to reduce spontaneous spikes in seizure activity via the NMDA receptor, while also decreasing the hyperexcitability of the neuronal surface [114,118,119]. In fact, it is well known that hypomagnesaemia, itself, can cause seizure activity with more severe deficiency [120].

Two recent reviews [114,121] have examined the literature on magnesium and epilepsy. Both reviews stress the lack of large-scale, randomized controlled trials that are essential to gaining insight into the potential role of magnesium as a treatment for epilepsy, in general, as well as more specifically, refractory epilepsy. Refractory epilepsy is of particular interest due to its lack of response to AEDs, usually resulting in the seizures and other symptoms going untreated.

In humans, magnesium deficiency has been found to result in seizures, as well as lower levels of magnesium being observed in epileptic patients when compared to healthy controls [114,121–128]. A recent meta-analysis that included 60 studies (40 on epilepsy and 25 on febrile seizures) found that magnesium levels were not significantly different in patients with epilepsy versus controls, or in patients with febrile seizures versus controls. Yet, that same study found that hair magnesium concentrations were significantly lower in both non-treated and treated epilepsy patients versus controls [129]. Another study reported lower magnesium levels in more severe cases of epilepsy and status epilepticus as compared to moderate and mild cases [124]. The relationship between disease severity and magnesium concentration is not an area that has been explored at length and could result in valuable information if more work focused on this potential association.

In regards to magnesium as a treatment, magnesium supplementation has been found to be beneficial for hypomagnesaemia, a known risk factor for seizures in both infants and adults [130,131]. Other conditions associated with symptomatic seizures, such as pre-eclampsia and eclampsia, have demonstrated an improvement as a result of magnesium supplementation, as well [132–134]. Additionally, studies that have examined subjects with a *TRPM6* gene mutation [135–137], juvenile onset Alpers syndrome [138], and a case of refractory status epilepticus in a subject with a normal MRI, have also reported therapeutic benefit from the administration of magnesium supplementation [114,121,139].

Despite the supporting evidence from these research studies, only one randomized controlled trial has been conducted on magnesium treatment for epilepsy, which focused on infantile spasms. The study found that intravenous administration of adrenocorticotropic hormone (ACTH) with magnesium supplementation for a three week period resulted in a significant reduction in seizures compared to receiving ACTH on its own. At eight weeks post administration, the group that received the magnesium supplementation had a 79% seizure-free rate compared to only a 53% seizure-free rate of the ACTH only group [140]. While this study offers promising results, there have been no other randomized controlled studies completed since the last review in 2015. A recent study investigated the interictal total serum magnesium concentrations along with serum ionized magnesium concentrations in 104 drug-resistant epileptic individuals. Data was collected at baseline and 14 years later, with results demonstrating that 60.6% (OR = 29.19) of the sample had low interictal ionized magnesium and total serum magnesium ratio [141].

More randomized controlled trials are needed to better understand the potential of magnesium as a treatment option for epilepsy. Such trials, with more accurate measuring of magnesium levels, would provide greater and more specific insight into the potential role of magnesium as a treatment (or adjunct treatment) for various types of epilepsy.

3.5. Parkinson's Disease

Parkinson's disease (PD) is a neurological disorder with symptoms such as loss of balance, muscle tension, slowed body movements, resting limb tremors, and cognitive impairment [142] caused by a selective loss of dopamine in the basal ganglia. Other factors that impact PD include mitochondrial dysfunction, oxidative stress, and protein dysfunction [143]. It has been suggested that excitotoxicity caused by excessive glutamatergic neurotransmission may mediate the dopaminergic cell loss seen in Parkinson's disease, making modulators of excitotoxicity an area of growing research interest [144]. Human research that investigates the potential role of magnesium in PD is scarce [145]. To our knowledge, no in-depth review articles focusing on magnesium and PD in humans exist. The most recently-published study was a multicenter hospital-based case-control study in Japan that examined dietary intake of metals in patients who were found to be within six years of onset for PD. The results of the study found that higher magnesium concentrations were associated with a reduced risk of PD [146].

Research examining magnesium levels in PD patients have yielded mixed results. Older research from the 1960s reported no differences in serum magnesium levels in PD patients compared to controls [147]; however, this research was likely limited by the types of magnesium testing available at that time. A more recent study found similar results, with no significant differences noted in hair magnesium levels between those with and without PD. Furthermore, no association between magnesium levels and disease duration or severity was observed [142]. In contrast, a study examining cerebrospinal fluid (CSF), blood, serum, urine, and hair magnesium levels of 18 controls and 91 PD patients found that CSF magnesium levels were inversely associated with disease duration and severity. The same study also concluded that PD patients with less than a year of the disease had higher magnesium levels than PD patients with more than eight years of the disease [148]. Finally, older studies comparing magnesium levels in brain areas of PD patients versus controls found that PD patients had lower magnesium levels in the cortex, white matter, basal ganglia, caudate nucleus, and brain stem as compared to controls [149,150]. It is essential to note that these studies utilized different methods to measure magnesium concentrations, which could be a factor in the contradictory results. Future research examining the role of magnesium in PD should include measurements of magnesium concentrations in the cerebral spinal fluid (CSF) (as a measure of magnesium in the central nervous system), rather than solely in the periphery. This measurement technique may be of use in other neurological disorders as well.

In short, human research of magnesium concentrations in PD is severely lacking, despite growing evidence implicating magnesium in animal studies. There is a need for more studies in PD patients focusing on magnesium concentrations in order to get a better consensus on the relationship between magnesium and PD. These few studies have provided a small window of insight into the possible role of magnesium as a treatment for PD; however, many more studies are needed before any conclusions can be drawn.

3.6. Alzheimer's Disease

Alzheimer's disease (AD) is a degenerative neurological disorder that is characterized by synaptic loss and cognitive impairments that include deterioration in learning and memory [1]. AD presents with accumulations of beta-amyloid and tau tangles, along with inflammation and atrophy [151]. Excitotoxicity, neuroinflammation, and mitochondrial dysfunction have all been implicated in Alzheimer's disease [152], thus, hypomagnesaemia could further impair neuronal function. Factors related to lower magnesium availability, such as malnutrition and poor nutrient intake, are also present in AD patients [153,154], making magnesium deficiency more likely. Research suggests that ionized magnesium [155], cerebral spinal fluid (CSF) magnesium, hair magnesium, plasma magnesium, and red blood cell magnesium concentrations are significantly reduced in AD patients compared to healthy and medical controls [154]. Additionally, postmortem brain examinations of AD brains have found decreased magnesium levels compared to healthy controls [154,156,157]. Magnesium depletion has been found in the hippocampus in patients with AD, providing more evidence that magnesium may be a target of treatment [156].

A systematic review analyzed 13 cross-sectional studies that included AD patients and healthy controls and/or medical controls [154]. The results demonstrated that AD patients had significantly lower magnesium concentrations in CSF [158,159] and in hair samples [160,161], but no such differences were found in serum [161–164], plasma [158,165,166], or ionized/ blood cell magnesium levels [165] compared to controls. Compared to medical controls, AD patients had reduced plasma [167] and ionized blood cell magnesium concentrations [168], but no differences in serum [155,169], or CSF concentrations [168]. Meanwhile, other research has found no differences between hair and serum magnesium levels in patients with AD compared to controls [170]. Hence, current research has found contradictory results on magnesium concentration levels and, thus, requires further investigation and standardized ways to measure magnesium levels. One specific study worth noting reported that ionized magnesium levels were significantly associated with cognitive function, but not with physical function, when comparing AD patients to age-matched controls [155]. Similar to Parkinson's disease, future AD research should include a greater focus on CNS magnesium concentrations from CSF measurements, as well as using magnetic resonance spectroscopy. The above findings suggest that AD patients may be commonly deficient in magnesium.

While previous reviews have demonstrated a link between magnesium deficiency and AD in humans, there is a distinct lack of research that looks at magnesium as a treatment for AD in humans. Research to date has focused mainly on dementia, as opposed to AD specifically, and has had mixed findings. One study observed low magnesium levels in patients with mild cognitive impairment and AD patients as compared to controls [171]. Yet, another study found that both low and high magnesium concentration levels were associated with a greater risk of all-cause dementia [172]. This is the only study that provides evidence for both high and low magnesium levels being related to the risk of dementia development. As the study insists, the replication of findings from large population-based research is essential for a better understanding of these findings. For dementia, focusing on magnesium treatment through diet has been shown to improve memory [173]. The PATH through Life Project found that higher magnesium intake was related to a reduced risk of developing mild cognitive impairment and mild cognitive disorders [173]. Similarly, one study in Japan found that the greater the magnesium intake, the lower the rates of all-cause dementia and vascular dementia. However, the same relationship was absent for AD patients [174]. It is important to remember that dementia has multiple causes, including that stemming from vascular origin. Magnesium is unique for its ability to affect vascular function in addition to neuronal function [1]. Thus, magnesium may be affecting cognitive function in multiple distinct ways. Future clinical trial research is needed in this area to add to the literature in examining whether magnesium should be an adjunct treatment option in AD and/or in other types of dementia.

3.7. Stroke

Stroke is a cerebrovascular accident that presents itself with symptoms such as slurred speech, paralysis/numbness, and difficulty walking. Stroke can be broken down into two types, ischemic (where blood flow is impeded, usually by a clot) and hemorrhagic (where a blood vessel ruptures, causing impaired blood flow in the brain) [175]. The induced hypoxia causes excitotoxicity and resultant cell death [176]. Magnesium's dual role in its ability to affect vascular function [177], as well as its ability to protect against excitotoxicity mediated by NMDA receptors [176], has made it an element of interest within the stroke research community. Studies examining risk of stroke and magnesium levels have yielded mixed results. Research has found no relationship between serum ionized magnesium levels and stroke risk, when based on ischemic stroke cases over a 16 years follow-up [178]. Similarly, another study reported that plasma magnesium levels were not associated with the risk of ischemic stroke in women, yet those with low ionized magnesium levels (<0.82 mmol/L) had a 57% higher risk of ischemic stroke, after controlling for potential confounds [179]. Yet, more recent studies have found that higher serum magnesium concentrations at the time of hospital admission were independently related to lower hematoma volume and lower intracerebral hemorrhage scores in patients with acute spontaneous intracerebral hemorrhage [180]. In a more general study of adults in the United States, very low serum magnesium concentrations were significantly related to increased risk of stroke mortality [181]. While magnesium levels and stroke risk have resulted in contradictory results, there is a clear suggestion of magnesium being protective against stroke.

Most of the research conducted on the association between risk of stroke and magnesium can be found in American, European, and Asian prospective cohort studies [182,183]. A recent publication on stroke reviewed multiple meta-analyses and reported a dose-dependent protective effect of magnesium against stroke [182]. Most of the meta-analyses reviewed found that each 100 mg/day increment of dietary magnesium intake provided between 2% and 13% protection against total stroke [183–186]. A recently updated meta-analysis by Fang et al. included 40 prospective cohort studies and found 22% protection against the risk of stroke when comparing people with the highest to the lowest categories of dietary magnesium intake [183]. These meta-analyses are noted in the review paper as exhibiting high homogeneity, low publication bias, and were careful to adjust for potential confounds [182]. Hence, these studies are highly reliable and support the notion of an inverse-dose dependent relationship between dietary magnesium intake and risk for total stroke. These meta-analyses suggest that increased magnesium intake, as well as higher levels of serum magnesium, appear to be beneficial in reducing total stroke risk.

It is important to note that there are many types of stroke, and that not all stroke subtypes have demonstrated a universal relationship with magnesium. For example, one meta-analysis [184] included 7 prospective studies and found that magnesium intake levels were inversely related to the risk of ischemic stroke [178,187–189]; however, this inverse relationship was absent for intracerebral hemorrhage or subarachnoid hemorrhage [184,187,188]. A later study investigating whether magnesium could reduce the risk of delayed cerebral ischemia in patients with aneurysmal subarachnoid hemorrhage, also found that magnesium was not beneficial and did not reduce the risk [190]. Such evidence suggests the possibility that different types of stroke have different relationships to magnesium, an important distinction to be made for understanding magnesium's role in the risk of stroke development.

Investigations on magnesium levels in stroke patients have suggested an association between low magnesium levels and poor outcomes post-stroke. A recent study confirms this notion, providing evidence that low serum magnesium levels at the time of hospital admission were independently related to in-hospital mortality of patients with acute ischemic stroke [191]. An earlier study reported that decreased CSF magnesium levels were observed in ischemic stroke patients compared to controls, and that a positive association existed between low CSF magnesium levels and mortality after 7 days [192]. In addition to ischemic stroke, an observational cohort study involving patients presenting with intracerebral hemorrhage found that three month post-observation, poor functional outcomes were associated with low magnesium levels at the time of hospital admission, even after adjusting for age and measures of disease severity. Furthermore, initial and final hematoma volumes, as well as hematoma growth, were all independently and inversely correlated with low admission serum magnesium levels [193]. It is important to address the major issue when studying hypomagnesemia in stroke patients, which is that the levels are measured post diagnosis, so a causal relationship cannot be assumed and consequently there is the possibility that the lower magnesium levels are a result of stroke and not a cause of stroke [182].

Despite what appears to be a protective effect of magnesium levels on stroke, magnesium as a treatment for stroke has yielded less clear results. A trial investigating acute stroke has found that intravenous magnesium administration within 12 h of stroke onset does not improve death or disability outcomes [194]. Similarly, a meta-analysis also reported no beneficial effect of magnesium on delayed cerebral ischemia when started early after an aneurysmal subarachnoid hemorrhage based on 5 trials [195–200].

Some studies have found magnesium sulfate to be beneficial for managing post-stroke outcomes [201,202]. A meta-analysis by Chen and Carter [203] investigated 8 controlled clinical trials, 4 of which provided evidence that magnesium sulfate reduces the risk of poor outcomes 3–6 months after aneurysmal subarachnoid hemorrhage when compared to controls [198,199,201,204]. The other studies reported that magnesium sulfate was not beneficial for treating aneurysmal subarachnoid hemorrhage [199,205,206]. The overall findings of the meta-analysis suggested that magnesium sulfate may be able to decrease the risk of poor functional outcome in subarachnoid hemorrhage.

In terms of overall stroke, Panahi et al. reviewed studies that demonstrate how magnesium sulfate has been found to improve scores on different measurement indices [196,201,207], neuroprotective properties [208,209], hospital stay length [207,210], and recovery outcomes [206,207]. An additional compound that has been studied as a potential treatment for stroke is an enriched salt that is made up of a combination of magnesium and potassium. In a double-blind randomized controlled trial study, the compound was found to improve neurologic deficits following a stroke when administered for a six month period [211].

In summary, there is research to suggest the use of magnesium to improve outcomes post-stroke. More research is needed to understand the potential protective role of maintaining adequate magnesium levels in the prevention of stroke occurrence.

4. Conclusions

In conclusion, the amount of quality data on the association of magnesium with various neurological disorders differs greatly. There is strong data for the role of magnesium in migraine and depression. There is also good potential for magnesium to be having an effect in chronic pain conditions, as well as commonly comorbid psychiatric disorders, such as anxiety and depression. Much more research is needed in regards to magnesium's effects on epilepsy, including clinical trials evaluating the use of magnesium as an adjunct treatment. Neurological disorders, like Parkinson's and Alzheimer's, would benefit greatly from additional research that include measures of CNS magnesium levels (via CSF measurements and MRS). Finally, there is some research to suggest a positive effect of magnesium for improving post-stroke outcomes, and as an important dietary strategy for potentially preventing stroke, though more prospective studies are needed in this regard.

Author Contributions: Conceptualization: K.F.H.; methodology: K.F.H., A.E.K. and G.L.S.: validation: K.F.H., A.E.K. and G.L.S.; Investigation: A.E.K. and G.L.S.; writing—original draft preparation: A.E.K., G.L.S. and K.F.H.; writing—review and editing: A.E.K., G.L.S. and K.F.H.; visualization: A.E.K., G.L.S. and K.F.H.; and supervision: K.F.H.

Conflicts of Interest: The authors declare no conflict of interest.

References

1. Grober, U.; Schmidt, J.; Kisters, K. Magnesium in prevention and therapy. *Nutrients* **2015**, *7*, 8199–8226. [CrossRef] [PubMed]

2. Vink, R.; Nechifor, M. *Magnesium in the Central Nervous System*; University of Adelaide Press: Adelaide, Australia, 2011; p. 342.

3. Stroebel, D.; Casado, M.; Paoletti, P. Triheteromeric nmda receptors: From structure to synaptic physiology. *Curr. Opin. Physiol.* **2018**, *2*, 1–12. [CrossRef] [PubMed]

4. Castilho, R.F.; Ward, M.W.; Nicholls, D.G. Oxidative stress, mitochondrial function, and acute glutamate excitotoxicity in cultured cerebellar granule cells. *J. Neurochem.* **1999**, *72*, 1394–1401. [CrossRef] [PubMed]

5. Olloquequi, J.; Cornejo-Cordova, E.; Verdaguer, E.; Soriano, F.X.; Binvignat, O.; Auladell, C.; Camins, A. Excitotoxicity in the pathogenesis of neurological and psychiatric disorders: Therapeutic implications. *J. Psychopharmacol.* **2018**, *32*, 265–275. [CrossRef] [PubMed]

6. Clerc, P.; Young, C.A.; Bordt, E.A.; Grigore, A.M.; Fiskum, G.; Polster, B.M. Magnesium sulfate protects against the bioenergetic consequences of chronic glutamate receptor stimulation. *PLoS ONE* **2013**, *8*, e79982. [CrossRef] [PubMed]

7. Lambuk, L.; Jafri, A.J.; Arfuzir, N.N.; Iezhitsa, I.; Agarwal, R.; Rozali, K.N.; Agarwal, P.; Bakar, N.S.; Kutty, M.K.; Yusof, A.P.; et al. Neuroprotective effect of magnesium acetyltaurate against NMDA-induced excitotoxicity in rat retina. *Neurotox. Res.* **2017**, *31*, 31–45. [CrossRef] [PubMed]

8. Kalia, L.V.; Kalia, S.K.; Salter, M.W. NMDA receptors in clinical neurology: Excitatory times ahead. *Lancet Neurol.* **2008**, *7*, 742–755. [CrossRef]

9. Rosanoff, A.; Weaver, C.M.; Rude, R.K. Suboptimal magnesium status in the United States: Are the health consequences underestimated? *Nutr. Rev.* **2012**, *70*, 153–164. [CrossRef] [PubMed]

10. Silberstein, S.; Loder, E.; Diamond, S.; Reed, M.L.; Bigal, M.E.; Lipton, R.B.; Group, A.A. Probable migraine in the United States: Results of the American migraine prevalence and prevention (AMPP) study. *Cephalalgia* **2007**, *27*, 220–229. [CrossRef] [PubMed]

11. Michael, J.; Aminoff, D.A.G.P.; David, A.; Greenburg, D.; Roger, P.; Simon, R. *Clinical Neurology*; McGraw-Hill: New York, NY, USA, 2009.

12. Nattagh-Eshtivani, E.; Sani, M.A.; Dahri, M.; Ghalichi, F.; Ghavami, A.; Arjang, P.; Tarighat-Esfanjani, A. The role of nutrients in the pathogenesis and treatment of migraine headaches. *Biomed. Pharmacother.* **2018**, *102*, 317–325. [CrossRef] [PubMed]

13. Goadsby, P.J.; Holland, P.R.; Martins-Oliveira, M.; Hoffmann, J.; Schankin, C.; Akerman, S. Pathophysiology of migraine: A disorder of sensory processing. *Physiol. Rev.* **2017**, *97*, 553–622. [CrossRef] [PubMed]

14. Hoffmann, J.; Charles, A. Glutamate and its receptors as therapeutic targets for migraine. *Neurotherapeutics* **2018**, 1–10. [CrossRef] [PubMed]

15. Welch, K.; Ramadan, N.M. Mitochondria, magnesium and migraine. *J. Neurol. Sci.* **1995**, *134*, 9–14. [CrossRef]

16. Peikert, A.; Wilimzig, C.; Köhne-Volland, R. Prophylaxis of migraine with oral magnesium: Results from a prospective, multi-center, placebo-controlled and double-blind randomized study. *Cephalalgia* **1996**, *16*, 257–263. [CrossRef] [PubMed]

17. Sarchielli, P.; Coata, G.; Firenze, C.; Morucci, P.; Abbritti, G.; Gallai, V. Serum and salivary magnesium levels in migraine and tension-type headache. Results in a group of adult patients. *Cephalalgia* **1992**, *12*, 21–27. [CrossRef] [PubMed]

18. Ramadan, N.; Halvorson, H.; Vande-Linde, A.; Levine, S.R.; Helpern, J.; Welch, K. Low brain magnesium in migraine. *Headache J. Head Face Pain* **1989**, *29*, 590–593. [CrossRef]

19. Bigal, M.; Bordini, C.; Tepper, S.; Speciali, J. Intravenous magnesium sulphate in the acute treatment of migraine without aura and migraine with aura. A randomized, double-blind, placebo-controlled study. *Cephalalgia* **2002**, *22*, 345–353. [CrossRef] [PubMed]

20. Cete, Y.; Dora, B.; Ertan, C.; Ozdemir, C.; Oktay, C. A randomized prospective placebo-controlled study of intravenous magnesium sulphate vs. metoclopramide in the management of acute migraine attacks in the emergency department. *Cephalalgia* **2005**, *25*, 199–204. [CrossRef] [PubMed]

21. Corbo, J.; Esses, D.; Bijur, P.E.; Iannaccone, R.; Gallagher, E.J. Randomized clinical trial of intravenous magnesium sulfate as an adjunctive medication for emergency department treatment of migraine headache. *Ann. Emerg. Med.* **2001**, *38*, 621–627. [CrossRef] [PubMed]

22. Frank, L.R.; Olson, C.M.; Shuler, K.B.; Gharib, S.F. Intravenous magnesium for acute benign headache in the emergency department: A randomized double-blind placebo-controlled trial. *Can. J. Emerg. Med.* **2004**, *6*, 327–332. [CrossRef]

23. Ginder, S.; Oatman, B.; Pollack, M. A prospective study of i.v. magnesium and i.v. prochlorperazine in the treatment of headaches. *J. Emerg. Med.* **2000**, *18*, 311–315. [CrossRef]

24. Choi, H.; Parmar, N. The use of intravenous magnesium sulphate for acute migraine: Meta-analysis of randomized controlled trials. *Eur. J. Emerg. Med.* **2014**, *21*, 2–9. [CrossRef] [PubMed]

25. Demirkaya, Ş.; Vural, O.; Dora, B.; Topçuoğlu, M.A. Efficacy of intravenous magnesium sulfate in the treatment of acute migraine attacks. *Headache J. Head Face Pain* **2001**, *41*, 171–177. [CrossRef]

26. Shahrami, A.; Assarzadegan, F.; Hatamabadi, H.R.; Asgarzadeh, M.; Sarehbandi, B.; Asgarzadeh, S. Comparison of therapeutic effects of magnesium sulfate vs. Dexamethasone/metoclopramide on alleviating acute migraine headache. *J. Emerg. Med.* **2015**, *48*, 69–76. [CrossRef] [PubMed]

27. Liu, R. Clinical effects of ozagrel combined with magnesium for treating migraine. *China Med. Eng.* **2013**, *21*, 93.

28. Tang, L.; Zhou, Y. Clinical effects of ozagrel combined with magnesium for treating migraine. *J. Prac. Med.* **2011**, *27*, 2531.

29. Wang, Y. Clinical study of intravenous magnesium for treating migraine. *J. Qiqihar Med. Coll.* **2013**, *31*, 89.

30. Xu, L.; XU, Y. Observation of the effect of intravenous magnesium combined with lidocaine for treating migraine. *Med. Inf.* **2010**, *23*, 2103.

31. Maizels, M.; Blumenfeld, A.; Burchette, R. A combination of riboflavin, magnesium, and feverfew for migraine prophylaxis: A randomized trial. *Headache J. Head Face Pain* **2004**, *44*, 885–890. [CrossRef] [PubMed]

32. Observation of Clinical Effects of Magnesium Valproate Combined with Venlafaxine Hcl in 54 Individuals with Migraine. Available online: https://wenku.baidu.com/view/280201f404a1b0717fd5ddfc.html (accessed on 5 June 2018).

33. Köseoglu, E.; Talaslıoglu, A.; Gönül, A.S.; Kula, M. The effects of magnesium prophylaxis in migraine without aura. *Magnes. Res.* **2008**, *21*, 101–108. [PubMed]

34. Esfanjani, A.T.; Mahdavi, R.; Mameghani, M.E.; Talebi, M.; Nikniaz, Z.; Safaiyan, A. The effects of magnesium, L-carnitine, and concurrent cagnesium–L-carnitine supplementation in migraine prophylaxis. *Biol. Trace Elem. Res.* **2012**, *150*, 42–48. [CrossRef] [PubMed]

35. Wang, S.; Shan, H. Effects of magnesium sulphate, ergotamine, and flunarizine hydrochloride on treating migraine. *Prev. Med.* **2001**, *12*, 366–367.

36. Yang, X.; Yang, J.; Yuan, R.; Xu, X.; Zhang, L. Randomized double blind controlled trial of magnesium valproate in migraine prophylaxis. *China Hosp. Pharm.* **2005**, *25*, 649–651.

37. Bian, X.; Zhu, Y.; Xia, J.; Ai, H.; Guo, Q.; Lu, L.; Zhang, Q. Clinical observation on potassium magnesium asparate oral soluation combined with flinarizine capsule for migraine prophylaxis. *J. Commun. Med.* **2013**, *11*, 6–7.

38. Lan, Q.; Yang, C. Clinical observation of magnesium propylvalerate on treating migraine. *Youjiang Med. Coll. Natl.* **1998**, *21*, 639–640.

39. Tang, X.; Lin, W.; Zheng, X.; Liu, C. Observation of effects of nimodipine and magnesium sulfate combination for treating migraine. *Qiqihar Med. Coll.* **1998**, *19*, 5–6.

40. Chiu, H.Y.; Yeh, T.H.; Huang, Y.C.; Chen, P.Y. Effects of intravenous and oral magnesium on reducing migraine: A meta-analysis of randomized controlled trials. *Pain Phys.* **2016**, *19*, E97–E112.

41. Baratloo, A.; Mirbaha, S.; Delavar Kasmaei, H.; Payandemehr, P.; Elmaraezy, A.; Negida, A. Intravenous caffeine citrate vs. magnesium sulfate for reducing pain in patients with acute migraine headache; a prospective quasi-experimental study. *Korean J. Pain* **2017**, *30*, 176–182. [CrossRef] [PubMed]

42. Von Luckner, A.; Riederer, F. Magnesium in migraine prophylaxis—Is there an evidence-based rationale? A systematic review. *Headache J. Head Face Pain* **2018**, *58*, 199–209. [CrossRef] [PubMed]

43. Crofford, L.J. Chronic pain: Where the body meets the brain. *Trans. Am. Clin. Climatol. Assoc.* **2015**, *126*, 167. [PubMed]

44. McBeth, J.; Jones, K. Epidemiology of chronic musculoskeletal pain. *Best Prac. Res. Clin. Rheumatol.* **2007**, *21*, 403–425. [CrossRef] [PubMed]

45. Fisher, K.; Coderre, T.J.; Hagen, N.A. Targeting the *N*-methyl-D-aspartate receptor for chronic pain management: Preclinical animal studies, recent clinical experience and future research directions. *J. Pain Symptom Manag.* **2000**, *20*, 358–373. [CrossRef]

46. Srebro, D.; Vuckovic, S.; Milovanovic, A.; Kosutic, J.; Savic Vujovic, K.; Prostran, M. Magnesium in pain research: State of the art. *Curr. Med. Chem.* **2017**, *24*, 424–434.

47. Banerjee, S.; Jones, S. *Magnesium as an Alternative or Adjunct to Opioids for Migraine and Chronic Pain: A Review of the Clinical Effectiveness and Guidelines*; Canadian Agency for Drugs and Technologies in Health: Ottawa, ON, Canada, 2017.

48. Fischer, S.G.; Collins, S.; Boogaard, S.; Loer, S.A.; Zuurmond, W.W.; Perez, R.S. Intravenous magnesium for chronic complex regional pain syndrome type 1 (CRPS-1). *Pain Med.* **2013**, *14*, 1388–1399. [CrossRef] [PubMed]

49. Van der Plas, A.A.; Schilder, J.C.; Marinus, J.; van Hilten, J.J. An explanatory study evaluating the muscle relaxant effects of intramuscular magnesium sulphate for dystonia in complex regional pain syndrome. *J. Pain* **2013**, *14*, 1341–1348. [CrossRef] [PubMed]

50. Yousef, A.; Al-deeb, A. A double-blinded randomised controlled study of the value of sequential intravenous and oral magnesium therapy in patients with chronic low back pain with a neuropathic component. *Anaesthesia* **2013**, *68*, 260–266. [CrossRef] [PubMed]

51. Venturini, M.A.; Zappa, S.; Minelli, C.; Bonardelli, S.; Lamberti, L.; Bisighini, L.; Zangrandi, M.; Turin, M.; Rizzo, F.; Rizzolo, A. Magnesium-oral supplementation to reduce pain in patients with severe peripheral arterial occlusive disease: The mag-paper randomised clinical trial protocol. *BMJ Open* **2015**, *5*, e009137. [CrossRef] [PubMed]

52. Wolfe, F.; Smythe, H.A.; Yunus, M.B.; Bennett, R.M.; Bombardier, C.; Goldenberg, D.L.; Tugwell, P.; Campbell, S.M.; Abeles, M.; Clark, P. The american college of rheumatology 1990 criteria for the classification of fibromyalgia. *Arthr. Rheumatol.* **1990**, *33*, 160–172. [CrossRef]

53. Bagis, S.; Karabiber, M.; As, I.; Tamer, L.; Erdogan, C.; Atalay, A. Is magnesium citrate treatment effective on pain, clinical parameters and functional status in patients with fibromyalgia? *Rheumatol. Int.* **2013**, *33*, 167–172. [CrossRef] [PubMed]

54. Littlejohn, G.; Guymer, E. Modulation of NMDA receptor activity in fibromyalgia. *Biomedicines* **2017**, *5*, 15. [CrossRef] [PubMed]

55. Abraham, G.E.; Flechas, J.D. Management of fibromyalgia: Rationale for the use of magnesium and malic acid. *J. Nutr. Med.* **1992**, *3*, 49–59. [CrossRef]

56. Magaldi, M.; Moltoni, L.; Biasi, G.; Marcolongo, R. Role of intracellular calcium ions in the physiopathology of fibromyalgia syndrome. *Boll. Della Soc. Ital. Biol. Sper.* **2000**, *76*, 1–4.

57. Eisinger, J.; Plantamura, A.; Ayavou, T. Glycolysis abnormalities in fibromyalgia. *J. Am. Coll. Nutr.* **1994**, *13*, 144–148. [CrossRef] [PubMed]

58. Eisinger, J.; Zakarian, H.; Pouly, E.; Plantamura, A.; Ayavou, T. Protein peroxidation, magnesium deficiency and fibromyalgia. *Magnes. Res.* **1996**, *9*, 313–316. [PubMed]

59. Romano, T.J.; Stiller, J.W. Magnesium deficiency in fibromyalgia syndrome. *J. Nutr. Med.* **1994**, *4*, 165–167. [CrossRef]

60. Clauw, D.; Ward, K.; Katz, P.; Rajan, S. Muscle intracellular magnesium levels correlate with pain tolerance in fibromyalgia (FM). *Arthr. Rheum.* **1994**, *37*, R29.

61. Sakarya, S.T.; Akyol, Y.; Bedir, A.; Canturk, F. The relationship between serum antioxidant vitamins, magnesium levels, and clinical parameters in patients with primary fibromyalgia syndrome. *Clin. Rheumatol.* **2011**, *30*, 1039–1043. [CrossRef] [PubMed]

62. Sendur, O.F.; Tastaban, E.; Turan, Y.; Ulman, C. The relationship between serum trace element levels and clinical parameters in patients with fibromyalgia. *Rheumatol. Int.* **2008**, *28*, 1117. [CrossRef] [PubMed]

63. Kasim, A.A. Calcium, magnesium and phosphorous levels in serum of Iraqi women with fibromyalgia. *Iraqi J. Pharm. Sci.* **2017**, *20*, 34–37.

64. Engen, D.J.; McAllister, S.J.; Whipple, M.O.; Cha, S.S.; Dion, L.J.; Vincent, A.; Bauer, B.A.; Wahner-Roedler, D.L. Effects of transdermal magnesium chloride on quality of life for patients with fibromyalgia: A feasibility study. *J. Integr. Med.* **2015**, *13*, 306–313. [CrossRef]

65. Calleo, J.; Amspoker, A.B.; Marsh, L.; Kunik, M.E. Mental health diagnoses and health care utilization in persons with dementia, Parkinson's disease, and stroke. *J. Neuropsychiatry Clin. Neurosci.* **2015**, *27*, e117–e121. [CrossRef] [PubMed]

66. Tsatali, M.; Papaliagkas, V.; Damigos, D.; Mavreas, V.; Gouva, M.; Tsolaki, M. Depression and anxiety levels increase chronic musculoskeletal pain in patients with alzheimer's disease. *Curr. Alzheimer Res.* **2014**, *11*, 574–579. [CrossRef] [PubMed]

67. Oh, K.; Cho, S.J.; Chung, Y.K.; Kim, J.M.; Chu, M.K. Combination of anxiety and depression is associated with an increased headache frequency in migraineurs: A population-based study. *BMC Neurol.* **2014**, *14*, 238. [CrossRef] [PubMed]

68. Riaza Bermudo-Soriano, C.; Perez-Rodriguez, M.M.; Vaquero-Lorenzo, C.; Baca-Garcia, E. New perspectives in glutamate and anxiety. *Pharmacol. Biochem. Behav.* **2012**, *100*, 752–774. [CrossRef] [PubMed]

69. Niciu, M.J.; Ionescu, D.F.; Richards, E.M.; Zarate, C.A., Jr. Glutamate and its receptors in the pathophysiology and treatment of major depressive disorder. *J. Neural Transm.* **2014**, *121*, 907–924. [CrossRef] [PubMed]

70. Pochwat, B.; Szewczyk, B.; Sowa-Kucma, M.; Siwek, A.; Doboszewska, U.; Piekoszewski, W.; Gruca, P.; Papp, M.; Nowak, G. Antidepressant-like activity of magnesium in the chronic mild stress model in rats: Alterations in the nmda receptor subunits. *Int. J. Neuropsychopharmacol.* **2014**, *17*, 393–405. [CrossRef] [PubMed]

71. Kessler, R.C.; Aguilar-Gaxiola, S.; Alonso, J.; Chatterji, S.; Lee, S.; Ormel, J.; Üstün, T.B.; Wang, P.S. The global burden of mental disorders: An update from the who world mental health (WMH) surveys. *Epidemiol. Psychiatr. Sci.* **2009**, *18*, 23–33. [CrossRef]

72. Boyle, N.B.; Lawton, C.; Dye, L. The effects of magnesium supplementation on subjective anxiety and stress-a systematic review. *Nutrients* **2017**, *9*, 429. [CrossRef] [PubMed]

73. Mocci, F.; Canalis, P.; Tomasi, P.; Casu, F.; Pettinato, S. The effect of noise on serum and urinary magnesium and catecholamines in humans. *Occup. Med.* **2001**, *51*, 56–61. [CrossRef]

74. Poleszak, E.; Szewczyk, B.; Kędzierska, E.; Wlaź, P.; Pilc, A.; Nowak, G. Antidepressant-and anxiolytic-like activity of magnesium in mice. *Pharmacol. Biochem. Behav.* **2004**, *78*, 7–12. [CrossRef] [PubMed]

75. Jacka, F.N.; Overland, S.; Stewart, R.; Tell, G.S.; Bjelland, I.; Mykletun, A. Association between magnesium intake and depression and anxiety in community-dwelling adults: The hordaland health study. *Aust. N. Z. J. Psychiatry* **2009**, *43*, 45–52. [CrossRef] [PubMed]

76. Islam, M.R.; Ahmed, M.U.; Mitu, S.A.; Islam, M.S.; Rahman, G.M.; Qusar, M.S.; Hasnat, A. Comparative analysis of serum zinc, copper, manganese, iron, calcium, and magnesium level and complexity of interelement relations in generalized anxiety disorder patients. *Biol. Trace Elem. Res.* **2013**, *154*, 21–27. [CrossRef] [PubMed]

77. Gendle, M.H.; O'Hara, K.P. Oral magnesium supplementation and test anxiety in university undergraduates. *J. Artic. Support Null Hypothesis* **2015**, *11*, 21–30.

78. Bourgeois, M. Rôle du magne-b6 dans les manifestations anxueuses en pratique medicale courante psychiatr. *Pract. Med* **1987**, *39*, 18–22.

79. Scharbach, H. Anxiété et magné-b6. *La Vie Médicale* **1988**, *69*, 867–869.

80. Caillard, V. *Sanofi Internal Report Mab6-26*; Paris, France. Unpublished work, 1992.

81. Caillard, V. *Sanofi Internal Report Mab6-32*; Paris, France. Unpublished work, 1996.

82. Cazaubiel, J.; Desor, D. Evaluation of the anti-stress effects of a fermented milk containing milk protein hydrolysate on healthy human subjects sensitive to the stress of everyday life. Proprietary data cited in scientific opinion of the panel on dietetic products, nutrition and allergies, No. 1924/20061. *Eur. Food Saf. Auth. J. Unpubl. Work* **2008**, *905*, 1–10.

83. Hanus, M.; Lafon, J.; Mathieu, M. Double-blind, randomised, placebo-controlled study to evaluate the efficacy and safety of a fixed combination containing two plant extracts (*Crataegus oxyacantha* and *Eschscholtzia californica*) and magnesium in mild-to-moderate anxiety disorders. *Curr. Med. Res. Opin.* **2004**, *20*, 63–71. [CrossRef] [PubMed]

84. Facchinetti, F.; Borella, P.; Sances, G.; Fioroni, L.; Nappi, R.E.; Genazzani, A.R. Oral magnesium successfully relieves premenstrual mood changes. *Obstet. Gynecol.* **1991**, *78*, 177–181.

85. Walker, A.F.; De Souza, M.C.; Vickers, M.F.; Abeyasekera, S.; Collins, M.L.; Trinca, L.A. Magnesium supplementation alleviates premenstrual symptoms of fluid retention. *J. Women Health* **1998**, *7*, 1157–1165. [CrossRef]

86. Walker, A.F.; Marakis, G.; Christie, S.; Byng, M. Mg citrate found more bioavailable than other mg preparations in a randomised, double-blind study. *Magnes. Res.* **2003**, *16*, 183–191. [PubMed]

87. Khine, K.; Rosenstein, D.L.; Elin, R.J.; Niemela, J.E.; Schmidt, P.J.; Rubinow, D.R. Magnesium (MG) retention and mood effects after intravenous mg infusion in premenstrual dysphoric disorder. *Biol. Psychiatry* **2006**, *59*, 327–333. [CrossRef] [PubMed]

88. De Souza, M.C.; Walker, A.F.; Robinson, P.A.; Bolland, K. A synergistic effect of a daily supplement for 1 month of 200 mg magnesium plus 50 mg vitamin b6 for the relief of anxiety-related premenstrual symptoms: A randomized, double-blind, crossover study. *J. Women Health Gend. Based Med.* **2000**, *9*, 131–139. [CrossRef] [PubMed]

89. Fathizadeh, N.; Ebrahimi, E.; Valiani, M.; Tavakoli, N.; Yar, M.H. Evaluating the effect of magnesium and magnesium plus vitamin B$_6$ supplement on the severity of premenstrual syndrome. *Iran. J. Nurs. Midwifery Res.* **2010**, *15*, 401. [PubMed]

90. Fard, F.E.; Mirghafourvand, M.; Mohammad-Alizadeh Charandabi, S.; Farshbaf-Khalili, A.; Javadzadeh, Y.; Asgharian, H. Effects of zinc and magnesium supplements on postpartum depression and anxiety: A randomized controlled clinical trial. *Women Health* **2017**, *57*, 1115–1128. [CrossRef] [PubMed]

91. Lakhan, S.E.; Vieira, K.F. Nutritional and herbal supplements for anxiety and anxiety-related disorders: Systematic review. *Nutr. J.* **2010**, *9*, 42. [CrossRef] [PubMed]

92. Eby, G.A.; Eby, K.L. Magnesium for treatment-resistant depression: A review and hypothesis. *Med. Hypotheses* **2010**, *74*, 649–660. [CrossRef] [PubMed]

93. Li, B.; Lv, J.; Wang, W.; Zhang, D. Dietary magnesium and calcium intake and risk of depression in the general population: A meta-analysis. *Aust. N. Z. J. Psychiatry* **2017**, *51*, 219–229. [CrossRef] [PubMed]

94. Rechenberg, K. Nutritional interventions in clinical depression. *Clin. Psychol. Sci.* **2016**, *4*, 144–162. [CrossRef]

95. Paul, I.A. Antidepressant activity and calcium signaling cascades. *Hum. Psychopharmacol. Clin. Exp.* **2001**, *16*, 71–80. [CrossRef] [PubMed]

96. Hollister, L.E.; Trevino, E.S.G. Calcium channel blockers in psychiatric disorders: A review of the literature. *Can. J. Psychiatry* **1999**, *44*, 658–664. [CrossRef] [PubMed]

97. Eby, G.A.; Eby, K.L. Rapid recovery from major depression using magnesium treatment. *Med. Hypotheses* **2006**, *67*, 362–370. [CrossRef] [PubMed]

98. Murck, H. Magnesium and affective disorders. *Nutr. Neurosci.* **2002**, *5*, 375–389. [CrossRef] [PubMed]

99. Nechifor, M. Magnesium in major depression. *Magnes. Res.* **2009**, *22*, 163–166.

100. Camardese, G.; De Risio, L.; Pizi, G.; Mattioli, B.; Buccelletti, F.; Serrani, R.; Leone, B.; Sgambato, A.; Bria, P.; Janiri, L. Plasma magnesium levels and treatment outcome in depressed patients. *Nutr. Neurosci.* **2012**, *15*, 78–84. [CrossRef] [PubMed]

101. Barragan-Rodriguez, L.; Rodriguez-Moran, M.; Guerrero-Romero, F. Depressive symptoms and hypomagnesemia in older diabetic subjects. *Arch. Med. Res.* **2007**, *38*, 752–756. [CrossRef] [PubMed]

102. Hasey, G.M.; D'Alessandro, E.; Cooke, R.G.; Warsh, J.J. The interface between thyroid activity, magnesium, and depression: A pilot study. *Biol. Psychiatry* **1993**, *33*, 133–135. [CrossRef]

103. Derom, M.-L.; Sayón-Orea, C.; Martínez-Ortega, J.M.; Martínez-González, M.A. Magnesium and depression: A systematic review. *Nutr. Neurosci.* **2013**, *16*, 191–206. [CrossRef] [PubMed]

104. Bhudia, S.K.; Cosgrove, D.M.; Naugle, R.I.; Rajeswaran, J.; Lam, B.K.; Walton, E.; Petrich, J.; Palumbo, R.C.; Gillinov, A.M.; Apperson-Hansen, C.; et al. Magnesium as a neuroprotectant in cardiac surgery: A randomized clinical trial. *J. Thorac. Cardiovasc. Surg.* **2006**, *131*, 853–861. [CrossRef] [PubMed]

105. Mehdi, S.; Atlas, S.E.; Qadir, S.; Musselman, D.; Goldberg, S.; Woolger, J.M.; Corredor, R.; Abbas, M.H.; Arosemena, L.; Caccamo, S. Double-blind, randomized crossover study of intravenous infusion of magnesium sulfate versus 5% dextrose on depressive symptoms in adults with treatment-resistant depression. *Psychiatry Clin. Neurosci.* **2017**, *71*, 204–211. [CrossRef] [PubMed]

106. Tarleton, E.K.; Littenberg, B.; MacLean, C.D.; Kennedy, A.G.; Daley, C. Role of magnesium supplementation in the treatment of depression: A randomized clinical trial. *PLoS ONE* **2017**, *12*, e0180067. [CrossRef] [PubMed]

107. Rajizadeh, A.; Mozaffari-Khosravi, H.; Yassini-Ardakani, M.; Dehghani, A. Effect of magnesium supplementation on depression status in depressed patients with magnesium deficiency: A randomized, double-blind, placebo-controlled trial. *Nutrition* **2017**, *35*, 56–60. [CrossRef] [PubMed]

108. Wang, J.; Um, P.; Dickerman, B.; Liu, J. Zinc, magnesium, selenium and depression: A review of the evidence, potential mechanisms and implications. *Nutrients* **2018**, *10*, 584. [CrossRef] [PubMed]

109. Ivanova, J.I.; Birnbaum, H.G.; Kidolezi, Y.; Qiu, Y.; Mallett, D.; Caleo, S. Economic burden of epilepsy among the privately insured in the US. *Pharmacoeconomics* **2010**, *28*, 675–685. [CrossRef] [PubMed]

110. Organization, W.H. *Atlas: Country Resources for Neurological Disorders 2004: Results of a Collaborative Study of the World Health Organization and the World Federation of Neurology*; World Health Organization: Geneva, Switzerland, 2004.

111. Metcalfe, A.; Jette, N. Medical and employment-related costs of epilepsy in the USA. *Expert Rev. Pharmacoecon. Outcomes Res.* **2010**, *10*, 645–647. [CrossRef] [PubMed]

112. Kwan, P.; Brodie, M.J. Early identification of refractory epilepsy. *N. Engl. J. Med.* **2000**, *342*, 314–319. [CrossRef] [PubMed]

113. Pati, S.; Alexopoulos, A.V. Pharmacoresistant epilepsy: From pathogenesis to current and emerging therapies. *Cleve Clin. J. Med.* **2010**, *77*, 457–567. [CrossRef] [PubMed]

114. Yuen, A.W.; Sander, J.W. Can magnesium supplementation reduce seizures in people with epilepsy? A hypothesis. *Epilepsy Res.* **2012**, *100*, 152–156. [CrossRef] [PubMed]

115. Alaimo, K.; McDowell, M.A.; Briefel, R.; Bischof, A.; Caughman, C.; Loria, C.; Johnson, C. Dietary intake of vitamins, minerals, and fiber of persons ages 2 months and over in the united states: Third national health and nutrition examination survey, phase 1, 1988–1991. *Adv. Data* **1994**, *258*, 1–28.

116. Ismail, Y.; Ismail, A.A.; Ismail, A.A. The underestimated problem of using serum magnesium measurements to exclude magnesium deficiency in adults; a health warning is needed for "normal" results. *Clin. Chem. Lab. Med.* **2010**, *48*, 323–327. [CrossRef] [PubMed]

117. Barker-Haliski, M.; White, H.S. Glutamatergic mechanisms associated with seizures and epilepsy. *Cold Spring Harb. Perspect. Med.* **2015**, *5*, a022863. [CrossRef] [PubMed]

118. Coan, E.; Collingridge, G. Magnesium ions block an N-methyl-D-aspartate receptor-mediated component of synaptic transmission in rat hippocampus. *Neurosci. Lett.* **1985**, *53*, 21–26. [CrossRef]

119. Isaev, D.; Ivanchick, G.; Khmyz, V.; Isaeva, E.; Savrasova, A.; Krishtal, O.; Holmes, G.L.; Maximyuk, O. Surface charge impact in low-magnesium model of seizure in rat hippocampus. *J. Neurophysiol.* **2011**, *107*, 417–423. [CrossRef] [PubMed]

120. Chen, B.B.; Prasad, C.; Kobrzynski, M.; Campbell, C.; Filler, G. Seizures related to hypomagnesemia: A case series and review of the literature. *Child Neurol. Open* **2016**, *3*, 2329048X16674834. [CrossRef] [PubMed]

121. Osborn, K.E.; Shytle, R.D.; Frontera, A.T.; Soble, J.R.; Schoenberg, M.R. Addressing potential role of magnesium dyshomeostasis to improve treatment efficacy for epilepsy: A reexamination of the literature. *J. Clin. Pharmacol.* **2016**, *56*, 260–265. [CrossRef] [PubMed]

122. Oladipo, O.; Ajala, M.; Okubadejo, N.; Danesi, M.; Afonja, O. Plasma magnesium in adult nigerian patients with epilepsy. *Niger. Postgrad. Med. J.* **2003**, *10*, 234–237. [PubMed]

123. Sinert, R.; Zehtabchi, S.; Desai, S.; Peacock, P.; Altura, B.; Altura, B. Serum ionized magnesium and calcium levels in adult patients with seizures. *Scand. J. Clin. Lab. Investig.* **2007**, *67*, 317–326. [CrossRef] [PubMed]

124. Gupta, S.K.; Manhas, A.S.; Gupta, V.K.; Bhatt, R. Serum magnesium levels in idiopathic epilepsy. *J. Assoc. Phys. India* **1994**, *42*, 456–457.

125. Sood, A.; Handa, R.; Malhotra, R.; Gupta, B. Serum, CSF, RBC & urinary levels of magnesium & calcium in idiopathic generalised tonic clonic seizures. *Indian J. Med. Res.* **1993**, *98*, 152–154. [PubMed]

126. Prebble, J. Primary infantile hypomagnesaemia: Report of two cases. *J. Paediatr. Child Health* **1995**, *31*, 54–56. [CrossRef] [PubMed]

127. Unachak, K.; Louthrenoo, O.; Katanyuwong, K. Primary hypomagnesemia in thai infants: A case report with 7 years follow-up and review of literature. *J. Med. Assoc. Thai.* **2002**, *85*, 1226–1231.

128. Visudhiphan, P.; Visudtibhan, A.; Chiemchanya, S.; Khongkhatithum, C. Neonatal seizures and familial hypomagnesemia with secondary hypocalcemia. *Pediatr. Neurol.* **2005**, *33*, 202–205. [CrossRef] [PubMed]

129. Saghazadeh, A.; Mahmoudi, M.; Meysamie, A.; Gharedaghi, M.; Zamponi, G.W.; Rezaei, N. Possible role of trace elements in epilepsy and febrile seizures: A meta-analysis. *Nutr. Rev.* **2015**, *73*, 760–779. [CrossRef] [PubMed]

130. Fagan, C.; Phelan, D. Severe convulsant hypomagnesaemia and short bowel syndrome. *Anaesth. Intens. Care* **2001**, *29*, 281.

131. Weisleder, P.; Tobin, J.A.; Kerrigan, J.F.; Bodensteiner, J.B. Hypomagnesemic seizures: Case report and presumed pathophysiology. *J. Child Neurol.* **2002**, *17*, 59–61. [CrossRef] [PubMed]

132. Chien, P.F.; Khan, K.S.; Arnott, N. Magnesium sulphate in the treatment of eclampsia and pre-eclampsia: An overview of the evidence from randomised trials. *BJOG Int. J. Obstet. Gynaecol.* **1996**, *103*, 1085–1091. [CrossRef]

133. Duley, L.; Gülmezoglu, A.M.; Henderson-Smart, D.J.; Chou, D. Magnesium sulphate and other anticonvulsants for women with pre-eclampsia. *Cochrane Libr.* **2010**, *11*, 100. [CrossRef] [PubMed]

134. Duley, L.; Henderson-Smart, D.J.; Walker, G.J.; Chou, D. Magnesium sulphate versus diazepam for eclampsia. *Cochrane Libr.* **2010**, *12*, 127–186. [CrossRef] [PubMed]

135. Kamate, M.; Singh, N.; Patil, S. Familial hypomagnesemia with secondary hypocalcemia mimicking neurodegenerative disorder. *Indian Pediatr.* **2015**, *52*, 521–522. [CrossRef] [PubMed]

136. Katayama, K.; Povalko, N.; Yatsuga, S.; Nishioka, J.; Kakuma, T.; Matsuishi, T.; Koga, Y. New trpm6 mutation and management of hypomagnesaemia with secondary hypocalcaemia. *Brain Dev.* **2015**, *37*, 292–298. [CrossRef] [PubMed]

137. Schlingmann, K.P.; Sassen, M.C.; Weber, S.; Pechmann, U.; Kusch, K.; Pelken, L.; Lotan, D.; Syrrou, M.; Prebble, J.J.; Cole, D.E. Novel TRPM6 mutations in 21 families with primary hypomagnesemia and secondary hypocalcemia. *J. Am. Soc. Nephrol.* **2005**, *16*, 3061–3069. [CrossRef] [PubMed]

138. Visser, N.A.; Braun, K.P.; Leijten, F.S.; van Nieuwenhuizen, O.; Wokke, J.H.; van den Bergh, W.M. Magnesium treatment for patients with refractory status epilepticus due to POLG1-mutations. *J. Neurol.* **2011**, *258*, 218–222. [CrossRef] [PubMed]

139. Pandey, M.; Gupta, A.; Baduni, N.; Vijfdar, H.; Sinha, S.; Jain, A. Refractory status epilepticus-magnesium as rescue therapy. *Anaesth. Intens. Care* **2010**, *38*, 962.

140. Zou, L.P.; Wang, X.; Dong, C.H.; Chen, C.H.; Zhao, W.; Zhao, R.Y. Three-week combination treatment with acth + magnesium sulfate versus acth monotherapy for infantile spasms: A 24-week, randomized, open-label, follow-up study in China. *Clin. Ther.* **2010**, *32*, 692–700. [CrossRef] [PubMed]

141. Gorica, D.; Slavica, D.D.; Vladan, D.; Nebojsa, Z.; Curcic, D.; Rankovic, A.; Branimir, R.; Vladimir, J. Interictal ionized magnesium/total serum magnesium ratio in serbian population with drug resistant epilepsy-whether is severe epilepsy in fact brain injury? *Neuropsychiatry* **2017**, *7*, 629–636. [CrossRef]

142. Forte, G.; Alimonti, A.; Violante, N.; Di Gregorio, M.; Senofonte, O.; Petrucci, F.; Sancesario, G.; Bocca, B. Calcium, copper, iron, magnesium, silicon and zinc content of hair in parkinson's disease. *J. Trace Elem. Med. Biol.* **2005**, *19*, 195–201. [CrossRef] [PubMed]

143. De Lau, L.M.; Breteler, M.M. Epidemiology of Parkinson's disease. *Lancet Neurol.* **2006**, *5*, 525–535. [CrossRef]

144. Ambrosi, G.; Cerri, S.; Blandini, F. A further update on the role of excitotoxicity in the pathogenesis of parkinson's disease. *J. Neural Transm.* **2014**, *121*, 849–859. [CrossRef] [PubMed]

145. Kurup, R.K.; Kurup, P.A. Hypothalamic digoxin-mediated model for Parkinson's disease. *Int. J. Neurosci.* **2003**, *113*, 515–536. [CrossRef] [PubMed]

146. Miyake, Y.; Tanaka, K.; Fukushima, W.; Sasaki, S.; Kiyohara, C.; Tsuboi, Y.; Yamada, T.; Oeda, T.; Miki, T.; Kawamura, N.; et al. Dietary intake of metals and risk of Parkinson's disease: A case-control study in Japan. *J. Neurol. Sci.* **2011**, *306*, 98–102. [CrossRef] [PubMed]

147. Schwab, R.S.; Poryali, A.; Ames, A. Normal serum magnesium levels in Parkinson's disease. *Neurology* **1964**, *14*, 855–856. [CrossRef] [PubMed]

148. Bocca, B.; Alimonti, A.; Senofonte, O.; Pino, A.; Violante, N.; Petrucci, F.; Sancesario, G.; Forte, G. Metal changes in csf and peripheral compartments of Parkinsonian patients. *J. Neurol. Sci.* **2006**, *248*, 23–30. [CrossRef] [PubMed]

149. Yasui, M.; Kihira, T.; Ota, K. Calcium, magnesium and aluminum concentrations in Parkinson's disease. *Neurotoxicology* **1992**, *13*, 593–600. [PubMed]

150. Uitti, R.J.; Rajput, A.H.; Rozdilsky, B.; Bickis, M.; Wollin, T.; Yuen, W.K. Regional metal concentrations in Parkinson's disease, other chronic neurological diseases, and control brains. *Can. J. Neurol. Sci.* **1989**, *16*, 310–314. [CrossRef] [PubMed]

151. Alzheimer's Association. 2018 alzheimer's disease facts and figures. *Alzheimer Dement.* **2018**, *14*, 367–429.

152. Zadori, D.; Veres, G.; Szalardy, L.; Klivenyi, P.; Vecsei, L. Alzheimer's disease: Recent concepts on the relation of mitochondrial disturbances, excitotoxicity, neuroinflammation, and kynurenines. *J. Alzheimers Dis.* **2018**, *62*, 523–547. [CrossRef] [PubMed]

153. Shatenstein, B.; Kergoat, M.-J.; Reid, I. Poor nutrient intakes during 1-year follow-up with community-dwelling older adults with early-stage Alzheimer dementia compared to cognitively intact matched controls. *J. Am. Diet. Assoc.* **2007**, *107*, 2091–2099. [CrossRef] [PubMed]

154. Veronese, N.; Zurlo, A.; Solmi, M.; Luchini, C.; Trevisan, C.; Bano, G.; Manzato, E.; Sergi, G.; Rylander, R. Magnesium status in Alzheimer's disease: A systematic review. *Am. J. Alzheimers Dis. Other Demen.* **2016**, *31*, 208–213. [CrossRef] [PubMed]

155. Barbagallo, M.; Belvedere, M.; Di Bella, G.; Dominguez, L.J. Altered ionized magnesium levels in mild-to-moderate Alzheimer's disease. *Magnes. Res.* **2011**, *24*, 115–121.

156. Andrasi, E.; Igaz, S.; Molnár, Z.; Mako, S. Disturbances of magnesium concentrations in various brain areas in alzheimer's disease. *Magnes. Res.* **2000**, *13*, 189–196. [PubMed]

157. Glick, J.L. Dementias: The role of magnesium deficiency and an hypothesis concerning the pathogenesis of alzheimer's disease. *Med. Hypotheses* **1990**, *31*, 211–225. [CrossRef]

158. Basun, H.; Forssell, L.; Wetterberg, L.; Winblad, B. Metals and trace elements in plasma and cerebrospinal fluid in normal aging and Alzheimer's disease. *J. Neural Transm. Parkinson Dis. Dement. Sect.* **1991**, *3*, 231–258.

159. Boström, F.; Hansson, O.; Gerhardsson, L.; Lundh, T.; Minthon, L.; Stomrud, E.; Zetterberg, H.; Londos, E. Csf mg and Ca as diagnostic markers for dementia with lewy bodies. *Neurobiol. Aging* **2009**, *30*, 1265–1271. [CrossRef] [PubMed]

160. Kobayashi, S.; Fujiwara, S.; Arimoto, S.; Koide, H.; Fukuda, J.; Shimode, K.; Yamaguchi, S.; Okada, K.; Tsunematsu, T. Hair aluminium in normal aged and senile dementia of alzheimer type. *Progress Clin. Biol. Res.* **1989**, *317*, 1095–1109. [CrossRef]

161. Shore, D.; Henkin, R.I.; Nelson, N.R.; Agarwal, R.P.; Wyatt, R.J. Hair and serum copper, zinc, calcium, and magnesium concentrations in alzheimer-type dementia. *J. Am. Geriatr. Soc.* **1984**, *32*, 892–895. [CrossRef] [PubMed]

162. Gustaw-Rothenberg, K.; Lerner, A.; Bonda, D.J.; Lee, H.-G.; Zhu, X.; Perry, G.; Smith, M.A. Biomarkers in Alzheimer's disease: Past, present and future. *Biomark. Med.* **2010**, *4*, 15–26. [CrossRef] [PubMed]

163. Singh, N.K.; Banerjee, B.; Bala, K.; Basu, M.; Chhillar, N. Polymorphism in cytochrome P450 2D6, glutathione S-transferases Pi 1 genes, and organochlorine pesticides in Alzheimer disease: A case–control study in north indian population. *J. Geriatr. Psychiatry Neurol.* **2014**, *27*, 119–127. [CrossRef] [PubMed]

164. Vural, H.; Demirin, H.; Kara, Y.; Eren, I.; Delibas, N. Alterations of plasma magnesium, copper, zinc, iron and selenium concentrations and some related erythrocyte antioxidant enzyme activities in patients with Alzheimer's disease. *J. Trace Elem. Med. Biol.* **2010**, *24*, 169–173. [CrossRef] [PubMed]

165. Borella, P.; Giardino, A.; Neri, M.; Andermarker, E. Magnesium and potassium status in elderly subjects with and without dementia of the Alzheimer type. *Magnes. Res.* **1990**, *3*, 283–289. [PubMed]

166. Brackenridge, C.; McDonald, C. The concentrations of magnesium and potassium in erythrocytes and plasma of geriatric patients with psychiatric disorders. *Med. J. Aust.* **1969**, *2*, 390. [PubMed]

167. Lemke, M.R. Plasma magnesium decrease and altered calcium/magnesium ratio in severe dementia of the Alzheimer type. *Biol. Psychiatry* **1995**, *37*, 341–343. [CrossRef]

168. Hozumi, I.; Hasegawa, T.; Honda, A.; Ozawa, K.; Hayashi, Y.; Hashimoto, K.; Yamada, M.; Koumura, A.; Sakurai, T.; Kimura, A. Patterns of levels of biological metals in CSF differ among neurodegenerative diseases. *J. Neurol. Sci.* **2011**, *303*, 95–99. [CrossRef] [PubMed]

169. Çilliler, A.E.; Öztürk, Ş.; Özbakır, Ş. Serum magnesium level and clinical deterioration in alzheimer's disease. *Gerontology* **2007**, *53*, 419–422. [CrossRef] [PubMed]

170. Koc, E.R.; Ilhan, A.; Ayturk, Z.; Acar, B.; Gurler, M.; Altuntas, A.; Karapirli, M.; Bodur, A.S. A comparison of hair and serum trace elements in patients with Alzheimer disease and healthy participants. *Turk. J. Med. Sci.* **2015**, *45*, 1034–1039. [CrossRef] [PubMed]

171. Balmus, I.M.; Strungaru, S.A.; Ciobica, A.; Nicoara, M.N.; Dobrin, R.; Plavan, G.; Stefanescu, C. Preliminary data on the interaction between some biometals and oxidative stress status in mild cognitive impairment and Alzheimer's disease patients. *Oxid. Med. Cell. Longev.* **2017**, *2017*, 1–7. [CrossRef] [PubMed]

172. Kieboom, B.C.T.; Licher, S.; Wolters, F.J.; Ikram, M.K.; Hoorn, E.J.; Zietse, R.; Stricker, B.H.; Ikram, M.A. Serum magnesium is associated with the risk of dementia. *Neurology* **2017**, *89*, 1716–1722. [CrossRef] [PubMed]

173. Cherbuin, N.; Kumar, R.; Sachdev, P.; Anstey, K.J. Dietary mineral intake and risk of mild cognitive impairment: The path through life project. *Front. Aging Neurosci.* **2014**, *6*, 4. [CrossRef] [PubMed]

174. Ozawa, M.; Ninomiya, T.; Ohara, T.; Hirakawa, Y.; Doi, Y.; Hata, J.; Uchida, K.; Shirota, T.; Kitazono, T.; Kiyohara, Y. Self-reported dietary intake of potassium, calcium, and magnesium and risk of dementia in the Japanese: The hisayama study. *J. Am. Geriatr. Soc.* **2012**, *60*, 1515–1520. [CrossRef] [PubMed]

175. Majid, A. Neuroprotection in stroke: Past, present, and future. *ISRN Neurol.* **2014**, *2014*, 515716. [CrossRef] [PubMed]

176. Lai, T.W.; Zhang, S.; Wang, Y.T. Excitotoxicity and stroke: Identifying novel targets for neuroprotection. *Prog. Neurobiol.* **2014**, *115*, 157–188. [CrossRef] [PubMed]

177. Laurant, P.; Touyz, R.M. Physiological and pathophysiological role of magnesium in the cardiovascular system: Implications in hypertension. *J. Hypertens.* **2000**, *18*, 1177–1191. [CrossRef] [PubMed]

178. Ohira, T.; Peacock, J.M.; Iso, H.; Chambless, L.E.; Rosamond, W.D.; Folsom, A.R. Serum and dietary magnesium and risk of ischemic stroke: The atherosclerosis risk in communities study. *Am. J. Epidemiol.* **2009**, *169*, 1437–1444. [CrossRef] [PubMed]

179. Adebamowo, S.N.; Jimenez, M.C.; Chiuve, S.E.; Spiegelman, D.; Willett, W.C.; Rexrode, K.M. Plasma magnesium and risk of ischemic stroke among women. *Stroke* **2014**, *45*, 2881–2886. [CrossRef] [PubMed]

180. Goyal, N.; Tsivgoulis, G.; Malhotra, K.; Houck, A.L.; Khorchid, Y.M.; Pandhi, A.; Inoa, V.; Alsherbini, K.; Alexandrov, A.V.; Arthur, A.S.; et al. Serum magnesium levels and outcomes in patients with acute spontaneous intracerebral hemorrhage. *J. Am. Heart Assoc.* **2018**, *7*, e008698. [CrossRef] [PubMed]

181. Zhang, X.; Xia, J.; Del Gobbo, L.C.; Hruby, A.; Dai, Q.; Song, Y. Serum magnesium concentrations and all-cause, cardiovascular, and cancer mortality among U.S. Adults: Results from the NHANES I epidemiologic follow-up study. *Clin. Nutr.* **2017**, 30304–30307. [CrossRef] [PubMed]

182. Rosique-Esteban, N.; Guasch-Ferré, M.; Hernández-Alonso, P.; Salas-Salvadó, J. Dietary magnesium and cardiovascular disease: A review with emphasis in epidemiological studies. *Nutrients* **2018**, *10*, 168. [CrossRef] [PubMed]

183. Fang, X.; Wang, K.; Han, D.; He, X.; Wei, J.; Zhao, L.; Imam, M.U.; Ping, Z.; Li, Y.; Xu, Y.; et al. Dietary magnesium intake and the risk of cardiovascular disease, type 2 diabetes, and all-cause mortality: A dose–response meta-analysis of prospective cohort studies. *BMC Med.* **2016**, *14*, 210. [CrossRef] [PubMed]

184. Larsson, S.C.; Orsini, N.; Wolk, A. Dietary magnesium intake and risk of stroke: A meta-analysis of prospective studies. *Am. J. Clin. Nutr.* **2011**, *95*, 362–366. [CrossRef] [PubMed]

185. Nie, Z.-L.; Wang, Z.-M.; Zhou, B.; Tang, Z.-P.; Wang, S.-K. Magnesium intake and incidence of stroke: Meta-analysis of cohort studies. *Nutr. Metab. Cardiovasc. Dis.* **2013**, *23*, 169–176. [CrossRef] [PubMed]

186. Adebamowo, S.N.; Spiegelman, D.; Flint, A.J.; Willett, W.C.; Rexrode, K.M. Intakes of magnesium, potassium, and calcium and the risk of stroke among men. *Int. J. Stroke* **2015**, *10*, 1093–1100. [CrossRef] [PubMed]

187. Iso, H.; Stampfer, M.J.; Manson, J.E.; Rexrode, K.; Hennekens, C.H.; Colditz, G.A.; Speizer, F.E.; Willett, W.C. Prospective study of calcium, potassium, and magnesium intake and risk of stroke in women. *Stroke* **1999**, *30*, 1772–1779. [CrossRef] [PubMed]

188. Larsson, S.C.; Virtanen, M.J.; Mars, M.; Männistö, S.; Pietinen, P.; Albanes, D.; Virtamo, J. Magnesium, calcium, potassium, and sodium intakes and risk of stroke in male smokers. *Arch. Int. Med.* **2008**, *168*, 459–465. [CrossRef] [PubMed]

189. Weng, L.-C.; Yeh, W.-T.; Bai, C.-H.; Chen, H.-J.; Chuang, S.-Y.; Chang, H.-Y.; Lin, B.-F.; Chen, K.-J.; Pan, W.-H. Is ischemic stroke risk related to folate status or other nutrients correlated with folate intake? *Stroke* **2008**, *39*, 3152–3158. [CrossRef] [PubMed]

190. Leijenaar, J.F.; Dorhout Mees, S.M.; Algra, A.; van den Bergh, W.M.; Rinkel, G.J.; Group, M.-I.S. Effect of magnesium treatment and glucose levels on delayed cerebral ischemia in patients with subarachnoid hemorrhage: A substudy of the magnesium in aneurysmal subarachnoid haemorrhage trial (MASH-II). *Int. J. Stroke* **2015**, *10* (Suppl. A100), 108–112. [CrossRef] [PubMed]

191. You, S.; Zhong, C.; Du, H.; Zhang, Y.; Zheng, D.; Wang, X.; Qiu, C.; Zhao, H.; Cao, Y.; Liu, C.F. Admission low magnesium level is associated with in-hospital mortality in acute ischemic stroke patients. *Cerebrovasc. Dis.* **2017**, *44*, 35–42. [CrossRef] [PubMed]

192. Bayir, A.; Kara, H.; Ak, A.; Cander, B.; Kara, F. Magnesium sulfate in emergency department patients with hypertension. *Biol. Trace Elem. Res.* **2009**, *128*, 38–44. [CrossRef] [PubMed]

193. Liotta, E.M.; Prabhakaran, S.; Sangha, R.S.; Bush, R.A.; Long, A.E.; Trevick, S.A.; Potts, M.B.; Jahromi, B.S.; Kim, M.; Manno, E.M.; et al. Magnesium, hemostasis, and outcomes in patients with intracerebral hemorrhage. *Neurology* **2017**, *89*, 813–819. [CrossRef] [PubMed]

194. Mozaffarian, D.; Benjamin, E.J.; Go, A.S.; Arnett, D.K.; Blaha, M.J.; Cushman, M.; Das, S.R.; de Ferranti, S.; Despres, J.P.; Fullerton, H.J.; et al. Heart disease and stroke statistics-2016 update: A report from the American heart association. *Circulation* **2016**, *133*, e38–e360. [CrossRef] [PubMed]

195. Mees, S.M.D.; Algra, A.; Vandertop, W.P.; van Kooten, F.; Kuijsten, H.A.; Boiten, J.; van Oostenbrugge, R.J.; Salman, R.A.-S.; Lavados, P.M.; Rinkel, G.J. Magnesium for aneurysmal subarachnoid haemorrhage (MASH-2): A randomised placebo-controlled trial. *Lancet* **2012**, *380*, 44–49. [CrossRef]

196. Saver, J.L.; Starkman, S.; Eckstein, M.; Stratton, S.J.; Pratt, F.D.; Hamilton, S.; Conwit, R.; Liebeskind, D.S.; Sung, G.; Kramer, I. Prehospital use of magnesium sulfate as neuroprotection in acute stroke. *N. Engl. J. Med.* **2015**, *372*, 528–536. [CrossRef] [PubMed]

197. Bradford, C.M.; Finfer, S.; O'Connor, A.; Yarad, E.; Firth, R.; McCallister, R.; Harrington, T.; Steinfort, B.; Faulder, K.; Assaad, N. A randomised controlled trial of induced hypermagnesaemia following aneurysmal subarachnoid haemorrhage. *Crit. Care Resusc.* **2013**, *15*, 119. [PubMed]

198. Van den Bergh, W.M.; van der Schaaf, I.; van Gijn, J. The spectrum of presentations of venous infarction caused by deep cerebral vein thrombosis. *Neurology* **2005**, *65*, 192–196. [CrossRef] [PubMed]

199. Wong, G.K.C.; Poon, W.S.; Chan, M.T.; Boet, R.; Gin, T.; Ng, S.C.; Zee, B.C. Intravenous magnesium sulphate for aneurysmal subarachnoid hemorrhage (IMASH): A randomized, double-blinded, placebo-controlled, multicenter phase III trial. *Stroke* **2010**, *41*, 921–926. [CrossRef] [PubMed]

200. Dorhout Mees, S.M.; Algra, A.; Wong, G.K.; Poon, W.S.; Bradford, C.M.; Saver, J.L.; Starkman, S.; Rinkel, G.J.; van den Bergh, W.M.; et al. Early magnesium treatment after aneurysmal subarachnoid hemorrhage: Individual patient data meta-analysis. *Stroke* **2015**, *46*, 3190–3193. [CrossRef] [PubMed]

201. Veyna, R.S.; Seyfried, D.; Burke, D.G.; Zimmerman, C.; Mlynarek, M.; Nichols, V.; Marrocco, A.; Thomas, A.J.; Mitsias, P.D.; Malik, G.M. Magnesium sulfate therapy after aneurysmal subarachnoid hemorrhage. *J. Neurosurg.* **2002**, *96*, 510–514. [CrossRef] [PubMed]

202. Van Norden, A.; Van Den Bergh, W.; Rinkel, G. Dose evaluation for long-term magnesium treatment in aneurysmal subarachnoid haemorrhage. *J. Clin. Pharm. Ther.* **2005**, *30*, 439–442. [CrossRef] [PubMed]

203. Chen, M.-D.; Rimmer, J.H. Effects of exercise on quality of life in stroke survivors: A meta-analysis. *Stroke* **2011**, *42*, 832–837. [CrossRef] [PubMed]

204. Chia, R.; Hughes, R.; Morgan, M.K. Magnesium: A useful adjunct in the prevention of cerebral vasospasm following aneurysmal subarachnoid haemorrhage. *J. Clin. Neurosci.* **2002**, *9*, 279–281. [CrossRef] [PubMed]

205. Akdemir, H.; Kulaksızoğlu, E.O.; Tucer, B.; Menkü, A.; Postalc, L.; Günald, Ö. Magnesium sulfate therapy for cerebral vasospasm after aneurysmal subarachnoid hemorrhage. *Neurosurg. Q.* **2009**, *19*, 35–39. [CrossRef]

206. Panahi, Y.; Mojtahedzadeh, M.; Najafi, A.; Ghaini, M.R.; Abdollahi, M.; Sharifzadeh, M.; Ahmadi, A.; Rajaee, S.M.; Sahebkar, A. The role of magnesium sulfate in the intensive care unit. *EXCLI J.* **2017**, *16*, 464. [PubMed]

207. Lampl, Y.; Gilad, R.; Geva, D.; Eshel, Y.; Sadeh, M. Intravenous administration of magnesium sulfate in acute stroke: A randomized double-blind study. *Clin. Neuropharmacol.* **2001**, *24*, 11–15. [CrossRef] [PubMed]

208. Hassan, A.E.; Chaudhry, S.A.; Grigoryan, M.; Tekle, W.G.; Qureshi, A.I. National trends in utilization and outcomes of endovascular treatment of acute ischemic stroke patients in the mechanical thrombectomy era. *Stroke* **2012**, *43*, 3012–3017. [CrossRef] [PubMed]

209. Singh, N.N.; Pan, Y.; Muengtaweeponsa, S.; Geller, T.J.; Cruz-Flores, S. Cannabis-related stroke: Case series and review of literature. *J. Stroke Cerebrovasc. Dis.* **2012**, *21*, 555–560. [CrossRef] [PubMed]

210. Afshari, D.; Moradian, N.; Rezaei, M. Evaluation of the intravenous magnesium sulfate effect in clinical improvement of patients with acute ischemic stroke. *Clin. Neurol. Neurosurg.* **2013**, *115*, 400–404. [CrossRef] [PubMed]
211. Pan, W.H.; Lai, Y.H.; Yeh, W.T.; Chen, J.R.; Jeng, J.S.; Bai, C.H.; Lin, R.T.; Lee, T.H.; Chang, K.C.; Lin, H.J.; et al. Intake of potassium- and magnesium-enriched salt improves functional outcome after stroke: A randomized, multicenter, double-blind controlled trial. *Am. J. Clin. Nutr.* **2017**, *106*, 1267–1273. [CrossRef] [PubMed]

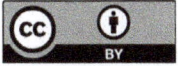

nutrients

MDPI

Article

TRPM6 is Essential for Magnesium Uptake and Epithelial Cell Function in the Colon

Francesca Luongo [1], Giuseppe Pietropaolo [1], Mathieu Gautier [2], Isabelle Dhennin-Duthille [2], Halima Ouadid-Ahidouch [2], Federica I. Wolf [1,*] and Valentina Trapani [1,*]

[1]   Istituto di Patologia Generale, Università Cattolica del Sacro Cuore, Fondazione Policlinico Universitario "Agostino Gemelli" IRCCS, I-00168 Rome, Italy; francesca.luongo@unicatt.it (F.L.); giuseppepietrop1993@libero.it (G.P.)
[2]   Laboratoire de Physiologie Cellulaire et Moléculaire-EA4667, UFR Sciences, Université de Picardie Jules Verne, F-80039 Amiens, France; mathieu.gautier@u-picardie.fr (M.G.); isabelle.dhennin-Duthille@u-picardie.fr (I.D.-D.); ha-sciences@u-picardie.fr (H.O.-A.)
*   Correspondence: federica.wolf@unicatt.it (F.I.W.); valentina.trapani@unicatt.it (V.T.)

Received: 28 May 2018; Accepted: 13 June 2018; Published: 18 June 2018

Abstract: Intestinal magnesium (Mg) uptake is essential for systemic Mg homeostasis. Colon cells express the two highly homologous transient receptor potential melastatin type (TRPM) 6 and 7 Mg^{2+} channels, but their precise function and the consequences of their mutual interaction are not clear. To explore the functional role of TRPM6 and TRPM7 in the colon, we used human colon cell lines that innately express both channels and analyzed the functional consequences of genetic knocking-down, by RNA interference, or pharmacological inhibition, by NS8593, of either channel. TRPM7 silencing caused an increase in Mg^{2+} influx, and correspondingly enhanced cell proliferation and migration, while downregulation of TRPM6 did not affect significantly either Mg^{2+} influx or cell proliferation. Exposure to the specific TRPM6/7 inhibitor NS8593 reduced Mg^{2+} influx, and consequently cell proliferation and migration, but Mg supplementation rescued the inhibition. We propose a model whereby in colon cells the functional Mg^{2+} channel at the plasma membrane may consist of both TRPM7 homomers and TRPM6/7 heteromers. A different expression ratio between the two proteins may result in different functional properties. Altogether, our findings confirm that TRPM6 cannot be replaced by TRPM7, and that TRPM6/7 complexes and TRPM6/7-mediated Mg^{2+} influx are indispensable in human epithelial colon cells.

Keywords: cell migration; cell proliferation; intestine; ion imaging; magnesium channel; magnesium homeostasis; MagT1; NS8593; TRPM7; wound healing

1. Introduction

Magnesium (Mg) is involved in virtually all major metabolic and signaling pathways in the cell, and disturbances of Mg homeostasis accompany a variety of diseases [1]. Despite recent advancements in understanding the critical role of Mg in health and disease, the molecular mechanisms governing cellular and systemic Mg balance remain debated. Systemic Mg homeostasis primarily depends on the concerted actions of the intestine responsible for Mg uptake from food, and the kidneys, that regulate urinary Mg excretion [1]. Classical physiological experiments with different animal species have identified two Mg transport systems in the intestinal epithelium: An active transcellular and a passive paracellular pathway [2,3]. The paracellular pathway, which is driven by the electrochemical gradient, is responsible for bulk Mg absorption and takes place mostly in the small intestine, whereas fine-tuning occurs in the cecum and colon via transcellular transport. The transcellular route consists of apical Mg entry, mediated by Mg permeable channels, and a basolateral extrusion step involving putative Na^+/Mg^{2+} exchangers.

Nutrients **2018**, *10*, 784

In the last two decades, several proteins have been proposed to facilitate Mg transport [4], but the biological roles of most of them continue to arouse dispute. The best-characterized transporters are the transient receptor potential melastatin (TRPM) 6 and 7 cation channels. Both TRPM6 and TRPM7 contain a transmembrane TRP channel segment fused to a cytosolic α-type serine/threonine protein kinase domain, but the functional relationship and the potential interplay between the channel and kinase moieties are still debated [5]. TRPM7 is ubiquitously expressed in human tissues and has been proposed as an indispensable cellular Mg entry pathway since TRPM7-deficient cell lines have intracellular Mg deficiency and severe cell growth defects [6,7]. The highly homologous TRPM6 channel has a more restricted expression: The highest levels are found in the distal convoluted tubule of the kidney and in the distal small intestine and colon, in murine as well as human tissues [8,9]. Interestingly, TRPM6 expression in the kidney and intestine is regulated by dietary Mg availability [8–11]. The critical role of TRPM6 for systemic Mg homeostasis became evident when loss-of-function mutations in the TRPM6 gene were discovered in patients with a rare form of hereditary hypomagnesemia (hypomagnesemia with secondary hypocalcemia, HSH) [12,13]. Although the etiology of low Mg levels in HSH was initially ascribed to renal Mg wasting, recent findings challenged this view suggesting that a defect in the intestinal Mg uptake might be of primary relevance [14]. Consequently, it is crucial to identify the key molecular players of intestinal Mg absorption and their regulation.

It is intriguing that transporting epithelia such as colon mucosa express both TRPM6 and TRPM7. Pioneering work showed that the two proteins are not redundant, and the functional ion channel at the plasma membrane is a multimeric complex consisting of either TRPM7 homotetramers or TRPM6/7 heterotetramers, each possessing different biophysical properties [15–17]. However, most findings were derived from heterologous expression models and resulted in considerable controversy on the relationship between the two channels and their exact functional role (for an up-to-date review, see Reference [5]). Recent data from our group seem to corroborate the view that TRPM6, rather than TRPM7, might have a central role in the colon; indeed, we showed that dietary Mg exerts a protective effect on colonic mucosa by upregulating TRPM6 expression in an in vivo model [18]. In the present work, we sought to scrutinize the exact role of each of the two sister channels in the colon. We decided to use human colon cell lines that innately express both channels, and, therefore, may well epitomize the physiological context. In our model cell lines, we dissected the contribution of each channel, by specifically RNA interference (RNAi) silencing either of them, and analyzing the functional consequences in terms of magnesium influx, proliferation, and migration. We present data suggesting that an alteration in the ratio between differently assorted tetramers might constitute a flexible way to modulate cation influx and affect related signaling pathways.

2. Materials and Methods

2.1. Cell Culture

Human colon carcinoma HT29, HCT116, and RKO cells were routinely grown in Dulbecco's modified Eagle's medium (DMEM) supplemented with 10% fetal bovine serum (FBS), 2 mM glutamine, 100 U/mL penicillin, and 100 μg/mL streptomycin in a 5% CO_2 humidified atmosphere at 37 °C. Human colon carcinoma Caco-2 cells were grown in the same medium supplemented with 20% FBS. To assess cell proliferation in conditions of different Mg availability, Mg-free DMEM (Invitrogen) was supplemented as for routine culture plus the desired amounts of $MgSO_4$. To obtain a transient downregulation of TRPM7, we used a short interfering RNA (siRNA) targeting the nucleotide sequence 5'-GTCTTGCCATGAAATACTC-3' (Dharmacon Research Inc., Chicago, IL, USA). For silencing TRPM6, predesigned siRNAs against human TRPM6 were purchased from Qiagen. Specific siRNAs were transfected into cells (50 ng per 400,000 cells) using HiPerFect Transfection Reagent (Qiagen Srl., Milan, Italy) following the manufacturer's protocol. Non-silencing, scrambled sequences were used as controls (CTRL). NS8593 hydrochloride salt was purchased from Sigma Aldrich; a stock solution was made in dimethyl sulfoxide (DMSO) and stored in aliquots at $-20\ °C$. To assess proliferation, cells were counted on a Thoma chamber in duplicate samples at given time points.

2.2. Western Blot

Cells were lysed in radioimmunoprecipitation assay (RIPA) buffer (50 mM Tris, pH = 8, 150 mM NaCl, 1 mM ethylenediaminetetraacetic acid (EDTA), 1% NP-40, 0.05% sodium deoxycholate, and 0.1% SDS) supplemented with protease inhibitors (10 µg/mL leupeptin, 20 µg/mL aprotinin, 1 mM phenylmethanesulfonyl fluoride, 1 mM NaVO$_4$, and 100 mM NaF). Protein concentrations were determined using the Bradford protein assay (Bio-Rad Laboratories Srl., Segrate (MI), Italy). Cell extracts (50 µg) were resolved by SDS-PAGE (8%), transferred to polyvinylidene fluoride (PVDF) membranes, and probed with rabbit monoclonal anti-TRPM7 (1:1000, Abcam Ltd., Cambridge, UK), rabbit polyclonal anti-TRPM6 (1:500, Biorbyt Ltd., Cambridge, UK), rabbit polyclonal anti-tubulin or actin (1:1000, Sigma-Aldrich Srl., Milan, Italy) primary antibodies. Horseradish peroxidase-conjugated secondary antibodies (GE Healthcare Srl., Milan, Italy) were detected by use of the ECL Prime Western Blotting Detection Reagent (GE Healthcare Srl, Milan, Italy) and the ChemiDoc XRS system (Bio-Rad Laboratories Srl., Segrate (MI) Italy).Densitometric analysis was performed by using the National Institutes of Health (NIH) ImageJ software.

2.3. Mg^{2+} Influx Measurements

Subconfluent cells grown on 35-mm microscopy dishes (µ-dish, ibidi GmbH, Martinsried, Germany) were loaded with 3 µM Mag-Fluo-4-AM (Thermo Fisher Scientific, Monza (MI), Italy), and imaged in a Na$^+$, Ca^{2+} and Mg^{2+}-free buffer at a confocal laser scanning microscope, as previously described [19]. Cytosolic fluorescence signals were recorded as time series of 5 min at a sampling frequency of 30 frames/min. The baseline was monitored for 30 s, then MgSO$_4$ was added drop wise to a final concentration of 20 mM. Changes in intracellular Mg levels at single cell level were estimated by the mean fluorescent increment ΔF/F [20]. Image analysis was performed by Leica Confocal Software on 10 representative cells in each microscopic field, and experiments were repeated independently at least three times.

2.4. Cell Cycle Analysis

Cells were fixed in 70% ethanol and stored at 4 °C until analysis. Prior to analysis, cell pellets were resuspended in 0.2 mg/mL of propidium iodide (PI) in Hank's balanced salt solution containing 0.6% NP-40 and RNase (1 mg/mL). The cell suspension was then filtered and analyzed for DNA content on a Coulter EPICS 753 flow cytometer, as previously described [21]. The percentage of cells in different phases of the cell cycle was determined using ModFit analysis software (version 5.2, Verity Software House Inc., Topsham, ME, USA).

2.5. Scratch Assay

A scratch assay was performed as previously reported [18]. Cells were seeded in culture inserts (ibidi GmbH, 70,000 cells/well insert) and cultured for 24 h to allow attachment. Insert removal created a 500-µm-wide cell-free gap between two confluent cell monolayers. Wound closure was monitored with an Eclipse TE2000-S microscope (Nikon Instruments Spa, Campo Bisenzio (FI), Italy) for up to 48 h, and images were analyzed using the NIH ImageJ software. Results were expressed as the percentage of the initial gap area that was covered by cells after the indicated time.

2.6. Statistical Analysis

All experiments were repeated independently three times. Prism software (version 5.01, GraphPad Software Inc., La Jolla, CA, USA) was used for all statistical analyses. Statistical significance was evaluated using unpaired Student's *t* test. Differences were considered statistically significant for a *p* value < 0.05, and significance levels were assigned as follows: * for *p* < 0.05, ** for *p* < 0.01.

3. Results

3.1. Cell Characterization

First, we assessed a panel of human colon cell lines (HT29, HCT116, RKO and Caco-2) for TRPM6 and TRPM7 protein expression using Western blot. As expected, all tested lines expressed both channels, though to various levels (Figure 1A,B). We focused on HT29 cells, which expressed the highest TRPM6 levels, but confirmed selected experiments in HCT116 cells. In HT29 cells, we also verified that proliferation was strictly dependent on extracellular Mg availability (Figure 1C).

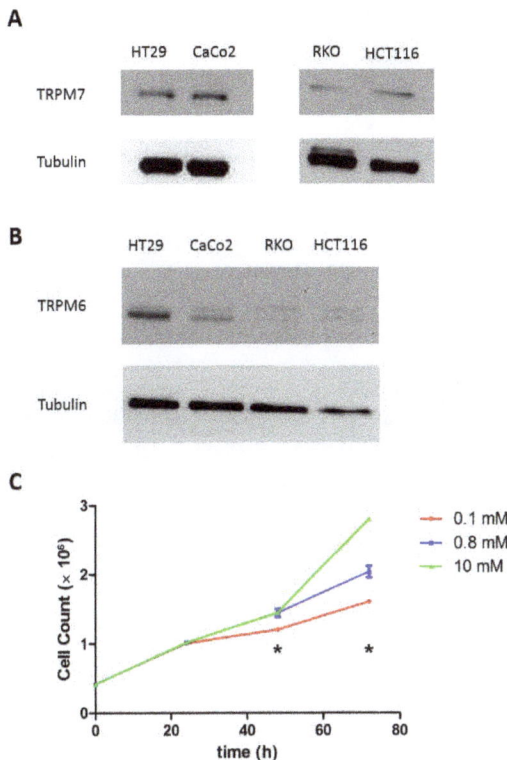

Figure 1. Human colon cells express both transient receptor potential melastatin type TRPM6 and TRPM7 and depend on extracellular Mg availability for growing. A representative Western blot (*n* = 3) is shown for (**A**) TRPM7 and (**B**) TRPM6 in a panel of human colon cell lines. Tubulin was used as a loading control. (**C**) HT29 cell proliferation in conditions of low (0.1 mM), normal (0.8 mM) and high (10 mM) Mg availability. Cells were grown in Mg-free Dulbecco's modified Eagle's medium (DMEM) supplemented as for routine culture plus the indicated amounts of $MgSO_4$ and counted at 24, 48 and 72 h in duplicates (*n* = 3). * *p* < 0.05 by unpaired Student's *t* test.

To downregulate specifically the expression of either channel, we used transient siRNA transfection and assessed mRNA and protein expression by real-time reverse transcriptase polymerase chain reaction (RT-PCR) and Western blot, respectively. Significant TRPM7 knock-down was achieved at the mRNA level and was confirmed at the protein level in both HT29 and HCT116 cells (Figure 2A,

Figures S1 and S2). TRPM7 silencing did not affect TRPM6 expression (Figure 2A). Transfection of TRPM6-specific siRNA resulted in knock-down of TRPM6 expression with no effects on TRPM7 expression in HT29 cells (Figure 2B). Similar results were obtained in HCT116 cells (not shown).

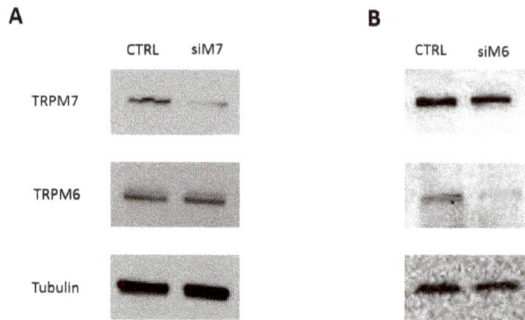

Figure 2. Specific short interfering RNA (siRNA) transfection efficiently downregulates TRPM7 and TRPM6 in human colon cells. HT29 cells were transfected with either (**A**) TRPM7 or (**B**) TRPM6-specific siRNA, and protein expression of both channels was evaluated by western blot 48 h after transfection. Non-silencing, scrambled sequences were used as controls (CTRL). Tubulin was used as a loading control. A representative blot is shown ($n = 3$). Note that TRPM7 silencing does not affect TRPM6 expression and vice versa. See Figure S1 in supplementary materials for complete blots, and Figure S2 in supplementary materials for mRNA expression by real time RT-PCR and additional data on HCT116 cells.

These data prove that RNAi can achieve specific and significant downregulation of each channel and allow the distinguishing of the contribution of TRPM6 vs. TRPM7 to given cell functions.

3.2. Contribution of TRPM7 to Colon Cell Functions

Next, we transfected cells with TRPM7-specific siRNA and evaluated the effects on cation influx and most closely related functions, such as proliferation and migration, in both HT29 and HCT116 cells. Results for HT29 cells are shown in Figure 3, while principal findings for HCT116 cells are reported in Figure S3. In preliminary experiments, TRPM7-silenced cells paradoxically exhibited a significant increase in constitutive divalent cation influx as assessed by the Mn^{2+} quenching technique (Figure S3A). Since the Mn^{2+} quenching assay does not discriminate the divalent species involved, to determine whether the transmembrane flux was due to an Mg^{2+} entry, we performed live imaging of cells loaded with the Mg-specific fluorescent probe Mag-Fluo-4. Fluorescence imaging confirmed that TRPM7-silenced cells had a higher Mg^{2+} uptake (Figure 3A). In addition, TRPM7-silenced cells showed a significantly faster proliferation rate, as assessed by cell counting (Figure 3B), and confirmed by a higher percentage of cells in the S phase of the cell cycle (Figure 3C). Finally, we performed a scratch assay to evaluate the effect of TRPM7 downregulation on wound healing capacity, which encompasses both proliferation and migration properties. We found that TRPM7-silenced cells closed the cell-free gap much more efficiently than control cells (Figure 3D,E).

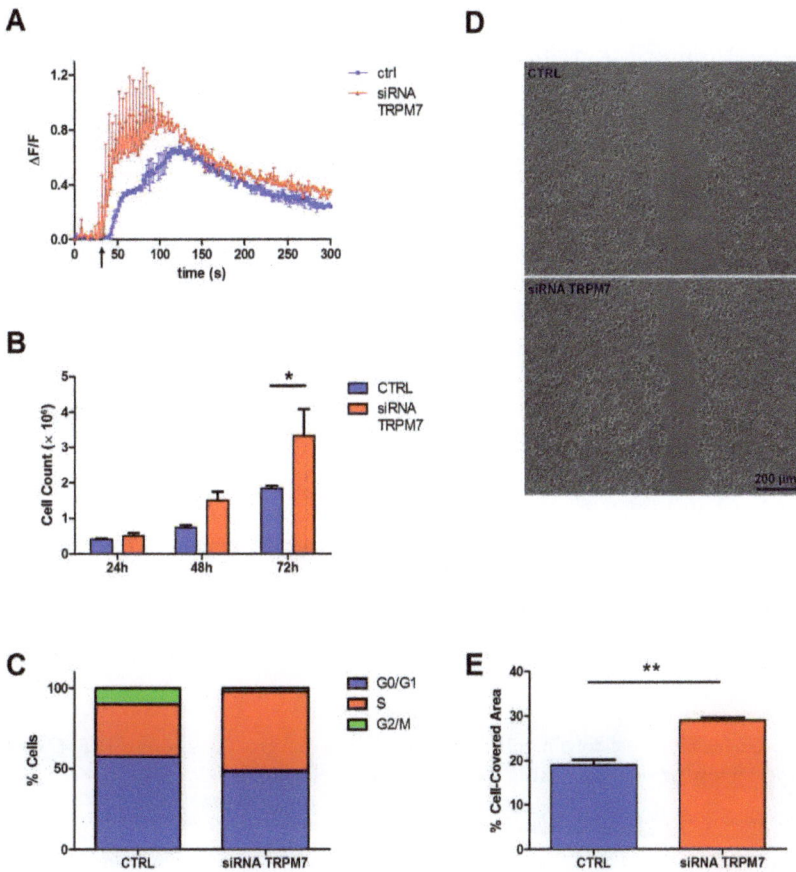

Figure 3. Contribution of TRPM7 to Mg^{2+} influx and Mg-dependent colon cell functions. HT29 cells were transiently silenced for TRPM7 as detailed in Materials and Methods. For HCT116 cells, see Figure S2. (**A**) Mg^{2+} influx capacity, as assessed 72 h after siRNA transfection. Mag-Fluo-4-loaded cells were challenged with 20 mM Mg (arrow) and time course of single-cell fluorescence was followed by live confocal imaging. The mean fluorescence ($\Delta F/F$) of 10 cells $\pm$ standard error (SE) from a representative experiment is reported ($n = 3$). (**B**) Cell proliferation. Cells were counted at the indicated times after siRNA transfection; mean $\pm$ SE of three independent experiments is shown. (**C**) Cell cycle distribution, as assessed 72 h after siRNA transfection. The percentage of cells in each phase was evaluated by flow cytometry; results are from a representative experiment ($n = 3$). (**D**) Cell migration. Cells were silenced and grown to confluence in well inserts for 24 h. Insert removal created a 500-μm-wide cell-free gap, whose closure was monitored by microscopy. Representative images of the wound after 24 h in CTRL and siRNA TRPM7 cells are shown. (**E**) Cell migration. Quantification of the cell-covered area from three independent wound healing assays. Results are expressed as the percentage of the initial gap area that was covered by cells after 24 h. * $p < 0.05$, ** $p < 0.01$ by unpaired Student's *t* test.

Altogether, these results provide a consistent picture whereby downregulation of TRPM7 in TRPM6-expressing colon cells paradoxically results in strengthening of the characteristics usually associated to TRPM7 expression in other tissues, namely cation entry, proliferation and migration.

3.3. Contribution of TRPM6 to Colon Cell Functions

We moved on to examine TRPM6 contribution to the same cellular functions by transfecting a TRPM6-specific siRNA in HT29 cells. In marked contrast to TRPM7-silenced cells, downregulation of TRPM6 did not appear to affect significantly Mg^{2+} influx, as measured by Mag-Fluo-4 imaging (Figure 4A). Correspondingly, proliferation rate of TRPM6-silenced cells did not differ considerably from that of control cells (Figure 4B).

A   **B**

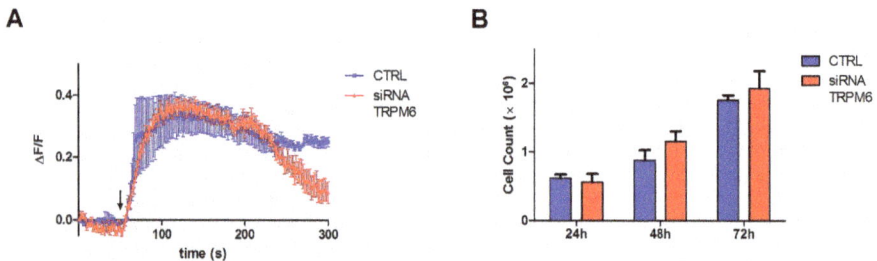

Figure 4. Contribution of TRPM6 to Mg^{2+} influx and cell proliferation in colon cells. HT29 cells were transiently silenced for TRPM6 and assessed at the indicate times after transfection. (**A**) Mg^{2+} influx capacity, as assessed 72 h after siRNA transfection. Mag-Fluo-4-loaded cells were challenged with 20 mM Mg (arrow) and time course of single-cell fluorescence was followed by live confocal imaging. The mean fluorescence ($\Delta F/F$) of 10 cells $\pm$ SE from a representative experiment is reported ($n = 3$). (**B**) Cell proliferation. Cells were counted in duplicates; mean $\pm$ SE of three independent experiments is shown.

We conclude that partial downregulation of TRPM6 on a background of normal TRPM7 expression is not sufficient to alter significantly Mg^{2+} entry and cell proliferation.

3.4. Contribution of TRPM6/7 Channels

In the light of the results reported in the previous sections, we hypothesized that the non-redundant role of TRPM6 and TRPM7 in colon cells might be due to the formation of heteromeric channels. It is known that, in cells expressing both TRPM6 and TRPM7, the functional ion channel at the plasma membrane may consist of both TRPM7 homomers and TRPM6/7 heteromers [5]. To support the idea that Mg^{2+} influx through TRPM6/7 channels is critical for colon cell function, we used pharmacological inhibition by NS8593, a specific TRPM6/7 inhibitor [22,23]. In the presence of 30 μM NS8593, colon cells exhibited a reduced Mg^{2+} influx capacity, as evidenced by a markedly delayed and slower uptake kinetics (Figure 5A). Correspondingly, NS8593-treated cells had a decreased proliferation rate (Figure 5B), and a lower percentage of cells in the S phase of the cell cycle (Figure 5C). Furthermore, NS8593 significantly inhibited wound healing capacity (Figure 5D,E). Importantly, inhibition by NS8593 on cell proliferation and migration was successfully rescued by Mg^{2+} supplementation (10 mM).

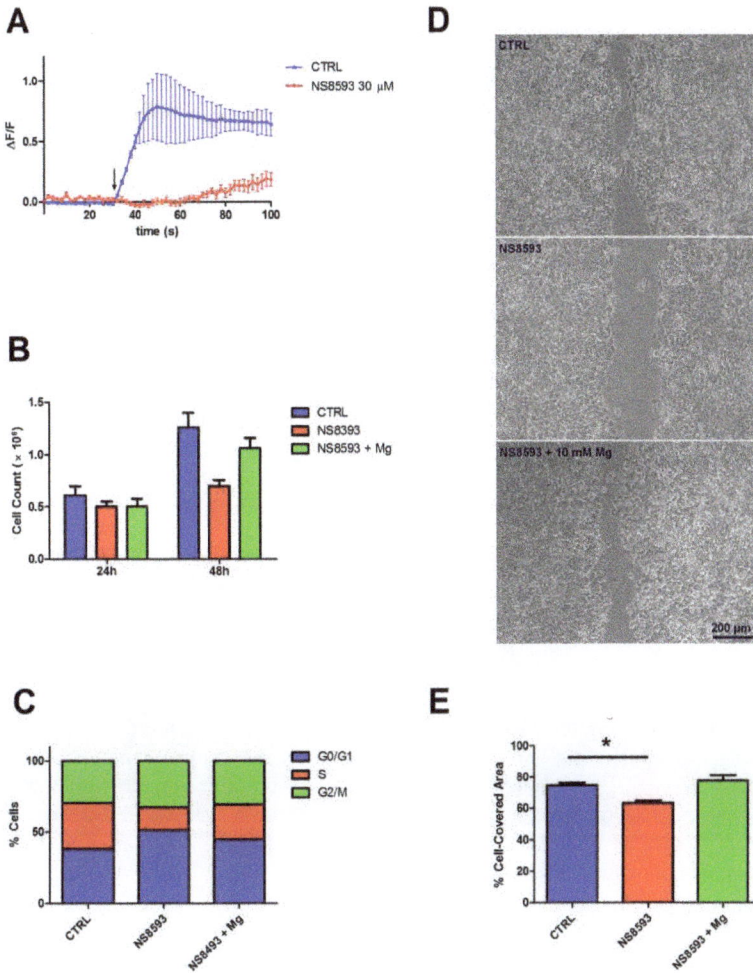

Figure 5. Contribution of TRPM6/7 channels to Mg^{2+} influx and cell proliferation. NS8593 was used at 30 μM. (**A**) Mg^{2+} influx capacity. Mag-Fluo-4-loaded cells were challenged with 20 mM Mg (arrow) in the presence of NS8593, and time course of single-cell fluorescence was followed by live confocal imaging. The mean fluorescence (ΔF/F) of 10 cells ± SE from a representative experiment is reported ($n = 3$). (**B**) Cell proliferation. Following NS8593 treatment, cells were counted at the indicated times; mean ± SE of three independent experiments is shown. (**C**) Cell cycle distribution. Percentage of cells in each phase was evaluated by flow cytometry 48 h after NS8593 treatment. Results are from a representative experiment ($n = 3$). (**D**) Cell migration. Cells were grown to confluence in inserts that were subsequently removed leaving a 500-μm-wide cell-free gap; NS8593 was added 4 h before insert removal. Wound closure was monitored by microscopy; representative images of the wound after 48 h in CTRL and NS8593-treated cells are shown. (**E**) Quantification of the cell-covered area ($n = 3$); results are expressed as the percentage of the initial gap area that was covered by cells after 48 h. * $p < 0.05$ by unpaired Student's *t* test.

Therefore, we conclude that in colon cells Mg^{2+} uptake and related cellular functions strictly depend on formation of TRPM6/7 heteromers, which are the physiological active form of the channel.

4. Discussion

In the present paper, we report the molecular characterization of Mg^{2+} uptake in colon cell lines and demonstrate that the presence of the TRPM6 channel is essential to guarantee intestinal Mg absorption and Mg-dependent epithelial functions. Surprisingly, we show that TRPM7 downregulation resulted in increased Mg^{2+} influx, and consequently faster cell proliferation and migration of colon cells (Figure 3). This is opposed to a vast body of literature indicating that in several other cell types TRPM7 expression is positively associated with proliferation and migration, in particular in tumor cells [24,25]. The most straightforward explanation for an increased Mg^{2+} influx in the face of a decreased TRPM7 expression would be that TRPM7 downregulation triggered an up-regulation in other Mg-transporting proteins, as previously demonstrated in different models [26,27]. Although we cannot rule out the involvement of still undisclosed players, we have convincing evidence that TRPM7-silenced cells displayed unchanged expression of the two major candidates, i.e., TRPM6 (Figure 2A) or MagT1 (Figure S1B). In contrast to TRPM7 knocking-down, TRPM6 silencing did not appear to affect significantly Mg^{2+} uptake and proliferation in colon cells (Figure 4).

To explain the apparent paradox in our results, we must take into account the coexistence of significant levels of both TRPM6 and TRPM7 in all tested cells. This implies that the functional ion channel at the plasma membrane may consist of both TRPM7 homomers and TRPM6/7 heteromers. The prevalence of either form may depend on the expression ratio between the two proteins, and may result in different functional properties.

It was originally proposed that native TRPM6 functions primarily as a subunit of heteromeric TRPM6/7 complexes [15], and this model has been corroborated by recent data [14,23,28]. The emerging picture is that TRPM6 and TRPM7 differentially contribute to regulatory characteristics of the heteromeric TRPM6/7 channel, so that the activity of the complex will hardly be affected by physiological intracellular concentrations of Mg^{2+} and Mg-ATP [23] or by osmotic changes [28]. This mechanism appears to be an indispensable prerequisite for efficient transcellular Mg^{2+} transport in intestinal cells, where a high and constant Mg^{2+} uptake should be uncoupled from cellular metabolism of Mg^{2+} and Mg-ATP [23], and should remain unaffected by frequent osmotic changes [28]. Such a functional fingerprint is probably not required in other cell types, which indeed only express TRPM7.

Our data fit perfectly in this model: Silencing either TRPM7 or TRPM6 is in fact a way to alter the relative abundance of the two proteins, and consequently will affect the ratio between differently assorted tetramers in favor of TRPM6/7 heteromers or TRPM7 homomers, respectively (Figure 6). We propose that TRPM7 downregulation tips the balance towards increased relative abundance of TRPM6/7 complexes, which are responsible for the observed increase in Mg^{2+} influx and Mg-dependent cell functions. Accordingly, in electrophysiological measurements current amplitudes of TRPM6/7 complexes were found to be higher than those of TRPM7 homomers [15,23,29]. In contrast, TRPM6 downregulation should favor TRPM7 homomerization and result in overall reduced Mg^{2+} influx and cell proliferation. Although we did not find a remarkable effect of TRPM6 downregulation (Figure 4), it must be noted that we only achieved a partial TRPM6 downregulation, which may be compatible with retaining sufficient levels of TRPM6/7 channels to foster Mg^{2+} entry and cell proliferation. However, when we used NS8593 as a potent and specific way to block channel activity regardless of its composition, we did obtain the expected reduction in Mg^{2+} uptake and cell growth (Figure 5). Furthermore, the observed inhibition was rescued by Mg supplementation, which proves that as long as sufficient Mg^{2+} entry occurs, cellular Mg homeostatic mechanisms are able to sustain cell proliferation and migration even with reduced TRPM6/7 function(s). Altogether, our findings confirm that TRPM6/7 complexes and TRPM6/7-mediated Mg^{2+} influx are absolutely necessary in human epithelial colon cells. More specifically, TRPM6 has an indispensable role in controlling Mg^{2+} entry and cell proliferation, and other ion channels, including the highly homologous TRPM7 channel, cannot replace its function.

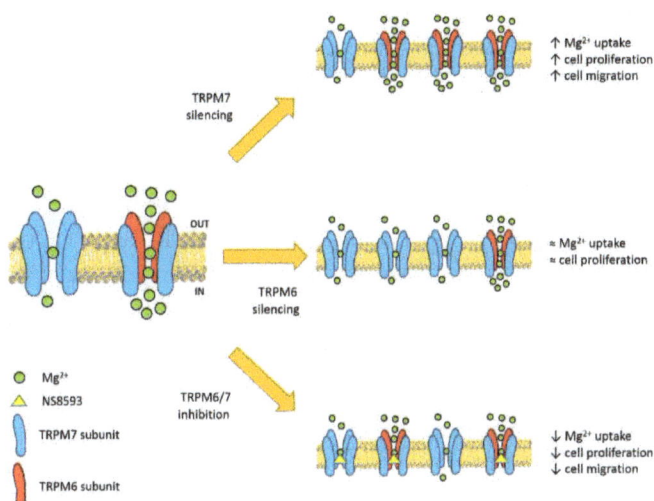

Figure 6. Suggested model for the role of TRPM6 in intestinal Mg absorption. Colon cancer cells express both TRPM7 and TRPM6, which can assemble into functional homomers or heteromers at the plasma membrane (left). The different regulation of TRPM7 and TRPM6/7 channels in physiological conditions determines higher Mg^{2+} fluxes through TRPM6/7 heteromers. Thus, the ratio between differently assorted tetramers affects cation influx and related signaling pathways (right panels). Partial TRPM7 silencing favors formation of TRPM6/7 channels, thereby increasing Mg^{2+} influx, and consequently cell proliferation and migration (upper right panel). In turn, partial TRPM6 knocking-down promotes assembly of TRPM7 homomers, which sustain basal Mg^{2+} influx and proliferation (middle right panel). Pharmacological inhibition of assembled channels decreases overall Mg^{2+} influx, and downstream functions (lower middle panel).

The main strength of our work is that we carried out our functional characterization in a completely naïve cell model, without resorting to heterologous expression systems. In the past, overexpression of recombinant proteins has greatly contributed to investigating TRPM6 and TRPM7 currents and regulation, but also generated conflicting and still unexplained results regarding TRPM6 [5]. Our results are limited to few prototypal human colon cell lines, and need further investigation before they can be generalized. In particular, the proof of concept of our hypothesis would require determination of the absolute expression levels of TRPM7 and TRPM6 as well as of the exact stoichiometric architecture of TRPM6/7 heteromers, which is technically very challenging.

Despite its limitations, our interpretation is completely in line with wider and more sophisticated studies demonstrating that TRPM6 is essential for intestinal magnesium absorption and systemic Mg balance. [14]. As for TRPM7, to the best of our knowledge, no studies investigated either mineral homeostasis in TRPM7-deficient adult mice or specific ablation of TRPM7 in the intestine. However, we would not expect to reproduce our results in a TRPM7 KO system, because the complete absence of TRPM7 would also impair TRPM6 proper localization and function [14,15]. Interestingly, heterozygous TRPM7 knock-in mice devoid of the kinase domain or activity display an altered systemic Mg homeostasis [7,30]. Although relative levels of TRPM7 homomers vs. TRPM6/7 heteromers might change in heterozygous mice, this situation cannot be exactly matched with our working model, since the current thinking is that the TRPM7 kinase moiety may function as a sensor of the organismal Mg status [30]. Overall, we cannot compare our in vitro data with any existing model. Nevertheless, the peculiarity, and paradoxically, the strength, of our model is that we only partially knock-down expression of either channel, thereby modulating the assortment of the functional complexes on a background of concurrent TRPM6 and TRPM7 expression.

5. Conclusions

In conclusion, our data confirm the existing view that maintenance of systemic Mg homeostasis requires a constant Mg supply that can be warranted only by TRPM6/7 heteromers in the intestine, and provide a simple and effective model to investigate the functional relationship between TRPM6 and TRPM7.

Supplementary Materials: The following are available online at http://www.mdpi.com/2072-6643/10/6/784/s1. Figure S1: Complete blots corresponding to the images shown in Figure 2A. Figure S2: Transient siRNA transfection efficiently downregulates *TRPM7* mRNA in human HT29 and HCT116 colon cells (**A**), and TRPM7 protein in HCT116 cells (**B**). Figure S3: Contribution of TRPM7 to Mg^{2+} influx and Mg-dependent cell functions in HCT116 cells. (**A**) Mn^{2+} quenching; (**B**) Mg^{2+} influx capacity; (**C**) Cell Proliferation; (**D**) Cell cycle distribution.

Author Contributions: Conceptualization: F.I.W. and V.T. Formal analysis: F.L. and V.T. Funding acquisition: H.O.-A. and F.I.W. Investigation: F.L., G.P., M.G., I.D.-D. and V.T. Resources: H.O.-A. and F.I.W. Supervision: H.O.-A., F.I.W. and V.T. Writing—original draft: V.T. Writing—review & editing: F.L., H.O.-A., F.I.W. and V.T.

Funding: F.L., G.P., F.I.W. and V.T. were supported by MIUR (D.3.2-2015). M.G., I.D.-D. and H.O.-A. were supported by the Ministère de l'Enseignement Supérieur et de la Recherche, by the Région Hauts-de-France" (Picardie) and Ligue Contre le Cancer (Septentrion).

Acknowledgments: Confocal imaging was performed at the LABCEMI (Laboratorio Centralizzato di Microscopia Ottica ed Elettronica), Università Cattolica del Sacro Cuore, Fondazione Policlinico Universitario "Agostino Gemelli" IRCCS, Rome, Italy.

Conflicts of Interest: The authors declare no conflict of interest.

References

1. De Baaij, J.H.; Hoenderop, J.G.; Bindels, R.J. Magnesium in man: Implications for health and disease. *Physiol. Rev.* **2015**, *95*, 1–46. [CrossRef] [PubMed]

2. Dai, L.J.; Ritchie, G.; Kerstan, D.; Kang, H.S.; Cole, D.E.; Quamme, G.A. Magnesium transport in the renal distal convoluted tubule. *Physiol. Rev.* **2001**, *81*, 51–84. [CrossRef] [PubMed]

3. Quamme, G.A. Recent developments in intestinal magnesium absorption. *Curr. Opin. Gastroenterol.* **2008**, *24*, 230–235. [CrossRef] [PubMed]

4. Quamme, G.A. Molecular identification of ancient and modern mammalian magnesium transporters. *Am. J. Physiol. Cell Physiol.* **2010**, *298*, C407–C429. [CrossRef] [PubMed]

5. Chubanov, V.; Mittermeier, L.; Gudermann, T. Role of kinase-coupled TRP channels in mineral homeostasis. *Pharmacol. Ther.* **2018**, *184*, 159–176. [CrossRef] [PubMed]

6. Schmitz, C.; Perraud, A.L.; Johnson, C.O.; Inabe, K.; Smith, M.K.; Penner, R.; Kurosaki, T.; Fleig, A.; Scharenberg, A.M. Regulation of vertebrate cellular Mg^{2+} homeostasis by TRPM7. *Cell* **2003**, *114*, 191–200. [CrossRef]

7. Ryazanova, L.V.; Rondon, L.J.; Zierler, S.; Hu, Z.; Galli, J.; Yamaguchi, T.P.; Mazur, A.; Fleig, A.; Ryazanov, A.G. TRPM7 is essential for Mg^{2+} homeostasis in mammals. *Nat. Commun.* **2010**, *1*, 109. [CrossRef] [PubMed]

8. Groenestege, W.M.; Hoenderop, J.G.; van den Heuvel, L.; Knoers, N.; Bindels, R.J. The epithelial Mg^{2+} channel transient receptor potential melastatin 6 is regulated by dietary Mg^{2+} content and estrogens. *J. Am. Soc. Nephrol.* **2006**, *17*, 1035–1043. [CrossRef] [PubMed]

9. Lameris, A.L.; Nevalainen, P.I.; Reijnen, D.; Simons, E.; Eygensteyn, J.; Monnens, L.; Bindels, R.J.; Hoenderop, J.G. Segmental transport of Ca^{2+} and Mg^{2+} along the gastrointestinal tract. *Am. J. Physiol. Gastrointest. Liver Physiol.* **2015**, *308*, G206–G216. [CrossRef] [PubMed]

10. Rondón, L.J.; Groenestege, W.M.; Rayssiguier, Y.; Mazur, A. Relationship between low magnesium status and TRPM6 expression in the kidney and large intestine. *Am. J. Physiol. Regul. Integr. Comp. Physiol.* **2008**, *294*, R2001–R2007. [CrossRef] [PubMed]

11. Van Angelen, A.A.; San-Cristobal, P.; Pulskens, W.P.; Hoenderop, J.G.; Bindels, R.J. The impact of dietary magnesium restriction on magnesiotropic and calciotropic genes. *Nephrol. Dial. Transplant.* **2013**, *28*, 2983–2993. [CrossRef] [PubMed]

12. Schlingmann, K.P.; Weber, S.; Peters, M.; Nejsum, L.N.; Vitzthum, H.; Klingel, K.; Kratz, M.; Haddad, E.; Ristoff, E.; Dinour, D.; et al. Hypomagnesemia with secondary hypocalcemia is caused by mutations in TRPM6, a new member of the TRPM gene family. *Nat. Genet.* **2002**, *31*, 166–170. [CrossRef] [PubMed]

13. Walder, R.Y.; Landau, D.; Meyer, P.; Shalev, H.; Tsolia, M.; Borochowitz, Z.; Boettger, M.B.; Beck, G.E.; Englehardt, R.K.; Carmi, R.; Sheffield, V.C. Mutation of TRPM6 causes familial hypomagnesemia with secondary hypocalcemia. *Nat. Genet.* **2002**, *31*, 171–174. [CrossRef] [PubMed]

14. Chubanov, V.; Ferioli, S.; Wisnowsky, A.; Simmons, D.G.; Leitzinger, C.; Einer, C.; Jonas, W.; Shymkiv, Y.; Bartsch, H.; Braun, A.; et al. Epithelial magnesium transport by TRPM6 is essential for prenatal development and adult survival. *Elife* **2016**, *5*, e20914. [CrossRef] [PubMed]

15. Chubanov, V.; Waldegger, S.; Mederos y Schnitzler, M.; Vitzthum, H.; Sassen, M.C.; Seyberth, H.W.; Konrad, M.; Gudermann, T. Disruption of TRPM6/TRPM7 complex formation by a mutation in the TRPM6 gene causes hypomagnesemia with secondary hypocalcemia. *Proc. Natl. Acad. Sci. USA* **2004**, *101*, 2894–2899. [CrossRef] [PubMed]

16. Schmitz, C.; Dorovkov, M.V.; Zhao, X.; Davenport, B.J.; Ryazanov, A.G.; Perraud, A.L. The channel kinases TRPM6 and TRPM7 are functionally nonredundant. *J. Biol. Chem.* **2005**, *280*, 37763–37771. [CrossRef] [PubMed]

17. Li, M.; Jiang, J.; Yue, L. Functional characterization of homo- and heteromeric channel kinases TRPM6 and TRPM7. *J. Gen. Physiol.* **2006**, *127*, 525–537. [CrossRef] [PubMed]

18. Trapani, V.; Petito, V.; Di Agostini, A.; Arduini, D.; Hamersma, W.; Pietropaolo, G.; Luongo, F.; Arena, V.; Stigliano, E.; Lopetuso, L.R.; et al. Dietary magnesium alleviates experimental murine colitis through upregulation of the transient receptor potential melastatin 6 channel. *Inflamm. Bowel Dis.* **2018**, in press. [CrossRef] [PubMed]

19. Trapani, V.; Arduini, D.; Luongo, F.; Wolf, F.I. EGF stimulates Mg^{2+} influx in mammary epithelial cells. *Biochem. Biophys. Res. Commun.* **2014**, *454*, 572–575. [CrossRef] [PubMed]

20. Trapani, V.; Schweigel-Röntgen, M.; Cittadini, A.; Wolf, F.I. Intracellular magnesium detection by fluorescent indicators. *Methods Enzymol.* **2012**, *505*, 421–444. [PubMed]

21. Wolf, F.I.; Trapani, V.; Simonacci, M.; Boninsegna, A.; Mazur, A.; Maier, J.A. Magnesium deficiency affects mammary epithelial cell proliferation: Involvement of oxidative stress. *Nutr. Cancer* **2009**, *61*, 131–136. [CrossRef] [PubMed]

22. Chubanov, V.; Mederos y Schnitzler, M.; Meißner, M.; Schäfer, S.; Abstiens, K.; Hofmann, T.; Gudermann, T. Natural and synthetic modulators of SK (K(ca)2) potassium channels inhibit magnesium-dependent activity of the kinase-coupled cation channel TRPM7. *Br. J. Pharmacol.* **2012**, *166*, 1357–1376. [CrossRef] [PubMed]

23. Ferioli, S.; Zierler, S.; Zaißerer, J.; Schredelseker, J.; Gudermann, T.; Chubanov, V. TRPM6 and TRPM7 differentially contribute to the relief of heteromeric TRPM6/7 channels from inhibition by cytosolic Mg^{2+} and Mg·ATP. *Sci. Rep.* **2017**, *7*, 8806. [CrossRef] [PubMed]

24. Trapani, V.; Arduini, D.; Cittadini, A.; Wolf, F.I. From magnesium to magnesium transporters in cancer: TRPM7, a novel signature in tumour development. *Magnes. Res.* **2013**, *26*, 149–155. [PubMed]

25. Gautier, M.; Perrière, M.; Monet, M.; Vanlaeys, A.; Korichneva, I.; Dhennin-Duthille, I.; Ouadid-Ahidouch, H. Recent advances in oncogenic roles of the TRPM7 chanzyme. *Curr. Med. Chem.* **2016**, *23*, 4092–4107. [CrossRef] [PubMed]

26. Deason-Towne, F.; Perraud, A.L.; Schmitz, C. The Mg^{2+} transporter MagT1 partially rescues cell growth and Mg^{2+} uptake in cells lacking the channel-kinase TRPM7. *FEBS Lett.* **2011**, *585*, 2275–2278. [CrossRef] [PubMed]

27. Cazzaniga, A.; Moscheni, C.; Trapani, V.; Wolf, F.I.; Farruggia, G.; Sargenti, A.; Iotti, S.; Maier, J.A.; Castiglioni, S. The different expression of TRPM7 and MagT1 impacts on the proliferation of colon carcinoma cells sensitive or resistant to doxorubicin. *Sci. Rep.* **2017**, *7*, 40538. [CrossRef] [PubMed]

28. Zhang, Z.; Yu, H.; Huang, J.; Faouzi, M.; Schmitz, C.; Penner, R.; Fleig, A. The TRPM6 kinase domain determines the Mg·ATP sensitivity of TRPM7/M6 heteromeric ion channels. *J. Biol. Chem.* **2014**, *289*, 5217–5227. [CrossRef] [PubMed]

29. Chubanov, V.; Schlingmann, K.P.; Wäring, J.; Heinzinger, J.; Kaske, S.; Waldegger, S.; Mederos y Schnitzler, M.; Gudermann, T. Hypomagnesemia with secondary hypocalcemia due to a missense mutation in the putative pore-forming region of TRPM6. *J. Biol. Chem.* **2007**, *282*, 7656–7667. [CrossRef] [PubMed]

30. Ryazanova, L.V.; Hu, Z.M.; Suzuki, S.; Chubanov, V.; Fleig, A.; Ryazanov, A.G. Elucidating the role of the TRPM7 alpha-kinase: TRPM7 kinase inactivation leads to magnesium deprivation resistance phenotype in mice. *Sci. Rep.* **2014**, *4*, 7599. [CrossRef] [PubMed]

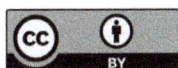

nutrients

MDPI

Article

A Pilot Randomized Trial of Oral Magnesium Supplementation on Supraventricular Arrhythmias

Pamela L. Lutsey [1,*], Lin Y. Chen [2], Anne Eaton [3], Melanie Jaeb [1], Kyle D. Rudser [3], James D. Neaton [3] and Alvaro Alonso [4]

[1] Division of Epidemiology & Community Health, School of Public Health, University of Minnesota, 1300 South 2nd Street, Suite 300, Minneapolis, MN 55454, USA; jaebx008@umn.edu
[2] Cardiovascular Division, Department of Medicine, University of Minnesota, Minneapolis, MN 55455, USA; chenx484@umn.edu
[3] Division of Biostatistics, School of Public Health, University of Minnesota, Minneapolis, MN 55455, USA; eato0055@umn.edu (A.E.); rudser@umn.edu (K.D.R.); jim@ccbr.umn.edu (J.D.N.)
[4] Department of Epidemiology, Rollins School of Public Health, Emory University, Atlanta, GA 30322, USA; alvaro.alonso@emory.edu
* Correspondence: Lutsey@umn.edu; Tel.: +1-612-624-5812; Fax: +1-612-624-0315

Received: 30 May 2018; Accepted: 6 July 2018; Published: 10 July 2018

Abstract: Low magnesium may increase the risk of atrial fibrillation. We conducted a double-blind pilot randomized trial to assess adherence to oral magnesium supplementation (400 mg of magnesium oxide daily) and a matching placebo, estimate the effect on circulating magnesium concentrations, and evaluate the feasibility of using an ambulatory heart rhythm monitoring device (ZioPatch) for assessing premature atrial contractions. A total of 59 participants were randomized; 73% were women, and the mean age was 62 years. A total of 98% of the participants completed the follow-up. In the magnesium supplement group, 75% of pills were taken, and in the placebo group, 83% were taken. The change in magnesium concentrations was significantly greater for those given the magnesium supplements than for those given the placebo (0.07; 95% confidence interval: 0.03, 0.12 mEq/L; $p = 0.002$). The ZioPatch wear time was approximately 13 of the requested 14 days at baseline and follow-up. There was no difference by intervention assignment in the change in log premature atrial contractions burden, glucose, or blood pressure. Gastrointestinal changes were more common among the participants assigned magnesium (50%) than among those assigned the placebo (7%), but only one person discontinued participation. In sum, compliance with the oral magnesium supplementation was very good, and acceptance of the ZioPatch monitoring was excellent. These findings support the feasibility of a larger trial for atrial fibrillation (AF) prevention with oral magnesium supplementation.

Keywords: magnesium; atrial fibrillation; glucose; randomized controlled trial

1. Introduction

Atrial fibrillation (AF) is a common cardiac arrhythmia characterized by irregular atrial electrical activity. In the United States (US), more than 3 million individuals had AF in 2010, and this figure is expected to more than double by 2050 [1–3]. Current AF treatments, including antiarrhythmic drugs and catheter ablation for rhythm restoration and oral anticoagulation for the prevention of thromboembolism, have suboptimal efficacy and carry significant risks [4]. The limitations of the available therapeutic approaches highlight the need for primary prevention interventions [5,6]. As highlighted in a 2009 National Heart, Lung, and Blood Institute (NHLBI) report [5] and stressed in a more recent Heart Rhythm Society-sponsored whitepaper [6], there is an urgent need to identify new and effective strategies for the primary prevention of AF.

Compelling evidence from numerous lines of inquiry suggests that low concentrations of serum magnesium may be causally associated with AF risk. First, magnesium supplementation is recommended as prophylaxis for the prevention of AF in patients undergoing cardiac surgery. A recent Cochrane systematic review and meta-analysis of randomized trials assessing the efficacy of magnesium supplementation for AF prevention in heart surgery reported an odds ratio of 0.55 (95% CI: 0.41, 0.73) for AF or supraventricular arrhythmia, comparing the magnesium intervention to the control [7]. Second, indirect evidence from three prospective epidemiologic studies provides some support for such intervention; each reported that individuals in the lowest versus the highest quantile of serum magnesium were 35–50% more likely to develop incident AF, after multivariable adjustment [8–10]. Finally, additional evidence for the effect of magnesium on the risk of arrhythmias is provided by a study of dietary magnesium restriction, in which 3 out of 14 women fed a low-magnesium diet developed AF, which resolved quickly after magnesium repletion [11].

Whether magnesium supplementation could have a role in the prevention of AF in the community has not been tested. Were magnesium supplementation shown to prevent AF and be safe over the long-term, it would be an ideal intervention for primary prevention, as it is easy to implement, inexpensive, and low concentrations are common. The population prevalence of low magnesium is not known but is believed to be high. Individuals at particularly high risk of hypomagnesemia are alcoholics, those who take certain diuretics, those with poorly controlled diabetes [12], and the elderly. In a study of nursing home residents, 33% were clinically deficient [13]. Intake of magnesium in the US population is also low, to the extent that the 2015 Dietary Guidelines Advisory Committee classified magnesium as a "shortfall nutrient", based on the finding that approximately 50% of Americans consume less than the estimated average requirement [14]. However, dietary magnesium intake and serum magnesium are poorly correlated; in the community-based Atherosclerosis Risk in Communities (ARIC) study, the Pearson's correlation coefficient was only 0.04 [9].

As part of the planning effort for a large randomized trial to prevent AF with magnesium supplementation, we conducted a double-blind, placebo-controlled randomized clinical trial of oral magnesium supplementation to assess supplement adherence, the side effects, the effect on serum magnesium concentration, and the feasibility of using an ambulatory monitoring device for the identification of arrhythmias.

2. Materials and Methods

The study was registered at Clinicaltrials.gov (# NCT02837328). The study protocol was approved by the University of Minnesota Institutional Review Board, and all participants provided written informed consent.

2.1. Study Participants

Participants of 55 years of age or older were recruited using fliers, the University of Minnesota StudyFinder website, invitations to individuals enrolled in the ResearchMatch research volunteer database, and invitations to University of Minnesota School of Public Health employees. The exclusion criteria included a prior history of heart disease (coronary heart disease, heart failure, AF), stroke, or known kidney disease; the use of type I or III antiarrhythmic drugs or digoxin; the current use of magnesium supplements; any prior history of allergy or intolerance to magnesium; lactose intolerance; and a prior history of inflammatory bowel disease or any severe gastrointestinal disorder. The use of multivitamins was allowable, because these typically contain relatively low dosages of Magnesium (e.g., 50 mg).

The eligible participants attended a baseline visit where measurements were conducted and a Zio® XT Patch (ZioPatch; iRhythm Technologies, Inc., San Francisco, CA, USA) heart rhythm monitor was applied by trained staff. After wearing the ZioPatch for 2 weeks, the participants were randomized 1:1 to either 400 mg of magnesium oxide or a placebo using block randomization within two strata of age (younger than 65 and 65 and older). The randomization was carried out separately for the two randomization strata. In each group, a randomization schedule was generated using randomly permuted blocks of random sizes. Block sizes of 2, 4, or 6 were permitted. The randomization was implemented using the blockrand package in R.

Following randomization, the participants were mailed the study intervention, which they took for a total of 12 weeks. Then, 10 weeks after beginning the study intervention, the participants took part in a follow-up clinic visit, and a second ZioPatch was applied. The participants continued the study intervention until the second ZioPatch was removed (2 weeks after the follow-up clinic visit). A participant flow diagram is provided in Figure 1.

Participant Flow Diagram

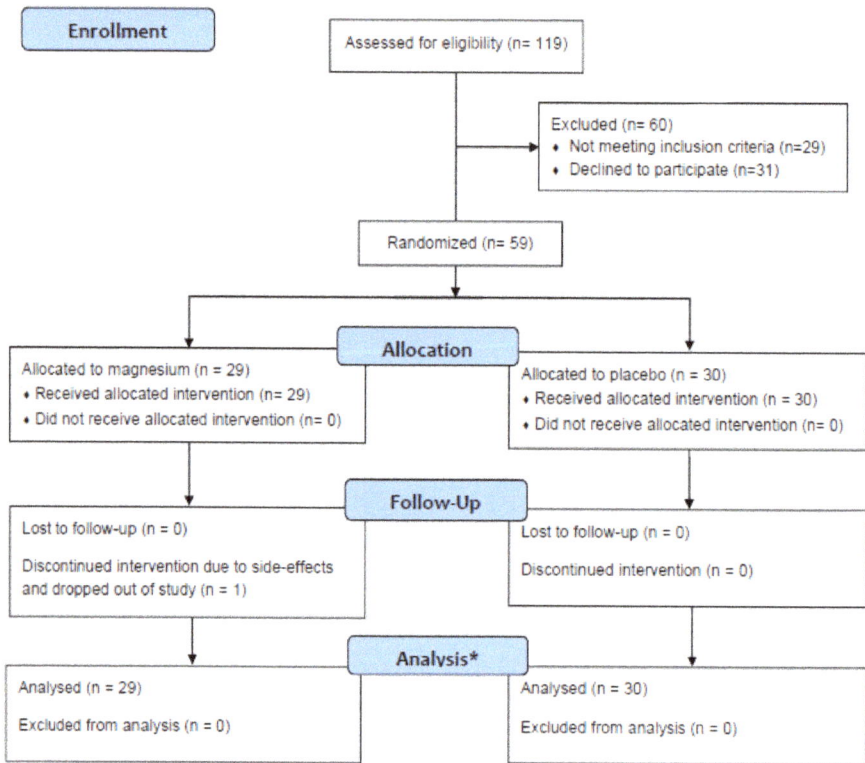

Figure 1. * Due to missing data on individual items, the total numbers of observations included in the linear models are 57, 57, 54, 54, 58, and 58 for the outcomes log premature atrial contraction (PAC) burden, PAC burden, serum magnesium, serum glucose, systolic blood pressure, and diastolic blood pressure, respectively.

2.2. Study Intervention and Blinding

The University of Minnesota Institute for Therapeutics Discovery and Drug Development produced the active study intervention (400 mg of magnesium oxide) and the matched placebo (lactose) according to Good Manufacturing Practices. The University of Minnesota Investigational Drug Service managed the bottling per the randomization scheme. The study participants and all the study staff were blinded to the treatment given.

2.3. Measurements

At the baseline and follow-up clinic visits, the participants completed questionnaires, and trained study staff conducted physiological measurements (i.e., anthropometry, blood pressure), phlebotomy, and applied the ZioPatch device. Treatment compliance was assessed by a pill count at the follow-up visit. At intervention days 21, 42, and 80, the participants were also emailed unique links to online questionnaires, administered via REDCap [15], which queried compliance and asked the following open-ended question about adverse effects: "Since starting the study, have you experienced anything out of the ordinary?" Participant blinding was also assessed on intervention day 80, the last day of the study.

The ZioPatch was used to identify premature atrial contractions (PACs). PACs are supraventricular arrhythmias associated with the future risk of AF [6,16,17] and are considered an intermediate phenotype of the arrhythmia, reflecting the underlying cardiac substrate that facilitates the development of AF [18]. The participants were asked to wear the ZioPatches for 2 weeks after each clinic visit. The information obtained from the ZioPatch devices was processed by the ZEUS algorithm, a comprehensive system that analyzes electrocardiographic data received from the device [19]. We counted as PACs isolated supraventricular ectopic beats, supraventricular ectopic couplet total count, and supraventricular ectopic triplet total count. The total PACs were then divided by the number of hours the ZioPatch recorded analyzable data, which yielded PACs per hour.

The participants were asked to fast for 8 h prior to blood draws. Serum magnesium and glucose were measured using the Roche Cobas 6000 at the University of Minnesota Advanced Research and Diagnostic Laboratory. Blood pressure was measured with the participant sitting, after a 5 min rest, with a random zero sphygmomanometer (Omron Digital Blood Pressure Monitor HEM-907XL; Omron Healthcare Inc., Kyoto, Japan). Three measurements were taken; all three measurements were averaged for use in analyses. Height and weight were measured with the participants in light clothing and shoes removed. Height was measured with a research stadiometer and weight with a scale.

2.4. Statistical Analysis

The goal of the pilot study was to assess adherence to the magnesium supplement and the feasibility of using the ZioPatch and to collect preliminary data on PACs, a predictor of AF. The targeted sample size of 60 was determined to detect a difference in the change in log PACs (follow-up minus baseline) between treatment groups of 0.79 standard deviation units with 80% power and 5% type I error (2-sided), assuming five participants would not complete the follow-up.

All analyses were intent-to-treat. Descriptive statistics are provided according to treatment assignment for baseline characteristics, adherence, magnesium concentrations, and other outcomes. The differences in baseline characteristics between groups were assessed using *t*-tests for continuous variables and Fisher's exact tests for categorical variables. Linear regression was used to evaluate whether change in outcomes differed according to treatment assignment, adjusting for the randomization stratification factor (age $\geq$65 vs. <65) and the baseline value of the outcome with robust variance estimates for confidence intervals and *p*-values. Post-hoc sensitivity analyses further adjusted for sex. As PAC burden is highly skewed, we pre-specified using log PAC burden for analysis and reported the ratio of geometric means. Pre-specified subgroup analyses were also performed, stratified by baseline magnesium concentration (< vs. $\geq$median). A two-sided *p*-value of <0.05 was used to indicate statistical significance. The analyses were conducted using R [20] version 3.4.0 (R Foundation, Vienna, Austria).

3. Results

3.1. Study Participants

Between March and June 2017, 59 participants were randomized: 29 were assigned to the magnesium supplement and 30 to the matching placebo. The participant characteristics were generally similar by treatment group, with the notable exception of sex; 86.2% of the participants in the treatment group were women, while in the placebo group, 60.0% were female (Table 1). The mean age of the participants was 61.5 ± 5.2 years. The baseline serum magnesium concentration was 1.74 ± 0.11 mEq/L in the participants assigned the magnesium supplements and 1.71 ± 0.10 in those assigned the placebo; 6.9% had magnesium concentrations below the threshold for clinical deficiency (<1.5 mEq/L), while 37.9% had concentrations below the threshold for subclinical deficiency (<1.7 mEq/L).

Table 1. Baseline participant characteristics * overall and stratified by intervention status.

	Overall	Magnesium (400 mg Daily)	Placebo	*p*-Value
N	59	29	30	
Demographics				
Age, years	61.5 ± 5.2	61.3 ± 5.3	61.6 ± 5.2	0.814
Age category				0.761
≥65 years	14 (23.7)	6 (20.7)	8 (26.7)	
<65 years	45 (76.3)	23 (79.3)	22 (73.3)	
Sex				0.039
Female	43 (72.9)	25 (86.2)	18 (60.0)	
Male	16 (27.1)	4 (13.8)	12 (40)	
Race				0.612
White	56 (94.9)	27 (93.1)	29 (96.7)	
Nonwhite	3 (5.1)	2 (6.9)	1 (3.3)	
Educational attainment				0.279
High school graduate or GED	1 (1.7)	0 (0)	1 (3.3)	
Some college	10 (16.9)	6 (20.7)	4 (13.3)	
College graduate	26 (44.1)	10 (34.5)	16 (53.3)	
Graduate school or professional school	22 (37.3)	13 (44.8)	9 (30)	
Physiologic characteristics				
Height, cm	167.9 (9.2)	167.1 (8.1)	168.7 (10.3)	0.491
Weight, kg	79.2 (18.2)	78.0 (18.0)	80.5 (18.7)	0.603
BMI, kg/m^2	27.9 ± 4.6	27.7 ± 4.9	28.0 ± 4.5	0.804
Serum magnesium, mEq/L	1.72 ± 0.11	1.74 ± 0.12	1.71 ± 0.10	0.308
Systolic blood pressure, mmHg	119 ± 16	119 ± 14	119 ± 18	0.933
Diastolic blood pressure, mmHg	71 ± 9	72 ± 9	71 ± 10	0.627
Antihypertensive medication	14 (24)	9 (31)	5 (17)	0.233
Serum glucose, mg/dL	98.9 ± 29.9	94.2 ± 10.6	103.2 ± 40.2	0.242
Sensitivity analysis **	95.2 ± 11.1	94.2 ± 10.6	96.2 ± 11.6	0.494
Glucose lowering medication	2 (3.4)	0 (0)	2 (6.7)	0.492
PAC burden, episodes/h	14.5 ± 58	8.5 ± 14	20.2 ± 80	0.437
Median (25th, 75th percentiles)	2.28 (1.22, 6.86)	3.64 (1.31, 7.57)	1.75 (1.12, 4.01)	
Log PAC burden, log(episodes/h)	1.15 ± 1.42	1.26 ± 1.35	1.04 ± 1.49	0.566
Median (25th, 75th percentiles)	0.82 (0.20, 1.92)	1.29 (0.27, 2.02)	0.55 (0.11, 1.39)	

GED, general education diploma; BMI, body mass index; PAC, premature atrial contractions; and SD, standard deviation. * mean ± SD or *n* (%). ** Omission of one participant with a baseline glucose value of 307 mg/dL.

Log PAC burden (episodes per hour) at baseline was 1.26 ± 1.35 in the treatment group and 1.15 ± 1.42 in the placebo group. At baseline, the average ZioPatch analyzable time in the intervention and placebo groups were 13.1 ± 1.7 and 12.9 ± 2.6 days, respectively, with 93.1% assigned to magnesium and 90.0% assigned to placebo wearing ≥12 days.

3.2. Follow-Up

A total of two participants, both in the intervention group, were missing ZioPatch information at follow-up; one participant dropped out of the study, and one was missing information due to a device malfunction.

3.3. Adherence and Magnesium Concentrations

Based on pill count, the participants in the magnesium group took 75.1% ± 17.8% of tablets, whereas those in the placebo group took 83.4% ± 5.9%. Self-reported information about the percent of missing pills and the reasons for missing pills is provided in Table 2. Of the participants, 60% in the Magnesium group reported missing at least 1 pill, as did 52% in the placebo group. The most common reason for missing pills was forgetting. However, five individuals in the Magnesium group marked the response "makes me sick" as the reason for not taking a pill, whereas no individuals in the placebo group reported missing pills for that reason.

Table 2. Self-reported compliance.

Compliance	% Reporting Missing Pills			Reason for Missing Pills, N			
				Forgot	Too Busy	Makes Me Sick	Other
Ever reported *							
Magnesium	60%			7	0	5	2
Placebo	52%			11	2	0	3
	% Reporting Missing Pills in:			Reason for Missing Pills, N			
Reported at Specific Follow-Up Visits **	Last 3 Days	Last 1 Week	Last 2 Weeks				
Intervention Day 21							
Magnesium	8%	12%	20%	2	0	2	1
Placebo	0%	7%	24%	7	1	0	0
Intervention Day 42							
Magnesium	22%	33%	39%	5	0	5	1
Placebo	15%	22%	31%	6	2	0	2
Intervention Day 80							
Magnesium	14%	27%	40%	5	0	1	0
Placebo	12%	23%	28%	6	1	0	1

* Over any time frame (i.e., last 3 days, last 1 week, last 2 weeks). ** Responses not mutually exclusive (e.g., the same individual could have reported forgetting to take pills at intervention days 21, 42, 80).

Over the 12-week follow-up period, those assigned magnesium supplementation had a significant increase in serum magnesium concentration as compared with those assigned the placebo (0.07 mEq/L; 95% CI: 0.03, 0.12; $p = 0.002$) (Table 3). In subgroup analyses, the change in magnesium concentration did not vary by baseline magnesium concentration (Table 4; p-interaction 0.24). Specifically, among the participants who at baseline were below the median serum magnesium concentration (i.e., 1.74 mEq/L), the effect of the magnesium versus the placebo on the change in the serum magnesium concentration was 0.05 (95% CI: 0.00, 0.10), whereas among those at or above the median at baseline, the effect was 0.12 (95% CI: 0.04, 0.20).

Table 3. Change in PACs and secondary endpoints (i.e., systolic blood pressure (SBP), diastolic blood pressure (DBP), serum glucose, serum magnesium) according to treatment group.

	Magnesium (400 mg Daily) Mean (SD)	Placebo Mean (SD)	Intervention Effect Coefficient * (95% CI)	p-Value
Primary outcome (episodes/h)				
Log PAC burden			0.94 (0.69, 1.3) **	0.73
Baseline	1.26 (1.4)	1.04 (1.49)		
Follow-up [†]	1.16 (1.41)	1.09 (1.53)		
Change	−0.06 (0.68)	0.05 (0.75)		
PAC burden			0.44 (−2.58, 3.46)	
Baseline	8.5 ± 14	20.2 ± 80		
Follow-up [†]	8.1 ± 12	14.6 ± 48		
Change	−0.6 ± 7	−5.6 ± 33		
Secondary outcomes				
Serum magnesium, mEq/L			0.07 (0.03, 0.12)	0.002
Baseline	1.74 (0.12)	1.71 (0.1)		
Follow-up [‡]	1.8 (0.13)	1.71 (0.11)		
Change	0.07 (0.09)	0 (0.1)		
Serum glucose, mg/dL				
Baseline	94.2 (10.6)	103.2 (40.2)	2.4 (−3.0, 7.7)	0.39
Follow-up [‡]	96.3 (12.2)	96.2 (13.7)		
Change	1.8 (7.5)	−7.1 (32.8)		
Serum glucose [¥], mg/dL				
Baseline	94.2 (10.6)	96.2 (11.6)	2.8 (−0.9, 6.4)	0.14
Follow-up [‡]	96.3 (12.2)	95 (12.4)		
Change	1.75 (7.5)	−1.21 (6.7)		
Systolic blood pressure, mmHg			2.9 (−1.8, 7.2)	0.18
Baseline	119 (14)	119 (18)		
Follow-up [‡]	118 (14)	115 (14)		
Change	−1 (10)	−4 (10)		
Diastolic blood pressure, mmHg			−0.5 (−3.5, 2.5)	0.74
Baseline	71.8 (8. 7)	70.6 (10.3)		
Follow-up [‡]	71.0 (8.8)	70.8 (8.7)		
Change	−0.5 (7.1)	0.2 (6.1)		

CI, confidence Interval; DBP, diastolic blood pressure; PAC, premature atrial contractions; SD, standard deviation; and SBP, systolic blood pressure. * Adjusted for age (≥65 or <65), and baseline concentration (e.g., when change in glucose is the outcome, models were adjusted for baseline glucose). The numbers of observations included in linear models are 57, 57, 54, 54, 53, 58, and 58 for the outcomes log PAC burden, PAC burden, serum magnesium, serum glucose, serum glucose excluding outlier, systolic blood pressure and diastolic blood pressure, respectively. ** Presented as a ratio of geometric means (i.e., exp(coefficient)). [†] ZioPatch was worn for a 2-week period, from the follow-up clinic visit (intervention week 10) through the end of the study (intervention week 12). [‡] Follow-up information obtained at clinic visit (intervention week 10). [¥] Outlier removed.

Table 4. Change in PACs and secondary endpoints (i.e., SBP, DBP, serum glucose, serum magnesium) according to treatment group, stratified by baseline serum magnesium concentration.

	Baseline Serum Magnesium Concentration				p-Interaction
Primary Outcome	<Median		≥Median		
	Intervention Effect Coefficient * (95% CI)	p-Value	Intervention Effect Coefficient * (95% CI)	p-Value	
Log PAC burden	0.89 (0.51, 1.54) **	0.67	0.91 (0.61, 1.35) **	0.64	0.88
Serum magnesium, mEq/L	0.05 (0, 0.10)	0.04	0.12 (0.04,0.20)	0.004	0.24
Serum glucose, magnesium/dL	−4.7 (−13.3, 4.0)	0.29	6.0 (2.0, 10.0)	0.03	0.06
Serum glucose, magnesium/dL [¥]	−3.2 (−9.0, 2.6)	0.28	6.0 (2.0, 10.0)	0.03	0.01
Systolic blood pressure, mmHg	4.8 (1.0, 8.5)	0.01	3.8 (−2.5, 10.2)	0.24	0.96
Diastolic blood pressure, mmHg	5.5 (0.6, 10.4)	0.03	2.4 (−5.6, 0.8)	0.14	0.009

CI, confidence Interval; DBP, diastolic blood pressure; PAC, premature atrial contractions; and SBP, systolic blood pressure. * Adjusted for age (≥65 or <65) and baseline concentration (e.g., when change in glucose is the outcome, models were adjusted for baseline glucose). [¥] Outlier removed. ** Ratio of geometric means.

3.4. Effect of Magnesium Supplementation on Trial Outcomes

Table 3 presents the study outcome values at baseline and follow-up, as well as age- and baseline value-adjusted differences in change according to intervention assignment. Spaghetti plots depicting individual change over the intervention period are provided in Figure 2. At follow-up, the ZioPatch average wear times were similar to the baseline, with 13.0 ± 1.8 days for the intervention group, 12.7 ± 2.3 days for the placebo group, and 92.6% assigned to magnesium and 73.3% assigned to placebo wearing ≥12 days. For the primary outcome, log PAC burden (episodes per hour), change over the intervention period was −0.06 (95% confidence interval (CI): −0.33, 0.20) for those randomized to the magnesium supplement and 0.05 (95% CI: −0.23, 0.33) for those randomized to the placebo. In the multivariable-adjusted models, there was no evidence of an intervention effect; the ratio of geometric means was 0.94 (0.69, 1.3), *p*-value = 0.73. Similarly, in subgroup analyses, the effect did not differ according to baseline magnesium concentration above versus below the median (Table 4; *p*-interaction = 0.88).

Magnesium supplementation was not significantly associated with change in serum glucose (2.4 (95% CI: −3.0, 7.7) mg/dL; *p* = 0.39). The lack of association remained in sensitivity analyses, excluding one participant with extremely high baseline glucose (2.8 (95% CI: −0.9, 6.4) mg/dL) and one participant who reported changing his/her diabetes medication status during the follow-up (2.0 (95%: −3.6, 7.5) mg/dL). The intervention was also not significantly associated with change in systolic or diastolic blood pressure overall (2.9 (95%: −1.4, 7.2) mmHg and −0.5 (95%: −3.5, 2.5) mmHg, respectively) or after excluding two participants who changed their blood pressure medication status between the baseline and follow-up visits.

In post-hoc analyses, where we additionally adjusted for sex, the results were similar. Also, no meaningful patterns emerged in additional subgroup analyses by age category and sex.

3.5. Safety and Tolerability of the Intervention

When asked an open-ended question about adverse events, the most commonly reported responses were related to gastrointestinal (GI) symptoms. Of the intervention group, 32% commented on GI changes at intervention day 21, 30% at day 42, and 33% at day 80. In the placebo group 7% commented on GI changes at intervention day 21, 4% at day 42, and 0% at day 80. When considering unique individuals, 50% assigned to magnesium and 7% assigned to placebo commented on GI changes at any point in the study. Specific GI comments, by intervention day, are provided in Table 5.

One person in the intervention group experienced side effects, which led the participant to discontinue blinded study treatment.

At the end of the study, when asked to which group they were assigned, among those assigned to the active treatment, 15% guessed magnesium supplements, 14.3% guessed placebo, and 35.7% reported not knowing (15 participants did not respond). Of those assigned to the placebo, 4.3% guessed magnesium supplements, 26.1% guessed placebo, and 69.6% reported not knowing (7 participants did not respond).

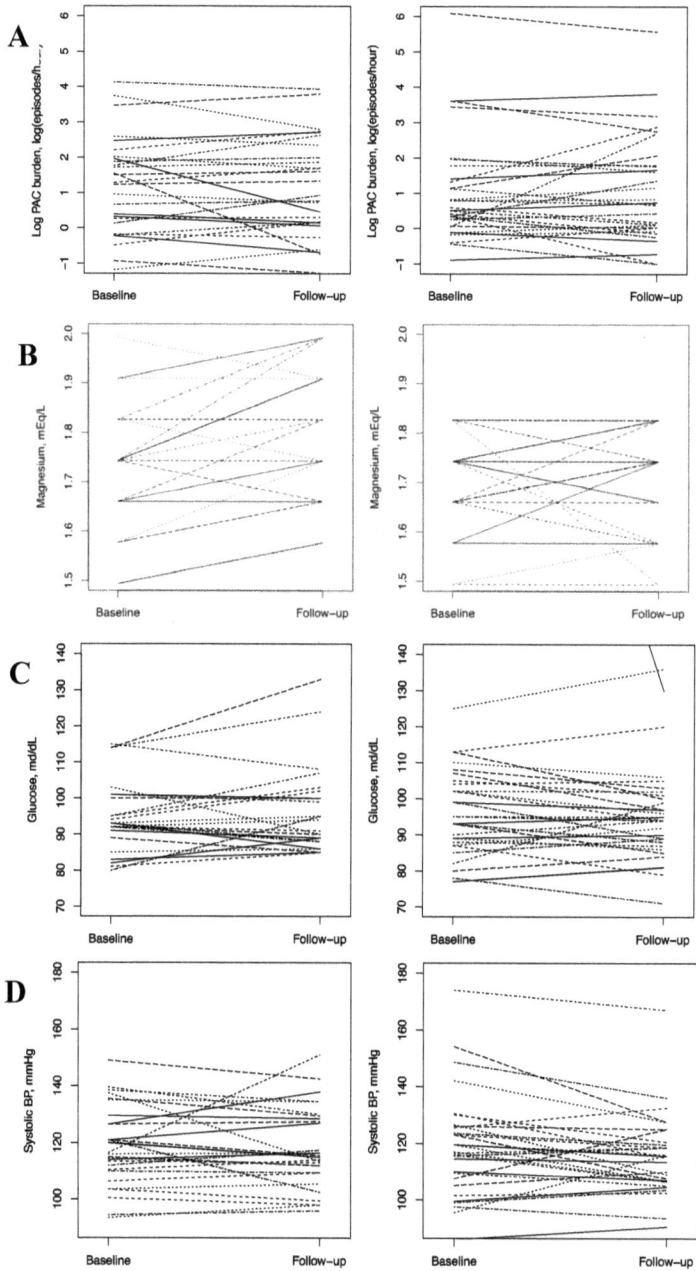

Figure 2. Spaghetti plots for change in (**A**) log PAC burden, (**B**) change in serum magnesium, (**C**) serum glucose *, and (**D**) SBP (systolic blood pressure). * One participant had a baseline glucose concentration of 307 mg/dL. The baseline value for this participant is outside the frame. PAC, premature atrial contractions; and BP, blood pressure.

Table 5. Gastrointestinal (GI)-related responses to the open-ended question, "Since starting the study, have you experienced anything out of the ordinary?" *.

Intervention Day #	Intervention	Comment
Day #21	Magnesium	Less solid stools
	Magnesium	Initially, I took the pill before bed with calcium and fish oil and a blood pressure med. It did not really make me sick, but I felt some bloating and cramping. I switched to taking it in the am, and that works better. That was the reason for missing.
	Magnesium	Diarrhea
	Magnesium	My stools have changed in consistency and color.
	Magnesium	I have had some diarrhea but that could be due to my innards. They have been unpredictable since my abdominal/colorectal surgeries.
	Magnesium	After 4 pills, I quit taking them due to intestinal issues. I was in the bathroom the third and fourth day and very crampy all day. I emailed and was told I could quit taking them.
	Magnesium	The first two days, I experienced brief bouts of diarrhea about 90 min after taking the pills. No problems since.
	Magnesium	Some diarrhea and gas
	Placebo	Sudden onset of nausea lasting about 30 s about an hour after taking the pill.
	Placebo	Increase in diarrhea but could be from the increase in nuts in my diet.
Day #42	Magnesium	Slightly often stools
	Magnesium	Diarrhea
	Magnesium	Slight nausea, slight pain in stomach, increased flatulence
	Magnesium	Upset Stomach
	Magnesium	The initial 4 pills made me sick. Also, I am currently stressed as my (spouse) is scheduled for (major) surgery next week.
	Magnesium	A little diarrhea an hour or so after taking the pill, but this only happened on the first two days.
	Magnesium	Had gastrointestional issues when taking the pill.
	Magnesium	Loose stools, some diarrhea, and cramps after taking pill in the morning.
	Placebo	Diarrhea, but could be due to increased nut intake,
Day #80	Magnesium	Some difficulty with digestion
	Magnesium	My fingernails have gotten must stronger, and my bowels were loose and somewhat sluggish.
	Magnesium	I have been a lot 'looser' since taking the pills.
	Magnesium	Upset stomach
	Magnesium	Small bouts of diarrhea the first two days of taking the pills; nothing since.

#, number .* Some details were modified slightly to reduce the likelihood of identifying a participant. Minor spelling and punctuation changes were made to improve clarity.

4. Discussion

In this pilot trial of 59 relatively healthy adults aged 55 and older, supplementation with 400 mg of magnesium daily over 12 weeks was safe and well tolerated and led to a change of 0.07 mEq/L in serum magnesium, which is substantial enough in magnitude that in a larger sample size it may translate to health outcomes. The intervention was not associated with change in PACs, but estimates of association had wide confidence intervals, and the study was not powered to identify important differences. Likewise, there was no association between supplemental magnesium and changes in glucose, systolic blood pressure, or diastolic blood pressure.

The mechanisms through which magnesium supplementation could reduce the risk of supraventricular arrhythmias and AF are not fully understood. However, magnesium is known to play a direct role in cardiac contractility [21]. Small studies in healthy individuals and in patients with cardiac disease have found that intravenous magnesium administration prolongs sinoatrial, intra-atrial, and atrioventricular node conduction and the atrial refractory period, which in turn may contribute to prevent the onset of AF [22–24]. Also, randomization to 148 mg of oral magnesium (and 296 mg of potassium) intake (vs. the placebo) had antiarrhythmic effects among 232 patients with frequent ventricular arrhythmias [25].

Blood pressure and diabetes are also established risk factors for AF [26,27], through which magnesium may lower AF risk. In the present pilot trial, changes in blood pressure and serum glucose did not differ significantly for those given the magnesium supplementation and those given the placebo. This is in contrast with the existing literature; however, our study was small, and confidence intervals around the treatment differences were wide. Meta-analyses of randomized controlled trials have consistently demonstrated that magnesium supplementation lowers blood pressure in a dose-dependent manner [28–30]. In the most recent meta-analysis, a median dose of 368 mg/d for a median duration of 3 months significantly reduced systolic blood pressure (BP) by 2.0 mm Hg (95% CI: 0.4, 3.6) and diastolic BP by 1.8 mm Hg (95% CI: 0.7, 2.8) [30]. Based partly on this evidence, in November 2016, a petition was filed with the Food and Drug Administration (FDA) for a qualified health claim for magnesium and reduced risk of high blood pressure (FDA-2016-Q-3770). A comparable meta-analysis of RCTs, including a total of 370 patients with type 2 diabetes, found that magnesium supplementation (median dosage 360 mg/day) reduced concentrations of fasting blood glucose (-10.1 mg/dL, 95% CI -19.8, -0.2) over a median intervention duration of 13 weeks [31]. These meta-analyses suggest that magnesium is causally related to hypertension and abnormal glucose homeostasis. However, their interpretation is complicated by the fact that the individual studies included in the meta-analyses were highly heterogeneous in terms of magnesium formulation and dosage and participant characteristics.

In terms of serum magnesium, the intervention of 400 mg of magnesium oxide daily was associated with a serum increase of 0.07 mEq/L. This finding is concordant with results from a meta-analysis of the effect of magnesium supplementation dosage on serum magnesium response. In the meta-analysis the median dose was 360 mg of magnesium/day, the intervention length was 12 weeks, and the response was 0.08 mEq/L [32]. In the meta-analysis there was evidence of an inverse relationship between the baseline magnesium concentration and responsiveness to the supplementation. A similar phenomenon was not observed in the present trial; however, in our sample, the baseline magnesium concentrations were quite high, and power was exceedingly low for subgroup comparisons.

The results from this study provide additional evidence about compliance with magnesium supplementation at the dosage of 400 mg of magnesium daily, as well as safety and tolerability. Among the participants randomized to magnesium, only 1 out of 29 participants (3.5%) ceased the intervention due to side effects. The compliance in this study was good, at 75% in the intervention group and 83% in the placebo group, according to pill counts. The low drop-out rate and high compliance provides support for the tolerability of this dosage. However, the fact that 50% in the intervention group commented on GI changes at some point in the follow-up should not be dismissed. Unfortunately, given the way side effects were assessed, it is not possible to quantify the severity of the GI complaints. Notably, several individuals only commented about GI changes in the first few days after taking the study treatment.

The primary limitation of this study is the small size, which led to an imbalance of some key potential confounding factors, such as sex. Among those randomized to magnesium, 86.2% were female, whereas among those randomized to the placebo, 60.0% were female. This is important, because AF risk is known to be greater among men [3]. However, the findings were similar in post-hoc sensitivity analyses where we adjusted for sex. An additional consideration is that the baseline serum concentrations of the trial participants were quite high; it is unclear how serum magnesium would have changed in a context of low baseline magnesium concentrations or how that may translate to change in other physiologic outcomes. Lastly, we assessed tolerability with a simple open-ended question, not a checklist of specific signs and symptoms graded for severity according to a standard toxicity table.

5. Conclusions

In sum, this small pilot double-blinded randomized controlled trial of supplementation with 400 mg of magnesium daily provides evidence to support the safety and tolerability of this intervention and for adherence to the ZioPatch heart rhythm monitoring device. Despite our study population being largely magnesium replete, a change in serum magnesium was observed. Magnesium supplementation was not associated with change in PACs, glucose, or blood pressure; however, this small pilot study was short-term and not powered to identify small-to-moderate clinically relevant differences. The results of this pilot study will guide the design of a larger trial to evaluate the effect of supplemental magnesium on arrhythmias.

Author Contributions: P.L.L. and A.A. conceived of the study. P.L.L., A.A., M.J., K.D.R., and J.D.N. designed the study. P.L.L., A.A., L.Y.C., and M.J. collected the data. A.E. conducted the data analysis. All authors were involved in the drafting and critical review of the manuscript.

Funding: McKnight Land-Grant Professorship funds (non-sponsored).

Acknowledgments: We thank the study participants, for taking part in this study.

Conflicts of Interest: The authors declare no conflicts of interest.

References

1. Go, A.S.; Hylek, E.M.; Phillips, K.A.; Chang, Y.C.; Henault, L.E.; Selby, J.V.; Singer, D.E. Prevalence of diagnosed atrial fibrillation in adults. National implications for rhythm management and stroke prevention: The Anticoagulation and Risk Factors in Atrial Fibrillation (ATRIA) study. *JAMA* **2001**, *285*, 2370–2375. [CrossRef] [PubMed]
2. Miyasaka, Y.; Barnes, M.E.; Gersh, B.J.; Cha, S.S.; Bailey, K.R.; Abhayaratna, W.P.; Seward, J.B.; Tsang, T.S.M. Secular trends in incidence of atrial fibrillation in Olmsted County, Minnesota, 1980 to 2000, and implications on the projections for future prevalence. *Circulation* **2006**, *114*, 119–125. [CrossRef] [PubMed]
3. Benjamin, E.J.; Virani, S.S.; Callaway, C.W.; Chang, A.R.; Cheng, S.; Chiuve, S.E.; Cushman, M.; Delling, F.N.; Deo, R.; de Ferranti, S.D.; et al. Heart Disease and Stroke Statistics—2018 Update: A Report From the American Heart Association. *Circulation* **2018**. [CrossRef] [PubMed]
4. January, C.T.; Wann, L.S.; Alpert, J.S.; Calkins, H.; Cigarroa, J.E.; Cleveland, J.C.; Conti, J.B.; Ellinor, P.T.; Ezekowitz, M.D.; Field, M.E.; et al. 2014 AHA/ACC/HRS guideline for the management of patients with atrial fibrillation: A report of the American College of Cardiology/American Heart Association Task Force on Practice Guidelines and the Heart Rhythm Society. *Circulation* **2014**, *130*, e199–e267. [CrossRef] [PubMed]
5. Benjamin, E.J.; Chen, P.-S.; Bild, D.E.; Mascette, A.M.; Albert, C.M.; Alonso, A.; Calkins, H.; Connolly, S.J.; Curtis, A.B.; Darbar, D.; et al. Prevention of atrial fibrillation: Report from an NHLBI workshop. *Circulation* **2009**, *119*, 606–618. [CrossRef] [PubMed]
6. Van Wagoner, D.R.; Piccini, J.P.; Albert, C.M.; Anderson, M.E.; Benjamin, E.J.; Brundel, B.; Califf, R.M.; Calkins, H.; Chen, P.-S.; Chiamvimonvat, N.; et al. Progress toward the prevention and treatment of atrial fibrillation: A summary of the Heart Rhythm Society Research Forum on the Treatment and Prevention of Atrial Fibrillation, Washington, DC, December 9–10, 2013. *Heart Rhythm* **2015**, *12*, e5–e29. [CrossRef] [PubMed]
7. Arsenault, K.A.; Yusuf, A.M.; Crystal, E.; Healey, J.S.; Morillo, C.A.; Nair, G.M.; Whitlock, R.P. Interventions for preventing post-operative atrial fibrillation in patients undergoing heart surgery. *Cochrane Database Syst. Rev.* **2013**, *1*, CD003611. [CrossRef] [PubMed]
8. Khan, A.M.; Lubitz, S.A.; Sullivan, L.M.; Sun, J.X.; Levy, D.; Vasan, R.S.; Magnani, J.W.; Ellinor, P.T.; Benjamin, E.J.; Wang, T.J. Low serum magnesium and the development of atrial fibrillation in the community: The Framingham Heart Study. *Circulation* **2013**, *127*, 33–38. [CrossRef] [PubMed]

9. Misialek, J.R.; Lopez, F.L.; Lutsey, P.L.; Huxley, R.R.; Peacock, J.M.; Chen, L.Y.; Soliman, E.Z.; Agarwal, S.K.; Alonso, A. Serum and dietary magnesium and incidence of atrial fibrillation in whites and in African Americans—Atherosclerosis Risk in Communities (ARIC) Study. *Circ. J.* **2013**, *77*, 323–329. [CrossRef] [PubMed]

10. Markovits, N.; Kurnik, D.; Halkin, H.; Margalit, R.; Bialik, M.; Lomnicky, Y.; Loebstein, R. Database evaluation of the association between serum magnesium levels and the risk of atrial fibrillation in the community. *Int. J. Cardiol.* **2016**, *205*, 142–146. [CrossRef] [PubMed]

11. Nielsen, F.H.; Milne, D.B.; Klevay, L.M.; Gallagher, S.; Johnson, L. Dietary magnesium deficiency induces heart rhythm changes, impairs glucose tolerance, and decreases serum cholesterol in post menopausal women. *J. Am. Coll. Nutr.* **2007**, *26*, 121–132. [CrossRef] [PubMed]

12. Wardlaw, G.M.; Byrd-Bredbenner, C.; Moe, G.; Berning, J.R.; Kelley, D.S. *Wardlaw's Perspectives in Nutrition*, 10th ed.; McGraw-Hill Education: New York, NY, USA, 2016.

13. Worwag, M.; Classen, H.G.; Schumacher, E. Prevalence of magnesium and zinc deficiencies in nursing home residents in Germany. *Magn. Res.* **1999**, *12*, 181–189.

14. Dietary Guidelines for Americans 2015–2020. Available online: https://health.gov/dietaryguidelines/2015/resources/2015-2020_Dietary_Guidelines.pdf (accessed on 2 October 2017).

15. Harris, P.A.; Taylor, R.; Thielke, R.; Payne, J.; Gonzalez, N.; Conde, J.G. Research Electronic Data Capture (REDCap)—A metadata-driven methodology and workflow process for providing translational research informatics support. *J. Biomed. Inform.* **2009**, *42*, 377–381. [CrossRef] [PubMed]

16. Dewland, T.A.; Vittinghoff, E.; Mandyam, M.C.; Heckbert, S.R.; Siscovick, D.S.; Stein, P.K.; Psaty, B.M.; Sotoodehnia, N.; Gottdiener, J.S.; Marcus, G.M. Atrial Ectopy as a Predictor of Incident Atrial Fibrillation A Cohort Study. *Ann. Intern. Med.* **2013**, *159*, 721–728. [CrossRef] [PubMed]

17. Chong, B.H.; Pong, V.; Lam, K.F.; Liu, S.; Zuo, M.L.; Lau, Y.F.; Lau, C.P.; Tse, H.F.; Siu, C.W. Frequent premature atrial complexes predict new occurrence of atrial fibrillation and adverse cardiovascular events. *Europace* **2012**, *14*, 942–947. [CrossRef] [PubMed]

18. Conen, D.; Adam, M.; Roche, F.; Barthelemy, J.C.; Felber Dietrich, D.; Imboden, M.; Kunzli, N.; von Eckardstein, A.; Regenass, S.; Hornemann, T.; et al. Premature atrial contractions in the general population: Frequency and risk factors. *Circulation* **2012**, *126*, 2302–2308. [CrossRef] [PubMed]

19. Turakhia, M.P.; Hoang, D.D.; Zimetbaum, P.; Miller, J.D.; Froelicher, V.F.; Kumar, U.N.; Xu, X.; Yang, F.; Heidenreich, P.A. Diagnostic utility of a novel leadless arrhythmia monitoring device. *Am. J. Cardiol.* **2013**, *112*, 520–524. [CrossRef] [PubMed]

20. R Development Core Team. *R: A Language and Environment for Statistical Computing*; R Foundation for Statistical Computing: Vienna, Austria, 2015.

21. Byrd-Bredbenner, C.; Moe, G.; Beshgetoor, D.; Berning, J. *Wardlaw's Perspectives in Nutrition*, 9th ed.; McGraw-Hill: New York, NY, USA, 2013; 259p.

22. Christiansen, E.H.; Frost, L.; Andreasen, F.; Mortensen, P.; Thomsen, P.E.; Pedersen, A.K. Dose-related cardiac electrophysiological effects of intravenous magnesium. A double-blind placebo-controlled dose-response study in patients with paroxysmal supraventricular tachycardia. *Europace* **2000**, *2*, 320–326. [CrossRef] [PubMed]

23. Rasmussen, H.S.; Thomsen, P.E. The electrophysiological effects of intravenous magnesium on human sinus node, atrioventricular node, atrium, and ventricle. *Clin. Cardiol.* **1989**, *12*, 85–90. [CrossRef] [PubMed]

24. Kulick, D.L.; Hong, R.; Ryzen, E.; Rude, R.K.; Rubin, J.N.; Elkayam, U.; Rahimtoola, S.H.; Bhandari, A.K. Electrophysiologic effects of intravenous magnesium in patients with normal conduction systems and no clinical evidence of significant cardiac disease. *Am. Heart J.* **1988**, *115*, 367–373. [CrossRef]

25. Zehender, M.; Meinertz, T.; Faber, T.; Caspary, A.; Jeron, A.; Bremm, K.; Just, H. Antiarrhythmic Effects of Increasing the Daily Intake of Magnesium and Potassium in Patients With Frequent Ventricular Arrhythmias fn1fn1This study was supported by Trommsdorff GmbH and Company, Alsdorf, Germany and Hexal AG, Holzkirchen, Germany. *J. Am. Coll. Cardiol.* **1997**, *29*, 1028–1034. [CrossRef]

26. Huxley, R.R.; Filion, K.B.; Konety, S.; Alonso, A. Meta-analysis of cohort and case-control studies of type 2 diabetes mellitus and risk of atrial fibrillation. *Am. J. Cardiol.* **2011**, *108*, 56–62. [CrossRef] [PubMed]

27. Roetker, N.S.; Chen, L.Y.; Heckbert, S.R.; Nazarian, S.; Soliman, E.Z.; Bluemke, D.A.; Lima, J.A.; Alonso, A. Relation of systolic, diastolic, and pulse pressure and aortic distensibility with atrial fibrillation (from the Multi-Ethnic Study of Atherosclerosis). *Am. J. Cardiol.* **2014**, *114*, 587–592. [CrossRef] [PubMed]

28. Jee, S.H.; Miller, E.R., 3rd; Guallar, E.; Singh, V.K.; Appel, L.J.; Klag, M.J. The effect of magnesium supplementation on blood pressure: A meta-analysis of randomized clinical trials. *Am. J. Hypertens.* **2002**, *15*, 691–696. [CrossRef]

29. Kass, L.; Weekes, J.; Carpenter, L. Effect of magnesium supplementation on blood pressure: A meta-analysis. *Eur. J. Clin. Nutr.* **2012**, *66*, 411–418. [CrossRef] [PubMed]

30. Zhang, X.; Li, Y.; Del Gobbo, L.C.; Rosanoff, A.; Wang, J.; Zhang, W.; Song, Y. Effects of Magnesium Supplementation on Blood Pressure: A Meta-Analysis of Randomized Double-Blind Placebo-Controlled Trials. *Hypertension* **2016**, *68*, 324–333. [CrossRef] [PubMed]

31. Song, Y.; He, K.; Levitan, E.B.; Manson, J.E.; Liu, S. Effects of oral magnesium supplementation on glycaemic control in type 2 diabetes: A meta-analysis of randomized double-blind controlled trials. *Diabet. Med.* **2006**, *23*, 1050–1056. [CrossRef] [PubMed]

32. Zhang, X.; Del Gobbo, L.C.; Hruby, A.; Rosanoff, A.; He, K.; Dai, Q.; Costello, R.B.; Zhang, W.; Song, Y. The circulating concentration and 24-h urine excretion of magnesium dose- and time-dependently respond to oral magnesium supplementation in a meta-analysis of randomized controlled trials. *J. Nutr.* **2016**, *146*, 595–602. [CrossRef] [PubMed]

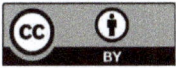

nutrients

MDPI

Communication

Bioaccessibility and Bioavailability of a Marine-Derived Multimineral, Aquamin-Magnesium

Valeria D. Felice [1,2,3,*], **Denise M. O'Gorman** [4], **Nora M. O'Brien** [2] **and Niall P. Hyland** [1,3]

1   Department of Pharmacology and Therapeutics and Department of Physiology, University College Cork, T12 K8AF Cork, Ireland; n.hyland@ucc.ie
2   School of Food and Nutritional Sciences, University College Cork, T12 K8AF Cork, Ireland; nob@ucc.ie
3   APC Microbiome Ireland, University College Cork, T12 K8AF Cork, Ireland
4   Marigot Ltd., P43 NN62 Cork, Ireland; denise.ogorman@marigot.ie
*   Correspondence: valeria.felice@marigot.ie; Tel.: +353-(0)21-420-5876

Received: 31 May 2018; Accepted: 11 July 2018; Published: 17 July 2018

Abstract: Introduction: Magnesium is an essential mineral involved in a range of key biochemical pathways. Several magnesium supplements are present on the market and their degree of bioavailability differs depending on the form of magnesium salt used. Aquamin-Mg is a natural source of magnesium, containing 72 additional trace minerals derived from the clean waters off the Irish coast. However, the in vitro bioaccessibility and bioavailability of Aquamin-Mg in comparison with other supplement sources of magnesium has yet to be tested. **Method:** Aquamin-Mg, magnesium chloride ($MgCl_2$) and magnesium oxide (MgO) were subjected to gastrointestinal digestion according to the harmonized INFOGEST in vitro digestion method and in vitro bioavailability tested using the Caco-2 cell model. Magnesium concentration was measured by atomic absorption spectrophotometry (AAS). **Results:** Magnesium recovery from both Aquamin-Mg and $MgCl_2$ was greater than for MgO. Magnesium from all three sources was transported across the epithelial monolayer with Aquamin-Mg displaying a comparable profile to the more bioavailable $MgCl_2$. **Conclusions:** Our data support that magnesium derived from a marine-derived multimineral product is bioavailable to a significantly greater degree than MgO and displays a similar profile to the more bioavailable $MgCl_2$ and may offer additional health benefits given its multimineral profile.

Keywords: Aquamin; multimineral supplement; magnesium bioavailability

---

1. Introduction

Magnesium is an essential mineral for the human body and is involved in a wide range of crucial physiological processes [1]. Magnesium can be obtained from the diet, being naturally present in foods such as green leafy vegetables, seeds, beans, whole grains, fish and nuts, amongst others. However, dietary magnesium intake has been shown to be insufficient in the Western population due to industrial food processing that reduces the nutrient contents including magnesium, as well as changes in dietary habits [2]. Deficiency in magnesium dietary intake may lead to hypomagnesemia which has been associated with several disorders including diabetes, osteoporosis and cardiovascular disease [3–5]. Early symptoms of hypomagnesemia are non-specific and include loss of appetite, nausea, vomiting, lethargy, fatigue and weakness with more pronounced hypomagnesemia characterised by increased neuromuscular excitability including muscle cramps, tremor, tetany and generalized seizures [6].

The market currently offers various supplement preparations to reach the recommended magnesium daily intake. These supplements differ in the type of magnesium salt used which can be either organic (i.e., magnesium citrate and magnesium aspartate) or inorganic (i.e., MgO and $MgCl_2$), their dosage and bioavailability. For example, magnesium from $MgCl_2$ has high bioavailability equivalent to organic magnesium supplements such as magnesium lactate and aspartate [7]. Moreover, these three sources of magnesium have significantly greater bioavailability than MgO [7]. Magnesium derived from magnesium hydroxide ($Mg(OH)_2$) (Mablet) has been shown to be absorbed into the circulation and, hence, bioavailable in healthy male adults [8]. In a previous study, the bioavailability of magnesium from formulations containing different combinations of magnesium salts displayed similar bioavailability, however the daily dose of magnesium differed [9].

Aquamin-Mg is a natural source of magnesium in the form of $Mg(OH)_2$ derived from the clean waters off the Irish coast. In addition to magnesium, Aquamin-Mg also contains 72 additional trace minerals (Marigot Ltd., Cork, Ireland, Table 1) with the same profile of Lithothamnion Aquamin which has previously been shown to be a highly bioavailable source of calcium [10].

Here we describe for the first time the in vitro bioaccessibility and bioavailability of Aquamin-Mg in comparison with two commercially available sources of magnesium, $MgCl_2$ and MgO.

Table 1. Mineral composition of Aquamin-Mg. (ppm, parts per million).

Mineral	ppm	Mineral	ppm
Aluminum	461	Molybdenum	1.78
Antimony	<0.5	Neodymium	2.810
Arsenic	1.811	Nickel	<0.5
Barium	1.83	Niobium	<0.5
Beryllium	<0.5	Osmium	0.002
Bismuth	<0.5	Palladium	0.301
Boron	186	Phosphorus	117
Cadmium	0.394	Platinum	0.002
Calcium	23,000	Potassium	88.21
Carbon	10,100	Praseodymium	0.697
Cerium	3.411	Rhenium	0.001
Cesium	0.008	Rhodium	0.010
Chloride	613.4	Rubidium	0.063
Chromium	5.83	Ruthenium	0.135
Cobalt	<0.5	Samarium	0.576
Copper	5.09	Scandium	1.050
Dysprosium	0.829	Selenium	<0.5
Erbium	0.613	Silicon	657
Europium	0.197	Silver	<0.5
Fluoride	1.1	Sodium	1467
Gadolinium	0.770	Strontium	84.7
Gallium	0.163	Sulfur	3335
Germanium	0.020	Tantalum	0.016
Gold	<0.5	Tellurium	<0.5
Hafnium	0.046	Terbium	0.140
Holmium	0.194	Thallium	<0.5
Indium	<0.001	Thorium	0.860
Iodine	9.1	Thulium	0.081
Iridium	0.002	Tin	0.179
Iron	1213	Titanium	18.5
Lanthanum	1.01	Tungsten	2.08
Lead	0.604	Vanadium	16.0
Lithium	<0.5	Ytterbium	0.498
Lutetium	0.116	Yttrium	7.38
Magnesium	404,400	Zinc	2.37
Manganese	486	Zirconium	<0.5
Mercury	0.009		

2. Methods

2.1. Harmonized INFOGEST in Vitro Digestion Protocol

To determine biaccessibility, the amount of magnesium subjected to digestion for each compound was calculated according to the recommended dietary allowance for men (RDA, 420 mg/day). 5.6 mg of magnesium from Aquamin-Mg, MgCl$_2$ and MgO were digested according to the harmonized INFOGEST in vitro digestion method published by Minekus and colleagues [11]. Four to five independent digestions were carried out for each compound (Aquamin-Mg, MgCl$_2$ and MgO). Aquamin-Mg, MgCl$_2$ and MgO were exposed to simulated gastric fluid (composition: 6.9 mM KCl, 0.9 mM KH$_2$PO$_4$, 25 mM NaHCO$_3$, 47.2 mM NaCl, 0.1 mM MgCl$_2$(H$_2$O)$_6$, 0.5 mM (NH$_4$)$_2$CO$_3$). Pepsin and calcium chloride were added to the mixture to achieve a final concentration of 2000 U/mL and 0.075 mM respectively. Hydrochloric acid (HCl, 6 M) was then used to acidify the mixture to pH 3 and water was added to reach a final volume of 20 mL. Samples were then incubated in a stirring water bath at 37 °C and 95 rpm for 2 h. The pH was checked after 1 hour and adjusted if necessary. The simulated intestinal fluid (composition: 6.8 mM KCl, 0.8 mM KH$_2$PO$_4$, 85 mM NaHCO$_3$, 38.4 mM NaCl, 0.33 mM MgCl$_2$(H$_2$O)$_6$) was then added together with pancreatin (the concentration was based on trypsin activity, 100 U/mL) and bile salts for a final concentration of 10 mM. Calcium chloride was also added to achieve a final concentration of 0.3 mM. Sodium hydroxide (NaOH, 1 M) was used to bring the pH to 7 and the necessary amount of water added to reach a final volume of 20 mL. Samples were incubated in a stirring water bath at 37 °C and 95 rpm for 2 h. The pH was checked after one hour and adjusted if necessary. A control sample containing all reagents included in the digestion protocol except the experimental powders was also subjected to the procedure. Upon completion of the incubation period, aliquots (1 mL) of each sample were frozen in liquid nitrogen. Prior to the analysis, one sample from each treatment was filtered using 0.2 µm cell culture sterile filters. The amount of magnesium recovered from these samples was then compared to non-filtered samples.

2.2. Caco-2 Cell Bioavailability Assay

Caco-2 cells are human epithelial colorectal adenocarcinoma cells that, upon differentiation, express numerous morphological and biochemical characteristics of small intestinal enterocytes. This in vitro model is widely used to study mineral bioavailability from different sources and their transport mechanisms [12].

For Caco-2 bioavailability experiments 60 mg of magnesium derived from Aquamin-Mg, MgCl$_2$ and MgO were subjected to the harmonized INFOGEST in vitro digestion protocol described above (data not shown), and unfiltered samples were used. 60 mg of magnesium was chosen in order to ensure that sufficient concentrations of magnesium could be achieved to perform the Caco-2 experiments. Three independent digestions were carried out for each compound (Aquamin-Mg, MgCl$_2$ and MgO) and these were subsequently used in the Caco-2 bioavailability assay. Caco-2 cells (supplied by the European Collection of Authenticated Cell Cultures (ECACC)) were cultured in Dulbecco's modified eagle's medium (DMEM) supplemented with 1% non-essential amino acids and 10% foetal bovine serum (FBS) and were stored in a humidified incubator at 37 °C and 5% CO$_2$. For all experiments, cells were seeded at a density of 1×10^5 cells/mL on 6-well Transwell plates with inserts of 24 mm diameter and differentiated for 21 days. Media was changed every other day.

2.3. Bioavailability of Magnesium from Aquamin-Mg, MgCl$_2$ and MgO Using Caco-2 Cells

On the day of the experiment, media was removed from all wells and 1 mL of fresh media was added to the luminal side and 2 mL to the basolateral side of each well. Transepithelial electrical resistance (TEER) was measured to confirm the integrity of the epithelial monolayer. Cells were then incubated with either Aquamin-Mg, MgCl$_2$- or MgO-derived magnesium in the luminal side (concentrations of 25, 50, 100 and 150 µg/mL) for 2 h at 37 °C. Samples from each independent digestion were used in a corresponding independent bioavailability study which was conducted in triplicate. Two controls were included in the assay, a blank sample, only containing media, and a digest sample, containing all reagents included in the digestion protocol except the experimental powders. At the end of the incubation time, TEER values were recorded again to ensure that the treatments did not have any effect on the integrity of the monolayer. Luminal and basolateral samples were collected and stored at 4 °C. Magnesium concentration of luminal and basolateral samples was measured by atomic absorption spectrophotometry (AAS). Three independent experiments were carried out. Each treatment was randomly assigned and was performed in duplicate.

2.4. Atomic Absorption Spectrophotometry (AAS)

The magnesium content of the digested samples, as well as luminal and basolateral samples was determined by AAS. Samples were diluted in Milli-Q water prior to analysis. Lanthanum chloride (0.1%) was also added to eliminate any phosphate interferences. A commercially available magnesium standard (Spectrosol from BDH Chemicals Ltd., Dublin, Ireland) was used. Standard solutions were prepared using Milli-Q water containing lanthanum chloride (0.1%) and ranged from 0 to 1 mg/L.

2.5. Statistical Analyses

Data are expressed as mean ± standard error of the mean (SEM). Statistical analysis was carried out using the Kruskal–Wallis test, followed by Dunn's multiple comparison test for the digestion study. For the bioavailability study, we calculated the residuals of the data to determine whether there were outliers and statistical analysis was performed using one-way analysis of variance (ANOVA) followed by Bonferroni post-hoc test. Values of $p < 0.05$ were considered statistically significant.

3. Results

3.1. Magnesium Recovery from Aquamin-Mg, MgCl$_2$ and MgO Following In Vitro Digestion

Aquamin-Mg-derived magnesium, showed an in vitro bioaccessibility more similar to highly soluble alternative such as MgCl$_2$ than to MgO (Aquamin-Mg, 122.6 ± 4.1 µg/mL, $n = 5$; MgCl$_2$, 115.4 ± 6.0 µg/mL, $n = 4$; MgO, 73.39 ± 10.20 µg/mL, $n = 4$; in unfiltered samples), which is characterised by low solubility (Figure 1, $p < 0.05$ Aquamin-Mg vs. MgO). To determine whether magnesium was lost during filtration for the Caco-2 cell culture experiments, magnesium concentration in filtered samples was also determined and these were lower for all the treatments relative to unfiltered samples (Aquamin-Mg, 99.3 ± 6.2 µg/mL, $n = 5$; MgCl$_2$, 92.2 ± 5.6 µg/mL, $n = 4$; MgO, 64.5 ± 9.3 µg/mL in filtered samples).

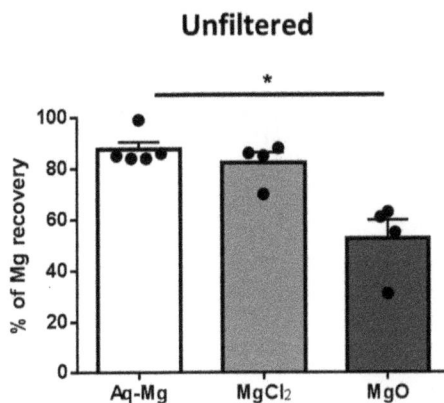

Figure 1. Magnesium recovery from Aquamin-Mg, MgCl$_2$ and MgO following in vitro digestion. The percentage of magnesium recovery from Aquamin-Mg was significantly higher than MgO (* $p < 0.5$, $n = 4$–5) in unfiltered samples.

3.2. Transepithelial Electrical Resistance (TEER)

As an indicator of cell viability we measured TEER at the start of each experiment and after treatment. The results from the transepithelial resistance measurements confirmed that after 21 days of culture, Caco-2 cells formed an integral monolayer. Moreover, none of the treatments, at any concentration tested, affected epithelial integrity following 2 h incubation at 37 °C (Figure 2).

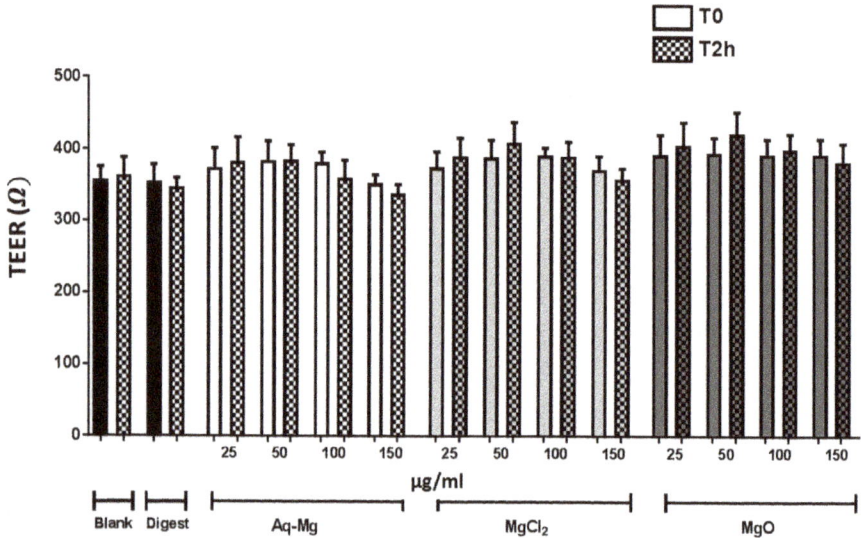

Figure 2. Transepithelial electrical resistance in Caco-2 cells following treatment with Aquamin-Mg, MgCl$_2$ and MgO. At time zero (T0) cells were differentiated in an integral monolayer. Transepithelial electrical resistance (TEER) values confirmed that the treatments did not compromise the integrity of the monolayer at any of the concentrations tested following 2 h incubation (T2h) (n = 3).

3.3. Bioavailability of Magnesium from Aquamin-Mg, MgCl$_2$ and MgO Using the Caco-2 Cell Model

Digestates were added to the luminal compartment. The reduced amount of magnesium from MgO is reflective of the reduced bioaccessibility (Figure 3a). These results are in accordance with the in vitro digestion data (60 mg; data not shown). When the concentration of magnesium was measured in the basolateral chamber, magnesium derived from Aquamin-Mg and MgCl$_2$ showed the same degree of bioavailability at all the concentrations tested, while only a small amount of magnesium from MgO was transported across the epithelium and thus bioavailable. Both Aquamin-Mg and MgCl$_2$ were significantly more bioavailable than MgO at the highest concentration tested (150 µg/mL) (Figure 3b, Table 2).

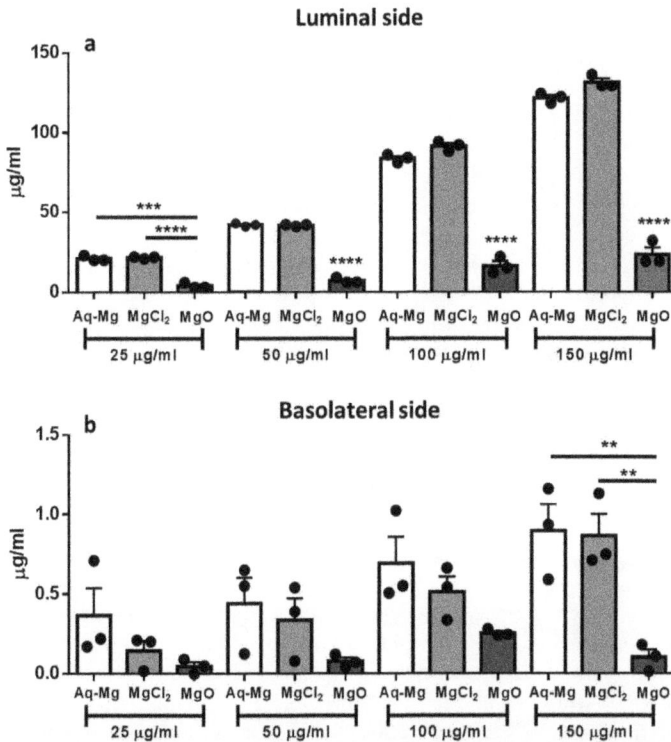

Figure 3. Bioavailability of magnesium from Aquamin-Mg, MgCl$_2$ and MgO using Caco-2 cells. (**a**) Magnesium derived from Aquamin-Mg, MgCl$_2$ and MgO applied into the luminal side. Following in vitro digestion, the amount of bioaccessible magnesium was significantly higher for Aquamin-Mg and MgCl$_2$ compared to MgO (*** $p < 0.001$ for Aquamin-Mg vs. MgO at 25 µg/mL, **** $p < 0.0001$ for MgCl$_2$ vs. MgO at 25 µg/mL and **** $p < 0.0001$ for Aquamin-Mg and MgCl$_2$ vs. MgO at 50, 100 and 150 µg/mL, $n = 3$); (**b**) Magnesium derived from Aquamin-Mg, MgCl$_2$ and MgO measured in the basolateral side after 2 h incubation at 37 °C. At the highest concentration tested, magnesium from Aquamin-Mg and MgCl$_2$ was significantly more bioavailable than MgO (** $p < 0.01$ for Aquamin-Mg and MgCl$_2$ vs. MgO at 150 µg/mL, $n = 3$).

Table 2. Magnesium derived from Aquamin-Mg, MgCl$_2$ and MgO measured in the basolateral side after 2 h incubation at 37 °C expressed as µg/mL ($n = 3$).

Magnesium Source	Sample Concentration (µg/mL)	Basolateral Side µg/mL Mean ± Standard Error of the Mean (SEM)
Aquamin-Mg	25	0.37 ± 0.17
	50	0.44 ± 0.16
	100	0.69 ± 0.16
	150	0.89 ± 0.17
MgCl$_2$	25	0.14 ± 0.06
	50	0.33 ± 0.13
	100	0.51 ± 0.09
	150	0.86 ± 0.13
MgO	25	0.05 ± 0.03
	50	0.08 ± 0.02
	100	0.25 ± 0.01
	150	0.10 ± 0.05

4. Discussion

The aim of these studies was to examine the bioaccessibility and bioavailability of magnesium from Aquamin-Mg compared to $MgCl_2$ and MgO using the Caco-2 cell model. In this model both active saturated and passive non-saturated pathways have been previously identified for magnesium transport [13]. The study from Thongon and Krishnamrain has indeed shown that in Caco-2 monolayers, magnesium transported from the apical to the basolateral side (representing magnesium absorption) against magnesium in the apical solution (representing magnesium concentration) was curvilinear as previously shown in humans [13,14]. Furthermore, the same study has shown that treatment with omeprazole selectively inhibited the non-saturable passive component, without affecting the saturable active component of magnesium transport which was abolished using the Transient Receptor Potential Cation Channel Subfamily M Member 6 (TRPM6) inhibitor Ruthenium Red (RR) [13]. This evidence shows that magnesium can be transported through both a paracellular and a transcellular pathway and that the Caco-2 monolayer is a suitable in vitro model of intestinal magnesium absorption. In the context of our findings, however, we cannot comment on which pathway was responsible for the apical to basolateral transport of magnesium and further research is warranted in order to elucidate these mechanisms. Our results show for the first-time, however, direct evidence that Aquamin-Mg-derived magnesium is highly bioaccessible following in vitro digestion and magnesium is transported across the intestinal epithelium in this well-established in vitro model. Moreover, the degree of bioaccessbility and bioavailability of Aquamin-Mg was comparable to $MgCl_2$ while being superior to MgO.

$MgCl_2$ and MgO represent a high bioavailable and low bioavailable source of magnesium respectively, and our in vitro data are in keeping with in vivo data demonstrating that the mean urinary excretion of magnesium in healthy volunteers was significantly higher for $MgCl_2$ than MgO [7]. Interestingly, in this study, $MgCl_2$ bioavailability was comparable to that of organic magnesium forms such as magnesium aspartate and magnesium lactate [7].

Magnesium in Aquamin-Mg is in the form of $Mg(OH)_2$. However, as well as magnesium, Aquamin-Mg also provides 72 additional trace minerals all derived from sea water (Marigot Ltd., Cork, Ireland, Table 1). In support of $Mg(OH)_2$ as a magnesium supplement, the pharmacokinetic profile of a single oral dose of $Mg(OH)_2$ in healthy male adults showed that the bioavailability of magnesium from $Mg(OH)_2$ was 15% [8]. Moreover, none of the participants recruited reported any side effect following supplementation suggesting that $Mg(OH)_2$ may be a clinically relevant option for oral magnesium supplementation [8]. In a second human study the degree of bioavailability of $Mg(OH)_2$ was compared to other sources of magnesium, including $MgCl_2$ measured as urinary elimination of magnesium [9]. In this study it was found that $Mg(OH)_2$ was required at a higher dose to reach the same level of bioavailability [9].

The solubility of magnesium in the gastrointestinal tract plays a key role in magnesium absorption. Our bioaccessiblity results demonstrate that magnesium from Aquamin-Mg is soluble as $MgCl_2$ and hence potentially available for absorption. Our bioavailability data support that $Mg(OH)_2$, derived from Aquamin-Mg, displays a similar profile and transport characteristics as magnesium derived from $MgCl_2$ at the same concentrations, suggesting that Aquamin-Mg represents a source of magnesium coupled with potential health benefits of a multimineral supplement. Currently, however, as Aquamin-Mg is not formulated as an oral supplement (tablets and capsules), further comparisons with other formulated magnesium supplements were not possible.

Moreover, Aquamin-Mg is composed of multiple minerals and whether these affect its bioaccessibility or bioavailability is difficult to determine.

5. Conclusions

In conclusion, our data suggests that Aquamin-Mg-derived magnesium is bioaccessible and bioavailable to a significantly greater degree than magnesium oxide while displaying a comparable profile to magnesium chloride. Nonetheless, our in vitro results are qualitatively consistent with the clinical study from Firoz and Graber showing that magnesium from $MgCl_2$ has significantly greater bioavailability than MgO. Further research is warranted to investigate the bioaccessibility and bioavailability of Aquamin-Mg in clinical studies.

Author Contributions: V.D.F., N.P.H., N.M.O. and D.M.O. conceived and designed the experiments. D.M.O. provided Aquamin-Mg. V.D.F. performed the experiments and V.D.F. and N.P.H. analysed the data. V.D.F. and N.P.H. wrote the manuscript; N.M.O., and D.M.O., edited the manuscript.

Funding: This research was funded by the Irish Research Council Enterprise Partnership Scheme (EPS) Postdoctoral Fellowship, grant number EPSPD/2015/52. Marigot Ltd. provided the mineral-rich algae extract Aquamin and their financial support. APC Microbiome Ireland is funded by SFI, through the Irish Government's National Development Plan (Grant 12/RC/2273).

Acknowledgments: Felice has received an Irish Research Council Enterprise Postdoctoral Fellowship. We would like also to acknowledge Marigot Ltd. who provided the mineral-rich algae extract Aquamin and their financial support. Thank you also to O'Callaghan, University College Cork, and Shane O'Connell (Marigot Ltd.), for their help in the preparation of this manuscript.

Conflicts of Interest: Felice and O'Gorman are employees of Marigot and Hyland and O'Brien have received research support from Marigot Ltd.

References

1. Saris, N.E.; Mervaala, E.; Karppanen, H.; Khawaja, J.A.; Lewenstam, A. Magnesium. An update on physiological, clinical and analytical aspects. *Clin. Chim. Acta* **2000**, *294*, 1–26. [CrossRef]
2. Marier, J.R. Magnesium content of the food supply in the modern-day world. *Magnesium* **1986**, *5*, 1–8. [PubMed]
3. Rosique-Esteban, N.; Guasch-Ferré, M.; Hernández-Alonso, P.; Salas-Salvadó, J. Dietary magnesium and cardiovascular disease: A review with emphasis in epidemiological studies. *Nutrients* **2018**, *10*, 168. [CrossRef] [PubMed]
4. Guerrero-Romero, F.; Jaquez-Chairez, F.O.; Rodríguez-Morán, M. Magnesium in metabolic syndrome: A review based on randomized, double-blind clinical trials. *Magnes. Res.* **2016**, *29*, 146–153. [PubMed]
5. Castiglioni, S.; Cazzaniga, A.; Albisetti, W.; Maier, J.A.M. Magnesium and osteoporosis: Current state of knowledge and future research directions. *Nutrients* **2013**, *5*, 3022–3033.
6. Grober, U.; Schmidt, J.; Kisters, K. Magnesium in prevention and therapy. *Nutrients* **2015**, *7*, 8199–8226. [CrossRef] [PubMed]
7. Firoz, M.; Graber, M. Bioavailability of US commercial magnesium preparations. *Magnes. Res.* **2001**, *14*, 257–262. [PubMed]
8. Dolberg, M.K.B.; Nielsen, L.P.; Dahl, R. Pharmacokinetic profile of oral magnesium hydroxide. *Basic Clin. Pharmacol. Toxicol.* **2017**, *120*, 264–269. [CrossRef] [PubMed]
9. Bøhmer, T.; Røseth, A.; Holm, H.; Weberg-Teigen, S.; Wahl, L. Bioavailability of oral magnesium supplementation in female students evaluated from elimination of magnesium in 24-hour urine. *Magnes. Trace Elem.* **1990**, *9*, 272–278.
10. Zenk, J.L.; Frestedt, J.L.; Kuskowski, M.A. Effect of Calcium Derived from Lithothamnion sp. on markers of calcium metabolism in premenopausal women. *J. Med. Food* **2018**, *21*, 154–158. [CrossRef] [PubMed]
11. Minekus, M.; Alminger, M.; Alvito, P.; Balance, S.; Bohn, T.; Bourlieu, C.; Carrière, F.; Boutrou, R.; Corredig, M.; Dupont, D.; et al. A standardised static in vitro digestion method suitable for food—An international consensus. *Food Funct.* **2014**, *5*, 1113–1124. [CrossRef]
12. Glahn, R. The use of Caco-2 cells in defining nutrient bioavailability: Application to iron bioavailability of foods. In *Designing Functional Foods*; McClements, D.J., Decker, E.A., Eds.; Woodhead Publishing: Cambridge, UK, 2009; pp. 340–361.

13. Thongon, N.; Krishnamra, N. Omeprazole decreases magnesium transport across Caco-2 monolayers. *World J. Gastroenterol.* **2011**, *17*, 1574–1583. [CrossRef] [PubMed]
14. Fine, K.D.; Ana, C.A.S.; Porter, J.L.; Fordtran, J.S. Intestinal absorption of magnesium from food and supplements. *J. Clin. Investig.* **1991**, *88*, 396–402. [CrossRef] [PubMed]

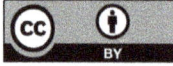

nutrients

MDPI

Article

Effects of Magnesium Supplementation on Unipolar Depression: A Placebo-Controlled Study and Review of the Importance of Dosing and Magnesium Status in the Therapeutic Response

Beata Ryszewska-Pokraśniewicz [1], Anna Mach [2,*], Michał Skalski [2], Piotr Januszko [2], Zbigniew M. Wawrzyniak [3], Ewa Poleszak [4], Gabriel Nowak [5,†], Andrzej Pilc [5] and Maria Radziwoń-Zaleska [2,†]

[1] Nowowiejski Hospital, 00-685 Warsaw, Poland; beataryszewska@wp.pl
[2] Department of Psychiatry, Medical University of Warsaw, 00-685 Warsaw, Poland; michal.skalski@wum.edu.pl (M.S.); piotr.januszko@wp.pl (P.J.); mariar@wum.edu.pl (M.R.-Z.)
[3] Faculty of Electronics and Information Technology, Warsaw University of Technology, 00-685 Warsaw, Poland; z.wawrzyniak@ise.pw.edu.pl
[4] Faculty of Pharmacy, Medical University of Lublin, 20-093 Lublin, Poland; ewa.poleszak@umlub.pl
[5] Institute of Pharmacology, Polish Academy of Sciences, 31-343 Kraków, Poland; nowak@if-pan.krakow.pl (G.N.); nfpilc@cyf-kr.edu.pl (A.P.)
*   Correspondence: anna.mach@wum.edu.pl; Tel.: +48-22-825-1236; Fax: +48-22-825-1315
†   These authors equally contributed to this study.

Received: 13 July 2018; Accepted: 31 July 2018; Published: 3 August 2018

Abstract: Animal studies using tests and models have demonstrated that magnesium exerts an antidepressant effect. The literature contains few studies in humans involving attempts to augment antidepressant therapy with magnesium ions. The purpose of our study was to assess the efficacy and safety of antidepressant treatment, in combination with magnesium ions. A total of 37 participants with recurrent depressive disorder who developed a depressive episode were included in this study. As part of this double-blind study, treatment with the antidepressant fluoxetine was accompanied with either magnesium ions (120 mg/day as magnesium aspartate) or placebo. During an 8-week treatment period, each patient was monitored for any clinical abnormalities. Moreover, serum fluoxetine and magnesium levels were measured, and pharmaco-electroencephalography was performed. The fluoxetine + magnesium and fluoxetine + placebo groups showed no significant differences in either Hamilton Depression Rating Scale (HDRS) scores or serum magnesium levels at any stage of treatment. Multivariate statistical analysis of the whole investigated group showed that the following parameters increased the odds of effective treatment: lower baseline HDRS scores, female gender, smoking, and treatment augmentation with magnesium. The parameters that increased the odds of remission were lower baseline HDRS scores, shorter history of disease, the presence of antidepressant-induced changes in the pharmaco-EEG profile at 6 h after treatment, and the fact of receiving treatment augmented with magnesium ions. The limitation of this study is a small sample size.

Keywords: unipolar depression; magnesium; pharmaco-electroencephalography; efficacy; remission

1. Introduction

According to the recent data from the World Health Organization, depression affects over 300 million people worldwide. By 2030, recurrent unipolar depressive disorders are projected to become the leading cause of the burden of disease worldwide, as calculated on the basis of Disability-Adjusted Life Years (DALYs) [1].

Despite having been studied for years, the etiology of depression is yet to be fully understood. More and more animal and clinical studies have suggested a role of the N-methyl-D-aspartate (NMDA) receptor complex and NMDA-mediated excitatory amino acid neurotransmission both in the pathophysiology and treatment of depression [2–5]. This concept seems to be confirmed by evidence of glutamate system abnormalities detected in the blood [6], cerebrospinal fluid [7], and brain tissue [8] of patients with depressive disorders. Modifying glutamatergic transmission by means of NMDA receptors is currently a promising target of antidepressant treatment [9].

The NMDA receptor complex is modified by multiple ligand binding sites. Recent years saw a number of experimental studies that confirmed an antidepressant effect of various NMDA receptor antagonists, such as ketamine, memantine, dextromethorphan, or MK-0657 [9]. However, the risk of severe side effects limits the use of these agents as antidepressant drugs [10].

One of the natural, inorganic modulators of the NMDA receptor complex are magnesium ions. They inhibit voltage-gated NMDA receptor channels at the same time inhibiting the flow of calcium ions. Moreover, they increase the expression of the GluN2B subunit of the NMDA receptor complex [11]. In the hippocampus, low magnesium levels in combination with high calcium and glutamate levels are believed to potentially cause functional changes in synapses, leading to the development of mood disorders, including depression [11,12]. There are several mechanisms responsible for antidepressant effects of magnesium. Apart from their direct NMDA-receptor antagonism, magnesium ions interact with other factors crucial in depression pathophysiology. Magnesium ions suppress hippocampal kindling and modulate protein kinase C [13]. Moreover, they affect P-glycoprotein (a protein responsible for blood-brain barrier permeability to glucocorticoids and other molecules), which alters the hypothalamic-pituitary-adrenal axis and damages the hippocampus [14]. Magnesium also plays a role in serotoninergic, noradrenergic, and dopaminergic neurotransmission [15] and it has an anti-inflammatory effect [16], which additionally increases its antidepressant potential.

Antidepressant properties of magnesium have been demonstrated in animal preclinical screen tests and models. Magnesium salts are active in the forced swim test (FST) as well as in olfactory bulbectomy and chronic mild stress models [17–20]. Furthermore, this bio-metal enhances antidepressant activity of standard antidepressants in the FST [15,21,22]. On the other hand, magnesium deficiency (induced by low-magnesium diet in laboratory animals) is related to depression-like behavior [23].

Multiple studies have demonstrated a relationship between depressive disorders and magnesium intake [24–27]. However, the data on the changes in magnesium levels in patients with depression are inconclusive. Some authors showed a positive correlation between magnesium levels and depression [28], whereas others showed a negative correlation [29]. Similar discrepancies were observed in the case of the severity of depression symptoms [30]. Nonetheless, Camardese et al. concluded that serum magnesium levels correlate with the response to treatment [31].

We would like to emphasize that the main goal in the treatment of a depressive episode is first to achieve a full therapeutic response and remission, followed by recurrence prevention, and ensuring the patient's return to normal functioning [32]. One of the major problems in treating depression is the effectiveness of therapy. Some patients fail to achieve a satisfactory response to treatment. Initial antidepressant treatment, with adequate dosing and treatment duration, leads to remission only in 50% of patients [33]. Moreover, 20–30% of patients achieve incomplete remission, with some depressive symptoms persisting for a long time. Another therapeutic problem is a delay in therapeutic effects. All currently approved monoaminergic antidepressants exhibit latency in the therapeutic response, which considerably increases the risk of suicide and self-harm. Thus, there are unceasing attempts to potentiate and speed up the therapeutic effect [32].

Due to the limited effectiveness of antidepressant treatment, there is a great need for developing novel, satisfactory therapies. To date, there have been few clinical studies on magnesium supplementation in depressive disorders, and their findings have been inconclusive [34–36]. Therefore, the purpose of our study was to assess the efficacy and safety of antidepressant treatment accompanied with magnesium supplements.

2. Materials and Methods

Our 8-week study included 37 patients (admitted either to the Department of Psychiatry, Medical University of Warsaw or to Nowowiejski Hospital in Warsaw) who met the inclusion criterion of an ICD-10-codable depressive episode or major depression as defined in DSM-IV. The exclusion criteria were delusional disorders, organic disorders, high risk of suicide requiring electroconvulsive therapy, absolute contraindications for selective serotonin re-uptake inhibitors (SSRIs), absolute contraindications for magnesium ions, alcohol and substance abuse, and baseline pharmaco-EEG abnormalities. Patients with severe depression (more than 19 points in the HDRS) were included in the study. Patients were recruited without age or gender restrictions—adults over 18 years old.

All patients received fluoxetine at a daily dose of 20–40 mg. This standard treatment was augmented, in a double-blind manner, with either placebo or magnesium. The magnesium supplements used in this study were 40-mg magnesium effervescent tablets or powder containing 40 mg of magnesium (equivalent to 3.30 mEq of magnesium aspartate) administered 3 times per day.

The study was conducted in accordance with the Declaration of Helsinki. The protocol was approved by the Institutional Review Board and Bioethics Committee at the Medical University of Warsaw (KB/96/2006; KB/227/2012). All participants gave informed written consent prior to participating in this study.

Study participants were recruited based on baseline assessments, which included a physical examination (conducted by the same psychiatrist as those conducted later, throughout the study), psychometric scale score, and pharmaco-electroencephalography. Individuals who qualified to take part in the study underwent a one-week wash-out period (except in cases of previous SSRI treatment, where wash-out was extended to 6 weeks).

All study group patients were examined by the same physician at pre-defined time points: prior to treatment initiation (time 0), 6 h after the first dose of the drug (maximum serum concentration of the drug), and subsequently at 24 h, 2 weeks, 4 weeks, 6 weeks, and 8 weeks after treatment initiation [37].

The psychometric scales used in this study were the 21-item Hamilton Depression Rating Scale (HDRS), Hamilton Anxiety Rating Scale (HARS), and Clinical Global Impression Scale (CGIS). Treatment was considered effective when there was a 50% reduction in the baseline HDRS score. The cut-off HDRS score that defined remission was 6 or less [38].

The presence and severity of side effects were assessed based on history-taking, changes in Side Effect Rating Scale (SERS) scores as compared to baseline, and laboratory assessments, which were conducted at the same time as psychometric assessments. Any drugs that could affect the levels of the antidepressant were avoided during the study. When necessary, zopiclone (7.5 mg) or zolpidem (10 mg) was allowed every other day.

A high-performance liquid chromatography (HPLC) system (Shimadzu Corporation, Analytical Instruments Division, Kyoto, Japan) was used in this study to measure serum fluoxetine (FLU) and norfluoxetine (NFLU) levels. The measurement method was based on the reports by El-Yazigi and Raines [39], Aymard [40], Meineke [41], and Komorowska [42].

The following therapeutic ranges were adopted [42,43]: fluoxetine 50–450 ng/mL, norfluoxetine 50–350 ng/mL, fluoxetine and norfluoxetine 50–550 ng/mL. Serum fluoxetine levels were measured at the Psychopharmacology Laboratory of the Department of Psychiatry, WUM. Serum magnesium levels were measured by ALAB Laboratories and analyzed with the use of Hulanicki's method [44]. The established ALAB reference range for serum magnesium levels (1.7–2.5 mg/dL) was adopted for this study. This was a double-blind study—with the principal investigator blinded to the magnesium levels in individual participants before study completion, as the laboratory reported only abnormalities in magnesium levels.

Pharmaco-EEG examinations were conducted prior to, and 6 and 24 h after, treatment initiation, and then at 2, 4, 6, and 8 weeks of treatment. The electroencephalograph used in this study was DigiTrack, version DTW (Elmico). Subsequently, EEG relative power spectra were calculated with NeuroGuide software using the fast Fourier transformation (FFT) algorithm. Adopting a 0.5-Hz resolution, we calculated the power spectra in delta (1.5–5.0 Hz), theta (5.5–8.0 Hz), alpha 1 (8.5–10.0 Hz), alpha 2 (10.5–12.0 Hz), beta 1 (12.5–18.5 Hz), beta 2 (19.0–20.5 Hz), and beta 3 (21.0–29.5 Hz) frequency bands. Arranged chronologically, *t*-test values for the individual bands formed a profile of EEG power spectrum changes over the treatment period.

Each of the graphs was classified by an expert, based on the presence or absence of an antidepressant-induced pharmaco-EEG profile. The following pharmaco-EEG profile, typical for tricyclic antidepressants (TCAs), was considered positive in fluoxetine-treated patients: an increase in high frequency beta waves (beta 3) [37,45,46].

All EEG examinations were performed at the Clinical Electroencephalography and Neurophysiology Laboratory of the Department of Psychiatry, WUM.

In the statistical analysis of our results, the Wilcoxon Rank-Sum Test for independent samples was used for the comparison of groups. Moreover, we used descriptive statistics and multivariate logistic regression models (GLIMMIX procedure), which allowed us to assess the odds ratios for an ineffective treatment and lack of remission with respect to each of the evaluated factors. The level of statistical significance was set at $p < 0.05$. All calculations were conducted with SAS 14.1.

3. Results

Seventeen (11 women [65%] and 6 men [35%]) out of the 37 participants included in the study received fluoxetine and magnesium, whereas 20 (10 women [50%] and 10 men [50%]) received fluoxetine and placebo. The mean age in the magnesium group ($n = 17$, group I) was 48.1 ± 15.5 years; the median age was 50 years; the age range was from 23 to 71 years, with 5 participants (29%) 60 years old or older. Body weight in this group ranged from 50.0 to 110.0 kg, with the mean of 71.2 ± 15.0 kg and median 70.0 kg. The mean height was 169.9 ± 10.0 cm (with the median of 168.0 cm and range of 158.0–192.0 cm). Mean disease duration at baseline was 5.6 ± 5.8 years (with the median of 4.0 years and range of 0.3–20.0 years). The mean age in the placebo group ($n = 20$, group II) was 49.7 ± 12.3 years; the median age was 52 years; the age range was from 24 to 65 years, with 6 participants (30%) 60 years old or older. The mean body weight in this group was 76.2 ± 16.1 kg (median 75.0 kg, range 48.0–112.0 kg). The mean height in this group was 171.9 ± 7.7 cm (median 173.5 cm, range 156.0–187.0 cm). Mean disease duration at baseline was 3.8 ± 4.5 years (median 2.0 years, range 0.4–16.0 years).

In group I, 10 participants (60%) were hospitalized once, 4 participants (23.5%) were hospitalized twice, one participant (5.9%) was hospitalized 3 times, one (5.9%) 4 times, and one participant (5.9%) was hospitalized more than 5 times. In group II, 15 participants (75.0%) were hospitalized once, 4 participants (20.0%) were hospitalized 2 times, one participant (5.0%) was hospitalized 5 times, and there were no participants hospitalized more than 5 times.

There were 2 non-smokers (11.8%) and 15 smokers (88.2%) in group I. The mean BMI in this group was 24.6 kg/m^2 (median 24.2 kg/m^2, range 19.1–35.5 kg/m^2). There were 5 non-smokers (25.0%) and 15 smokers (75.0%) in group II. The mean BMI in this group was 25.8 kg/m^2 (median 24.8 kg/m^2, range 17.6–37.4 kg/m^2).

Prior to treatment initiation, the mean HDRS score in group I (fluoxetine and magnesium) was 30.5 ± 6.0 (median 29; range 21–44) (Table 1). Other scales used in this study yielded the following scores prior to treatment initiation: HARS (mean score 20.1 ± 4.8, median 19, range 13–28), CGI (mean score 2.9 ± 0.7, median 3, range 2–4), and SERS (mean score 10.5 ± 3.4, median 10, range 6–18).

Table 1. Effect of magnesium or placebo supplementation on Hamilton Depression Rating Scale (HDRS) scores in patients treated with fluoxetine.

| | Group I: Magnesium | | | | | Group II: Placebo | | | | | |
Variable	N	Mean	SD	Med	Min	Max	N	Mean	SD	Med	Min	Max	*p*-Value
HDRS_0	17	30.5	6	29	21	44	20	27.5	5.5	28	18	38	0.1120
HDRS_6H	17	30.4	5.8	29	21	43	20	27.5	5.5	28	18	38	0.1197
HDRS_24H	17	30.4	5.8	29	21	43	20	27.4	5.4	28	18	38	0.1059
HDRS_2W	17	24.5	5.6	24	13	36	20	21.8	7.5	23	9	36	0.2237
HDRS_4W	17	18.5	5.9	17	10	31	17	17.2	6.4	17	5	28	0.5605
HDRS_6W	17	14.6	6.9	13	5	29	16	13.4	6.6	14	2	28	0.6100
HDRS_8W	17	10.7	7.9	8	1	29	15	10.4	6.8	10	1	28	0.9080

N—number of patients; SD—standard deviation; Med—Median; Min—minimum; Max—maximum HDRS: Hamilton Depression Rating Scale; HDRS_0—scores before treatment; H—hours; W—week. The Wilcoxon Rank-Sum Test for independent samples was used for the comparison of groups.

Prior to treatment initiation, the mean HDRS score in group II (fluoxetine and placebo) was 27.5 ± 5.5 (median 28; range 18–38) (Table 1). Other scales yielded the following scores at baseline: HARS scores: mean 18.5 ± 3.8, median 19, range 8–25; CGI scores: mean 3.1 ± 0.7, median 3, range 2–5; SERS scores: mean 11.3 ± 3.5, median 11, range 5–20.

There were no differences between groups at each examined time points in either HDRS (Table 1) or in CGI, HARS, and SERS scores (data not shown).

After 8 weeks of treatment, there was a 50% improvement in HDRS scores in 15 participants (88%) from group I and in 11 participants (73%) from group II. There was no significant difference between the groups in terms of treatment efficacy.

Remission, which had been pre-defined as HDRS score reduction to 6 points or less, was achieved in 6 participants (35%) from group I and in 4 participants (27%) from group II. There was no significant difference between the groups in terms of remission rates.

The two study groups (I and II) showed no significant differences in terms of HDRS score changes during treatment (Figure 1). The two study groups (I and II) showed no significant differences in terms of serum magnesium levels during treatment (Figure 2).

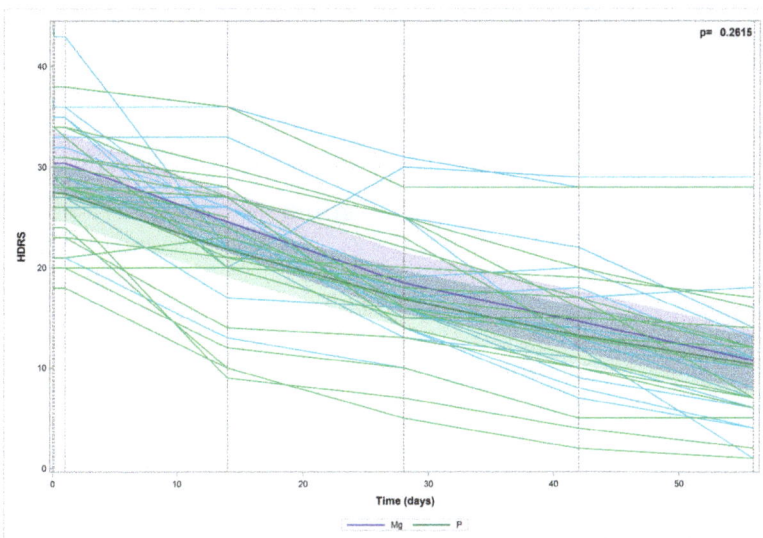

Figure 1. Hamilton Depression Rating Scale (HDRS) scores over time—the measured data and trend.

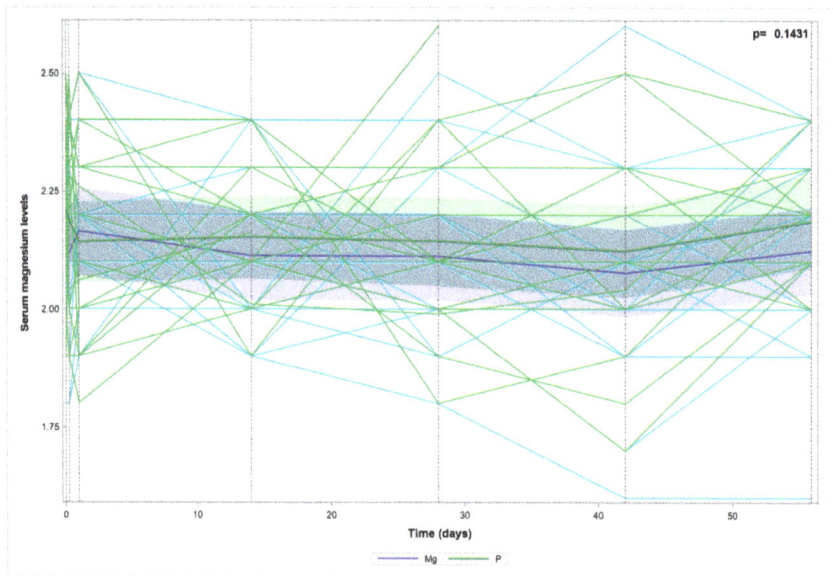

Figure 2. Serum magnesium levels over time—the measured data and trend.

Models of multivariate analysis were used to calculate odds ratios for both remission (model 1) and treatment efficacy (model 2) using the compared values of each evaluated parameter.

Model 1 (Table 2), which was used to analyze the odds of remission, included the following parameters: the baseline HDRS score; disease duration; pharmaco-EEG profile (obtained 6 h after treatment initiation) showing evidence of TCA use (yes vs. no); and the type of treatment (magnesium vs. placebo).

Table 2. Odds ratio values for the parameters evaluated in this model—the odds ratio for remission.

Parameter	Values	Odds Ratio	95% LCL	95% UCL	*p*-Value
HDRS-0	$[x + 1]$ vs. $[x]$	0.8982	0.7503	1.0752	0.2422
Duration of disease	$[x + 1]$ vs. $[x]$	0.8001	0.5842	1.0956	0.1643
PROF-1	0 vs. 1	0.4151	0.1637	1.0527	0.0641
Mg-P	Mg vs. P	1.5545	0.6206	3.8938	0.3464

LCL lower confidence limit; UCL upper confidence limit.

Figure 3 shows the odds ratios (ORs) for remission (with 95% confidence intervals) for the individual parameters. A statistically significant parameter would have its OR = 1.0 value positioned completely beyond the confidence interval. An odds ratio equal to 1.0 means that both compared values of the given parameter yield identical odds of remission.

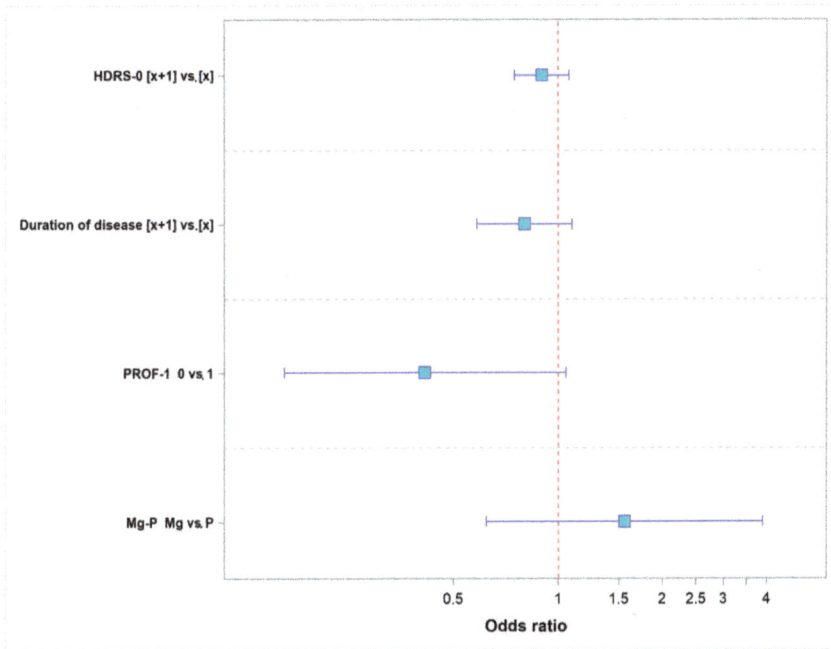

Figure 3. Odds ratio values for remission.

We found that an increase in the HDRS score by 1 point as compared to baseline, disease duration longer by 1 year, and a lack of antidepressant-induced changes in the pharmaco-EEG profile at 6 h after treatment decrease the odds of remission. The use of magnesium to augment the effect of treatment increases the odds of remission.

Model 2 (Table 3)—which was used to analyze treatment efficacy, included the following parameters: the baseline HDRS score; the patients' gender; smoking status; and the type of treatment (magnesium vs. placebo). Figure 4 shows the increase in the baseline HDRS score by 1 point and being a non-smoker ($p = 0.0034$) reduced the odds of effective treatment. The female sex and the use of magnesium to potentialize the effect of fluoxetine increased the odds of effective treatment.

Table 3. Odds ratio values for the parameters evaluated in this model—the odds of achieving 50% improvement in HDRS scores (efficacy).

Parameter	Values	Odds Ratio	95% LCL	95% UCL	*p*-Value
HDRS-0	[$x + 1$] vs. [x]	0.8614	0.7093	1.0461	0.1321
Gender	F vs. M	2.1942	0.6840	7.0392	0.1864
Smoking status	0 vs. 1	0.1242	0.0181	0.8530	0.0339
Mg-P	Mg vs. P	2.5869	0.7510	8.9111	0.1320

LCL, lower confidence limit; UCL, upper confidence limit.

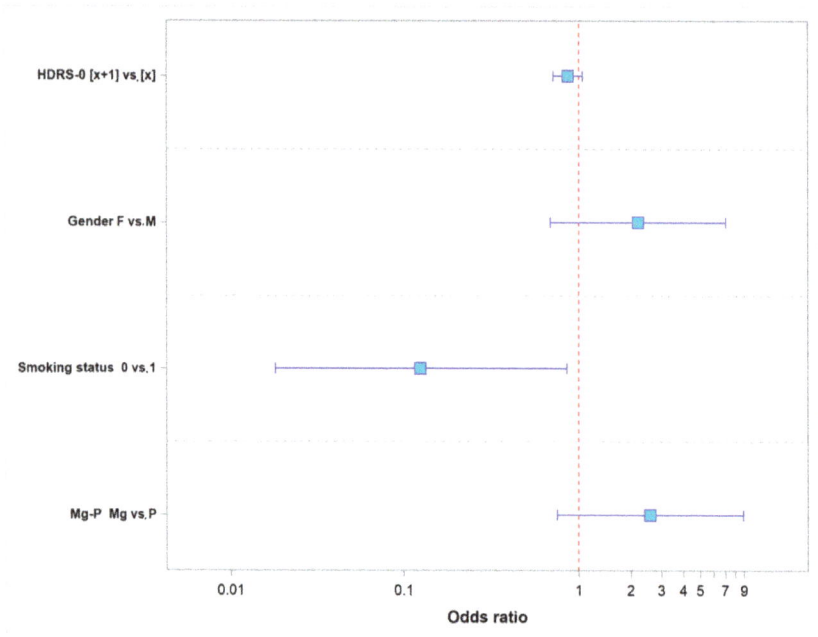

Figure 4. Odds ratio values for treatment efficacy.

4. Discussion

Our study evaluated the efficacy and safety of antidepressant treatment augmented with magnesium. Despite the fact that the fluoxetine-and-magnesium group showed higher rates of 50% improvement in HDRS scores at week 8 than the fluoxetine-and-placebo group, the difference was not statistically significant. Similar, though also non-significant, results were obtained while evaluating remission. Moreover, the magnesium and placebo groups showed no significant differences in terms of the efficacy and safety of treatment at any evaluated time point.

Our findings are unlike those reported in some earlier studies. Tarleton et al. demonstrated a decrease in depression symptoms already after a two-week period of magnesium supplementation at 248 mg per day. Their study employed the PHQ-9 for the diagnosis of depression [47], with 126 participants with mild-to-moderate depression symptoms included in the study. Their results showed no relationship with the participants' age, gender, baseline disease severity, or antidepressant treatment [48]. Earlier reports by Tarleton et al. also showed a relationship between low magnesium intake (<184 mg/day) and depression [26]. This observation was also supported by a Finnish study including exclusively males (2320 participants). That study demonstrated that adequate magnesium intake may prevent depression [27]. In light of the available studies, the reports of major depression cases described by Eby et al. seem very interesting, as they showed a rapid (within under 7 days) recovery in response to treatment with magnesium (in the form of glycinate and taurinate) at 125–300-mg administered with every meal and before sleep [35]. Moreover, another two-week randomized study in a group of 23 elderly patients with newly diagnosed depression, associated with type 2 diabetes and hypomagnesemia, showed treatment with magnesium chloride (450 mg/day) to be equally effective as that with imipramine (50 mg/day) [49].

Nonetheless, our findings were consistent with those of some other authors. Mehdi et al. observed no changes in HDRS scores following magnesium supplementation in a group of participants (*n* = 12) with mild-to-moderate treatment-resistant depression [50]. Similar results were observed in a randomized clinical study in a group of female patients with postpartum depression, where an 8-week treatment with magnesium at 320 mg/day failed to reduce the symptoms of depression evaluated with the Edinburgh Postnatal Depression Scale [51]. Moreover, a large Spanish study conducted in a Mediterranean population (15,836 participants) showed no conclusive evidence to support the claim that an increased magnesium intake might be associated with a lower risk of developing depression [52]. Due to these conflicting findings, the efficacy of magnesium in antidepressant treatment is still unknown.

Table 4 presents a compilation of clinical studies on the use of magnesium in the treatment of depressive disorders as well as data on the study methods used.

Table 4. Effect of magnesium (Mg) supplementation in human depression.

Depression Type	Type of Study	N	Dose of Mg^{+2} mg/day p.o.	Salt	Effect	References
Major depression	Case	4	125–300	Glycinate taurinate	+	[28]
Depression (early, type 2 diabetes, hypomagnesemia)	Randomized Mg vs. IMI	23	450	Chloride	+	[42]
Depression Gitelman's syndrome, (hypomagnesemia)	Case	1	300–900 plus intravenous 1200	Oxide sulfate	+	[46]
Major depression (hypomagnesemia)	Placebo	60	300	Oxide	+	[47]
Major depression	Placebo cross-over	112	248	Chloride	+	[41]
Postpartum depression	Placebo	66	87	Sulfate	−	[44]
Major depression	Placebo	37	120	Aspartate	−	present study
Major depression (TRD)	Monotherapy	12	Intravenous 1000	Sulfate	−	[43]

N—number of patients; + positive effect of Mg supplementation; − no effect of Mg supplementation.

We would like to emphasize the fact that the tools for assessing depression symptoms which were used in the studies cited above were non-uniform, with the following being the most commonly used questionnaires: the Human Population Laboratory (HPL) Depression Scale [27], Patient Health Questionnaire (PHQ-9), Yasavage and Brink Scale [49], and Hamilton Depression Rating Scale (HDRS) [50]. It seems obvious that these psychometric instruments differ in terms of accuracy, reliability, or standardization. Therefore, the selection of an appropriate questionnaire may determine the study findings. Consistent with our observations, a study by Mehdi et al. showed no significant changes in HDRS scores following magnesium supplementation; however, increased serum magnesium levels correlated with a clinical improvement measured with the PHQ-9 [50]. The questionnaire used in our study is currently considered to be the gold standard among psychometric tools used to assess the severity of depression. Additionally, it helps precisely monitor the patient's condition during antidepressant treatment. The HDRS is an observer-rated instrument, which means that the assessment is conducted by an experienced physician who knows the standards in symptom severity assessment. Unlike self-administered questionnaires used by other investigators, the HDRS is considered to be a more objective and accurate tool. The methods of assessing a response to treatment in our study additionally included looking for antidepressant-induced changes in pharmaco-EEG profiles at various time points. Our results showed no statistically significant differences between the study groups. The discrepancies between our findings and the ones reported by other authors may be also due to a varied duration of magnesium supplementation and different assessment time points.

Other factors that may affect treatment efficacy include both the dosage and form of magnesium supplements. In all the studies mentioned above where oral magnesium supplementation was shown to decrease depression symptoms magnesium doses ranged from 125 to 900 mg/day. In all these cases the dosage was higher than that used in our study. Currently, there are a number of available magnesium formulations. The key criterion that makes these formulations different is their bioavailability. Due to the fact that only some (30–40%) of the ingested magnesium is absorbed by the body, it is very important to conduct magnesium supplementation using formulations characterized by better absorption. Magnesium aspartate, citrate, lactate, and chloride are considered to have a higher bioavailability in comparison with that of either magnesium oxide or sulfate [11]. In the present study dose of magnesium (120 mg Mg^{2+}/day) was chosen as the acceptable (and widely applied) in Poland (indicated by Pharmindex—polish drug encyclopedia). Despite the fact that we used magnesium aspartate characterized by high bioavailability and a structure similar to that of magnesium compounds found in a normal diet, we observed no significant improvement in depression symptoms. Moreover, since our study was conducted exclusively in a Polish population, we cannot exclude the potential effects of genetic and environmental factors.

Despite the well-documented relationship between magnesium and depression, its mechanisms are still unknown. Thus, the role of magnesium in antidepressant treatment augmentation is difficult to elucidate. A study by Camardese et al. demonstrated a more pronounced response to antidepressant treatment in patients with higher magnesium levels [31]. Another study showed a marked increase in intracellular magnesium levels following treatment with either amitriptyline or sertraline. It is precisely this increase in intracellular magnesium levels that has been suggested to be partially responsible for the effect of antidepressant drugs [53].

Experimental pre-clinical studies on animal models demonstrated that the antidepressant effect of magnesium is a result of its role in serotoninergic neurotransmission [54]. The potential synergism between magnesium and antidepressants warrants further studies on antidepressant treatment potentialization.

Further studies are necessary to discover whether magnesium supplementation can justify the use of antidepressants at lower doses or help avoid the necessity of combination regimens.

We would like to emphasize our multivariate analysis results that identified the parameters that increased the odds of remission and treatment efficacy. The parameters increasing the odds of remission (i.e., HDRS score of <6) included lower baseline HDRS scores, shorter history of disease, the presence of antidepressant-induced pharmaco-EEG profile at 6 h after drug administration, and treatment augmentation with magnesium ions. The parameters increasing the odds of treatment efficacy were lower baseline HDRS scores, female gender, being a smoker, and treatment augmentation with magnesium ions. It seems obvious that an earlier diagnosis and lower symptom severity are favorable prognostic factors. The benefits of magnesium supplementation have been widely discussed. One of the arguments explaining the better treatment efficacy in females observed in our study may be other authors' reports of generally lower magnesium levels in females [55,56]. Pregnancy and chronic use of oral contraceptives are known to lead to hypomagnesemia [57]. Moreover, magnesium supplementation has been shown to prevent the development of postpartum depression [35].

We would like to emphasize that one of the parameters shown to significantly increase the odds of effective treatment was the fact of being a smoker. Nicotine is known to directly affect mood in humans. The relationship between depression and smoking has been extensively studied, and the findings demonstrated antidepressant properties of nicotine [58–60]. Smokers with a history of depression who refrain from smoking have a higher risk of developing another depressive episode [61]. Salin-Pascual et al. observed an improvement in the mood of non-smoking participants with major depression following the use of nicotine patches [62]. This effect is most likely associated with dopaminergic reward system activation [63] and serotoninergic neurotransmission [60]. The results of our study demonstrate potentially antidepressant effects of nicotine. However, our findings need to be confirmed in a larger number of patients.

Despite the fact that our study did not conclusively demonstrate an increased efficacy of antidepressant treatment augmented with magnesium, magnesium supplementation helped predict treatment efficacy and remission. Further studies are necessary to assess whether magnesium supplementation may be a valuable complement to standard antidepressant treatments.

5. Conclusions

The magnesium and placebo groups showed no statistically significant differences in terms of HDRS scores, serum magnesium levels, treatment safety and efficacy, or pharmaco-EEG profiles. Nonetheless, supplementation with magnesium ions is one of the parameters that help increase the chances of treatment efficacy and remission. The limitation of this study is the small sample size.

Author Contributions: M.S., G.N. and M.R.-Z. conceived and designed the experiments; B.R.-P., A.M., P.J. and M.R.-Z. performed the experiments; A.M., M.S., Z.M.W., E.P., G.N., A.P. and M.R.-Z. analyzed the data; P.J., A.M. and M.S. contributed reagents/materials/analysis tools; B.R.-P., A.M., G.N. and M.R.-Z. wrote the paper.

Funding: This study was partially financed from a grant from the National Science Center [Narodowe Centrum Nauki] (NCN2012/07/B/NZ7/04375) and statutory founds from Medical University of Warsaw and Institute of Pharmacology PAS, Kraków.

Conflicts of Interest: All authors declare no conflict of interest.

References

1. World Health Organization. Available online: http://www.who.int/en/news-room/fact-sheets/detail/depression (accessed on 15 May 2018).
2. Deutschenbaur, L.; Beck, J.; Kiyhankhadiv, A.; Mühlhauser, M.; Borgwardt, S.; Walter, M.; Hasler, G.; Sollberger, D.; Lang, U.E. Role of calcium, glutamate and NMDA in major depression and therapeutic application. *Prog. Neuro-Psychopharmacol. Biol. Psychiatry* **2016**, *64*, 325–333. [CrossRef] [PubMed]
3. Poleszak, E.; Wlaź, P.; Socała, K.; Wrobel, A.; Szewczyk, B.; Kasperek, R.; Nowak, G. Interaction of glycine/NMDA receptor ligands and antidepressant drugs in the forced swim test. *Pharmacol. Rep.* **2010**, *62*, 58. [CrossRef]
4. Nowak, G.; Papp, M.; Paul, I.A. The NMDA receptor complex and the action of antidepressant drugs in the CMS model of depression. *Eur. J. Pharm. Sci.* **1996**, *4*, S53. [CrossRef]
5. Wlaź, P.; Kasperek, R.; Wlaź, A.; Szumiło, M.; Wróbel, A.; Nowak, G.; Poleszak, E. NMDA and AMPA receptors are involved in the antidepressant-like activity of tianeptine in the forced swim test in mice. *Pharmacol. Rep.* **2011**, *63*, 1526–1532. [PubMed]
6. Küçükibrahimoğlu, E.; Saygin, M.Z.; Caliskan, M.; Kaplan, O.K.; Unsal, C.; Gören, M.Z. The change in plasma GABA, glutamine and glutamate levels in fluoxetine- or S-citalopram-treated female patients with major depression. *Eur. J. Clin. Pharmacol.* **2009**, *65*, 571–577. [CrossRef] [PubMed]
7. Frye, M.A.; Tsai, G.E.; Huggins, T.; Coyle, J.T.; Post, R.M. Low Cerebrospinal Fluid Glutamate and Glycine in Refractory Affective Disorder. *Biol. Psychiatry* **2007**, *61*, 162–166. [CrossRef] [PubMed]
8. Hashimoto, K.; Sawa, A.; Iyo, M. Increased Levels of Glutamate in Brains from Patients with Mood Disorders. *Biol. Psychiatry* **2007**, *62*, 1310–1316. [CrossRef] [PubMed]
9. Machado-Vieira, R.; Henter, I.D.; Zarate, C.A., Jr. New targets for rapid antidepressant action. *Prog. Neurobiol.* **2017**, *152*, 21–37. [CrossRef] [PubMed]
10. Sanacora, G.; Wilkinson, S.; Schalkwyk, G.V. 201. Measuring Dissociative Effects of NMDA Receptor Antagonists in the Treatment of Depression. *Biol. Psychiatry* **2017**, *81*, S83. [CrossRef]
11. Serefko, A.; Szopa, A.; Poleszak, E. Magnesium and depression. *Magnes. Res.* **2016**, *29*, 112–119. [CrossRef]
12. Poleszak, E.; Wlaz, P.; Kedzierska, E.; Nieoczym, D.; Wrobel, A.; Fidecka, S.; Pilc, A.; Nowak, G. NMDA/glutamate mechanism of antidepressant-like action of magnesium in forced swim test in mice. *Pharmacol. Biochem. Behav.* **2007**, *88*, 158–164. [CrossRef] [PubMed]
13. Murck, H. Ketamine, magnesium and major depression—From pharmacology to pathophysiology and back. *J. Psychiatr. Res.* **2013**, *47*, 955–965. [CrossRef] [PubMed]
14. Gould, T.D.; Manji, H.K. Glycogen synthase kinase-3: A putative molecular target for lithium mimetic drugs. *Neuropsychopharmacol. Off. Publ. Am. Coll. Neuropsychopharmacol.* **2005**, *30*, 1223–1237. [CrossRef] [PubMed]

15. Cardoso, C.C.; Lobato, K.R.; Binfare, R.W.; Ferreira, P.K.; Rosa, A.O.; Santos, A.R.; Rodrigues, A.L. Evidence for the involvement of the monoaminergic system in the antidepressant-like effect of magnesium. *Prog. Neuro-Psychopharmacol. Biol. Psychiatry* **2009**, *33*, 235–242. [CrossRef] [PubMed]

16. King, D.E.; Mainous, A.G., 3rd; Geesey, M.E.; Ellis, T. Magnesium intake and serum C-reactive protein levels in children. *Magnes. Res.* **2007**, *20*, 32–36. [PubMed]

17. Decollogne, S.; Tomas, A.; Lecerf, C.; Adamowicz, E.; Seman, M. NMDA receptor complex blockade by oral administration of magnesium: Comparison with MK-801. *Pharmacol. Biochem. Behav.* **1997**, *58*, 261–268. [CrossRef]

18. Poleszak, E.; Szewczyk, B.; Kedzierska, E.; Wlaz, P.; Pilc, A.; Nowak, G. Antidepressant- and anxiolytic-like activity of magnesium in mice. *Pharmacol. Biochem. Behav.* **2004**, *78*, 7–12. [CrossRef] [PubMed]

19. Pochwat, B.; Szewczyk, B.; Sowa-Kucma, M.; Siwek, A.; Doboszewska, U.; Piekoszewski, W.; Gruca, P.; Papp, M.; Nowak, G. Antidepressant-like activity of magnesium in the chronic mild stress model in rats: Alterations in the NMDA receptor subunits. *Int. J. Neuropsychopharmacol.* **2014**, *17*, 393–405. [CrossRef] [PubMed]

20. Pochwat, B.; Sowa-Kucma, M.; Kotarska, K.; Misztak, P.; Nowak, G.; Szewczyk, B. Antidepressant-like activity of magnesium in the olfactory bulbectomy model is associated with the AMPA/BDNF pathway. *Psychopharmacology* **2015**, *232*, 355–367. [CrossRef] [PubMed]

21. Poleszak, E.; Wlaz, P.; Szewczyk, B.; Kedzierska, E.; Wyska, E.; Librowski, T.; Szymura-Oleksiak, J.; Fidecka, S.; Pilc, A.; Nowak, G. Enhancement of antidepressant-like activity by joint administration of imipramine and magnesium in the forced swim test: Behavioral and pharmacokinetic studies in mice. *Pharmacol. Biochem. Behav.* **2005**, *81*, 524–529. [CrossRef] [PubMed]

22. Serefko, A.; Szopa, A.; Wlaź, P.; Nowak, G.; Radziwoń-Zaleska, M.; Skalski, M.; Poleszak, E. Magnesium in depression. *Pharmacol. Rep.* **2013**, *65*, 547–554. [CrossRef]

23. Singewald, N.; Sinner, C.; Hetzenauer, A.; Sartori, S.B.; Murck, H. Magnesium-deficient diet alters depression- and anxiety-related behavior in mice—Influence of desipramine and Hypericum perforatum extract. *Neuropharmacology* **2004**, *47*, 1189–1197. [CrossRef] [PubMed]

24. Jacka, F.N.; Overland, S.; Stewart, R.; Tell, G.S.; Bjelland, I.; Mykletun, A. Association between magnesium intake and depression and anxiety in community-dwelling adults: The Hordaland Health Study. *Aust. N. Z. J. Psychiatry* **2009**, *43*, 45–52. [CrossRef] [PubMed]

25. Huang, J.H.; Lu, Y.F.; Cheng, F.C.; Lee, J.N.; Tsai, L.C. Correlation of magnesium intake with metabolic parameters, depression and physical activity in elderly type 2 diabetes patients: A cross-sectional study. *Nutr. J.* **2012**, *11*, 41. [CrossRef] [PubMed]

26. Tarleton, E.K.; Littenberg, B. Magnesium intake and depression in adults. *J. Am. Board Fam. Med.* **2015**, *28*, 249–256. [CrossRef] [PubMed]

27. Yary, T.; Lehto, S.M.; Tolmunen, T.; Tuomainen, T.P.; Kauhanen, J.; Voutilainen, S.; Ruusunen, A. Dietary magnesium intake and the incidence of depression: A 20-year follow-up study. *J. Affect Disord.* **2016**, *193*, 94–98. [CrossRef] [PubMed]

28. Linder, J.; Brismar, K.; Beck-Friis, J.; Saaf, J.; Wetterberg, L. Calcium and magnesium concentrations in affective disorder: Difference between plasma and serum in relation to symptoms. *Acta Psychiatr. Scand.* **1989**, *80*, 527–537. [CrossRef] [PubMed]

29. Barragan-Rodriguez, L.; Rodriguez-Moran, M.; Guerrero-Romero, F. Depressive symptoms and hypomagnesemia in older diabetic subjects. *Arch. Med. Res.* **2007**, *38*, 752–756. [CrossRef] [PubMed]

30. Derom, M.-L.; Sayón-Orea, C.; Martínez-Ortega, J.M.; Martínez-González, M.A. Magnesium and depression: A systematic review. *Nutr. Neurosci.* **2013**, *16*, 191–206. [CrossRef] [PubMed]

31. Camardese, G.; De Risio, L.; Pizi, G.; Mattioli, B.; Buccelletti, F.; Serrani, R.; Leone, B.; Sgambato, A.; Bria, P.; Janiri, L. Plasma magnesium levels and treatment outcome in depressed patients. *Nutr. Neurosci.* **2012**, *15*, 78–84. [CrossRef] [PubMed]

32. Bauer, M.; Bschor, T.; Pfennig, A.; Whybrow, P.C.; Angst, J.; Versiani, M.; Möller, H.-J. World Federation of Societies of Biological Psychiatry (WFSBP) Guidelines for Biological Treatment of Unipolar Depressive Disorders in Primary Care. *World J. Biol. Psychiatry Off. J. World Fed. Soc. Biol. Psychiatry* **2007**, *8*, 67–104. [CrossRef] [PubMed]

33. Trevino, K.; McClintock, S.M.; McDonald Fischer, N.; Vora, A.; Husain, M.M. Defining treatment-resistant depression: A comprehensive review of the literature. *Ann. Clin. Psychiatry Off. J. Am. Acad. Clin. Psychiatr.* **2014**, *26*, 222–232.

34. Radziwoń-Zaleska, M.; Ryszewska-Pokraśniewicz, B.; Skalski, M.; Skrzeszewski, J.; Drozdowicz, E.; Nowak, G.; Pilc, A.; Bałkowiec-Iskra, E. Therapeutic drug monitoring of depression—Amplification by magnesium ions. *Pharmacol. Rep.* **2015**, *67*, 36. [CrossRef]

35. Eby, G.A.; Eby, K.L. Rapid recovery from major depression using magnesium treatment. *Med. Hypotheses* **2006**, *67*, 362–370. [CrossRef] [PubMed]

36. Derom, M.L.; Martinez-Gonzalez, M.A.; Sayon-Orea Mdel, C.; Bes-Rastrollo, M.; Beunza, J.J.; Sanchez-Villegas, A. Magnesium intake is not related to depression risk in Spanish university graduates. *J. Nutr.* **2012**, *142*, 1053–1059. [CrossRef] [PubMed]

37. Radziwoń-Zaleska, M.; Matsumoto, H.; Skalski, M.; Androsiuk, W.; Dziklińska, A.; Grobel, I.; Kunicki, P. Monitored therapy of depression. *Farmakoterapia w Psychiatrii i Neurologii* **1998**, *3*, 5–12.

38. Hamilton, M. A rating scale for depression. *J. Neurol. Neurosurg. Psychiatry* **1960**, *23*, 56–62. [CrossRef] [PubMed]

39. El-Yazigi, A.; Raines, D.A. Concurrent liquid chromatographic measurement of fluoxetine, amitryptyline, imipramine, and their active metabolites norfluoxetine, nortyptyline, and desipramine in plasma. *Ther. Drug. Monit.* **1993**, *15*, 305–309. [CrossRef] [PubMed]

40. Aymard, G.; Livi, P.; Pham, Y.T.; Diquet, B. Sensitive and rapid method for the simultaneous quantification of five antidepressants with their respective metabolites in plasma using high-performance liquid chromatography with diode-array detection. *J. Chromatogr. B Biomed. Sci. Appl.* **1997**, *700*, 183–189. [CrossRef]

41. Meineke, I.; Schreeb, K.; Kress, I.; Gundert-Remy, U. Routine measurement of fluoxetine and norfluoxetine by high-performance liquid chromatography with ultraviolet detection in patients under concomitant treatment with tricyclic antidepressants. *Ther. Drug Monit.* **1998**, *20*, 14–19. [CrossRef] [PubMed]

42. Komorowska, E. *Walidacja i Zastosowanie Metody Oznaczania Fluoksetyny Techniką HPLC*; Akademia Medyczna w Warszawie, Wydział Farmaceutyczny: Warszawa, Poland, 2002.

43. Baldessarini, R.J. Drugs and treatment of psychiatric disorders: Depression and mania. W. In *Goodman & Gilman's The Pharmacological Basis of Therapeutic*; McGraw-Hills Co.: New York, NY, USA, 1996; pp. 431–461.

44. Hulanicki, A.; Lewenstam, A.; Maj-Żurawska, M. *Magnesium; Clinical Significance and Analytical Determination; Reviews on Analytical Chemistry, Euroanalysis VIII*; Littlejohn, D., Thorburn Burns, D., Eds.; RSC: Cambridge, CA, USA, 1994; pp. 317–325.

45. Szelenberger, W. Farmakoelektroencefalografia: Aktualny stan wiedzy i perspektywy. *Psychiatr. Polska* **1990**, *24*, 52–57.

46. Skalski, M.; Szelenberger, W.; Radziwoń-Zaleska, M.; Matsumoto, H. Zastosowanie metody farmakoelektroencefalografii (farmako—EEG) w monitorowaniu terapii depresji. *Farmakoterapia w Psychiatrii i Neurologii* **1995**, *4*, 60–70.

47. Kroenke, K.; Spitzer, R.L.; Williams, J.B. The PHQ-9: Validity of a brief depression severity measure. *J. Gen. Intern. Med.* **2001**, *16*, 606–613. [CrossRef] [PubMed]

48. Tarleton, E.K.; Littenberg, B.; MacLean, C.D.; Kennedy, A.G.; Daley, C. Role of magnesium supplementation in the treatment of depression: A randomized clinical trial. *PLoS ONE* **2017**, *12*, e0180067. [CrossRef] [PubMed]

49. Barragan-Rodriguez, L.; Rodriguez-Moran, M.; Guerrero-Romero, F. Efficacy and safety of oral magnesium supplementation in the treatment of depression in the elderly with type 2 diabetes: A randomized, equivalent trial. *Magnes. Res.* **2008**, *21*, 218–223. [PubMed]

50. Mehdi, S.M.; Atlas, S.E.; Qadir, S.; Musselman, D.; Goldberg, S.; Woolger, J.M.; Corredor, R.; Abbas, M.H.; Arosemena, L.; Caccamo, S.; et al. Double-blind, randomized crossover study of intravenous infusion of magnesium sulfate versus 5% dextrose on depressive symptoms in adults with treatment-resistant depression. *Psychiatry Clin. Neurosci.* **2017**, *71*, 204–211. [CrossRef] [PubMed]

51. Fard, F.E.; Mirghafourvand, M.; Mohammad-Alizadeh Charandabi, S.; Farshbaf-Khalili, A.; Javadzadeh, Y.; Asgharian, H. Effects of zinc and magnesium supplements on postpartum depression and anxiety: A randomized controlled clinical trial. *Women Health* **2017**, *57*, 1115–1128. [CrossRef] [PubMed]

52. Martínez-González, M.Á.; Sánchez-Villegas, A. Magnesium intake and depression: The SUN cohort. *Magnes. Res.* **2016**, *29*, 102–111. [PubMed]

53. Nechifor, M. Magnesium in major depression. *Magnes. Res.* **2009**, *22*, 163s–166s. [PubMed]

54. Poleszak, E. Modulation of antidepressant-like activity of magnesium by serotonergic system. *J. Neural Transm.* **2007**, *114*, 1129–1134. [CrossRef] [PubMed]

55. George, M.S.; Rosenstein, D.; Rubinow, D.R.; Kling, M.A.; Post, R.M. CSF magnesium in affective disorder: Lack of correlation with clinical course of treatment. *Psychiatry Res.* **1994**, *51*, 139–146. [CrossRef]

56. Herzberg, L.; Bold, A.M. Sex difference in mean serum-magnesium levels in depression. *Lancet* **1972**, *1*, 1128–1129. [CrossRef]

57. Stanton, M.F.; Lowenstein, F.W. Serum magnesium in women during pregnancy, while taking contraceptives, and after menopause. *J. Am. Coll. Nutr.* **1987**, *6*, 313–319. [CrossRef] [PubMed]

58. Brown, R.A.; Abrantes, A.M.; Strong, D.R.; Niaura, R.; Kahler, C.W.; Miller, I.W.; Price, L.H. Efficacy of sequential use of fluoxetine for smoking cessation in elevated depressive symptom smokers. *Nicotine Tob. Res. Off. J. Soc. Res. Nicotine Tob.* **2014**, *16*, 197–207. [CrossRef] [PubMed]

59. Kenney, B.A.; Holahan, C.J.; North, R.J.; Holahan, C.K. Depressive symptoms and cigarette smoking in American workers. *Am. J. Health Promot. AJHP* **2006**, *20*, 179–182. [CrossRef] [PubMed]

60. Vázquez-Palacios, G.; Bonilla-Jaime, H.; Velázquez-Moctezuma, J. Antidepressant effects of nicotine and fluoxetine in an animal model of depression induced by neonatal treatment with clomipramine. *Prog. Neuro-Psychopharmacol. Biol. Psychiatry* **2005**, *29*, 39–46. [CrossRef] [PubMed]

61. Glassman, A.H.; Covey, L.S.; Stetner, F.; Rivelli, S. Smoking cessation and the course of major depression: A follow-up study. *Lancet* **2001**, *357*, 1929–1932. [CrossRef]

62. Salín-Pascual, R.J.; Galicia-Polo, L.; Drucker-Colín, R.; de la Fuente, J.R.; Drucker-Colín, R.; Salín-Pascual, R.J. Effects of transderman nicotine on mood and sleep in nonsmoking major depresssed patients. *Psychopharmacology* **1995**, *121*, 476–479. [CrossRef] [PubMed]

63. Cosci, F.; Nardi, A.E.; Griez, E.J. Nicotine effects on human affective functions: A systematic review of the literature on a controversial issue. *CNS Neurol. Disord. Drug Targets* **2014**, *13*, 981–991. [CrossRef] [PubMed]

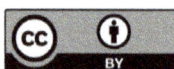

MDPI
St. Alban-Anlage 66
4052 Basel
Switzerland
Tel. +41 61 683 77 34
Fax +41 61 302 89 18
www.mdpi.com

Nutrients Editorial Office
E-mail: nutrients@mdpi.com
www.mdpi.com/journal/nutrients